FRACTURED INTENTIONS:
A History of Central State Hospital for the Insane

by
Nicole R. Kobrowski, MS Adult Ed.

Unseenpress.com, Inc.
Westfield, Indiana

Copyright ©2014 By Nicole Kobrowski
All rights reserved.

No part of this book may be reproduced, transmitted in any form or by any means, known or unknown, electronic or mechanical, including photocopying, recording, or by an information storage and retrieval system-except by a reviewer who may quote brief passages in a review to be printed in a magazine, newspaper or on the Web- without permission in writing from the publisher.

For information or copies contact:
Unseenpress.com, Inc.
PO Box 687
Westfield, IN 46074

Library of Congress Cataloging-in-Publication Data

Kobrowski, Nicole
    Fractured Intentions: A History of Central State Hospital/Nicole Kobrowski
    1. Central State Hospital Indiana; 2. Psychiatric hospitals-Indiana-Central State Hospital-Indiana;
    3. Hospitals Indiana; 4. Mental Health; 5. Indiana History; 4. Indiana Travel. I. Title

Library of Congress Control Number: 2008930458
Includes bibliographical references and index.
ISBN-13: 978-0-9774130-6-5
ISBN-0-9774130-6-3

Printed in the United States of America

Published by
Forgotten History
an imprint of Unseenpress.com, Inc.
PO Box 687
Westfield, IN 46074

Although the authors and publisher have made every effort to ensure the accuracy and completeness of information contained in this book, we assume no responsibility for errors, inaccuracies, omissions or any inconsistency herein. We also disclaim any liability in connection with the use of this book. The publishers and author do not condone, advise, or recommend visiting this site without obtaining permission.
Any slights of people, places or organizations are unintentional.

The Unseenpress.com, Inc. website is
http://www.unseenpress.com/

Cover design by Brittany Norris and Unseenpress.com, Inc.
Text layout and design by Unseenpress.com, Inc.
Cover photograph by Nicole R. Kobrowski

DEDICATION

This book is dedicated to the patients of
Central State Hospital and
the voices of mentally ill.
May they be heard and find
compassion, help, answers, and relief.

This book is also dedicated to
the many staff members
who were dedicated to the true care
of the patients.
The progress made with them
would not have been possible
without you.

Forward

Since the beginning of time, treatment for persons with mental illness has run the gamut from being hotly contested to ignorance. In some cultures, they have been viewed with reverence as shaman-like people, able to interpret perceived spiritual signs and in others, have been demonized and seen as carriers of evil spirits.

Mental illness is a common affliction among the poverty stricken as well as the affluent and needs to be seen not as a result of poor living skills, but as a disorder as common as diabetes, cancer and heart disease, with the resulting correct treatments to allow those persons to live as all do, with freedoms and choices.

Those suffering from depression or anxiety- a plethora of people- were exposed to countless questions about their inability to "cheer up", judgments from their family and friends, and left with feelings of hopelessness.

Persons with Bipolar Disorder or Schizophrenia were even more unsuccessfully treated. They were scrutinized as "crazy" and were feared, for the most part, because of their symptoms. Oftentimes, those persons committed suicide and were subject to all sorts of mistreatments, from being locked up, as in jail, to being tortured by their caretakers and the public at large.

Most of the time, these persons became outcasts, facing poverty, disease, hunger, homelessness and a certain early death. These stressors, of course, only contributed to their symptoms of mental illness, and paradoxically confirmed society's conviction that these people did not belong in acceptable society.

Hence, institutions were developed to house those with mental illness in an effort to isolate them from society. Initial intentions were not to treat them but to protect society from these. This devolved into inhumane treatments of those with mental disorders.

Written documentation (although poorly done) and anecdotal evidence provides the rest of the story. Vilified, demonized and cast out, the mentally ill were left to the devices of "experts" who provided treatment in the form of medications (poorly tested, often misdiagnosed, and inadequately monitored), ice baths, ECT and various other forms of accepted and innovated treatment.

Although it is widely held that there should be state-run institutions for those with little resources, the monitoring and treatment of mentally ill persons needs to be vigilant and careful, allowing for personal choice and freedoms. In addition, perhaps with the influence of this book, there needs to be more money applied to the treatment of mental illness, not just for the person afflicted, but for that person's family and support system.

It has only been in recent decades through advanced scientific research and study that alternative treatments such as appropriate medications, talk therapy, and community support have kept the mentally ill from being ostracized. In addition to the scientific advances, better training and education has occurred, allowing caretakers to be mindful of symptoms and appropriate treatments. Ms. Kobrowski's book details in excellent form the history of Central State Hospital from the beginning of the institution to the timely death of it and should be seen as an exposure to the ill treatment of persons with mental illness and a caution against reverting back to this sort of treatment.

Mary Jo Sparke, LCSW
January, 2015

PROLOGUE

My purposes for writing this book were varied. I wanted to contribute to changing the perception about what the hospital was. I wanted to correct some foolish myths. I enjoy writing and this was a fantastic idea. I would like people have a better understanding of Central State Hospital, mental health, and how mental healthcare has progressed over the last 250 years. I hope this book helps people think about where mental healthcare is going as well. I feel there is much more to do outside of drug therapy. I hope that people in the mental healthcare field find better ways to treat and possibly cure mental illness. Finally, I hope that there is a better dialogue about mental health after people read this book.

To understand Central State Hospital, you have to put the hospital into the context of what remains and what can be teased from various sources. I used many books about the history of mental health to supplement my knowledge of the system and medicine. Much of the correspondence between the hospital and others does not exist. A handful of files regarding patient issues exist. For any patient records after 1900 (even though HIPPA is 75 years), the State Archives requires that you provide proof of kinship. An incomplete set of annual reports exists as does a few accounts of early patient and staff experiences. I also conducted my own interviews with former employees and others.

When the hospital opened, photography wasn't a widely used medium. There are very view photos that exist before 1900. The State Archives and the Indiana Historical Society have the majority of known photos available for viewing by the public. The newspapers largely did not keep copies of the photos and tracking down the photographers after so many years has been nearly fruitless. What other pictures exist reside in private collections and certainly only represent a small fraction of the 146 years that the institution was opened. Sanborn maps help pinpoint buildings and tunnel locations along with my own knowledge about the institution.

I went into this book wanting to find out everything I could. As of this writing, I am saturated with knowledge but still have dozens of questions. I hoped in a small way to right some of the mysteries in some of the brief histories about Central State. In one of the surviving account, where the history focused on a brief overview of several state hospital institutions, three questions were left to answer, despite the research done by the author, Superintendent Clifford L. Williams, M.D. He charged that there were "discrepancies" in the following questions and that "time" didn't allow for these items to be addressed.

Those "discrepancies" were where was the first "Crazy House", who were the first eight patients (in Central State Hospital) and when did Dorothea Dix study in Indiana.

I've been able to answer two of those questions. In the book, I gave a list of the first patients at Central State Hospital for the Insane. The first asylum was at the south east corner of Vermont Street, Massachusetts Avenue and Alabama Street. Of course, the building currently at the site was not the first asylum, but its placement is interesting. Massachusetts Avenue used to go all the way to the Circle where the old governor's mansion used to sit. Indianapolis itself was laid out as "squares" much as other cities are. But in the early 1800s, not as many people lived in Indianapolis and having the local asylum only three blocks away from the governor's mansion is a stark comparison with the 2 miles it eventually came.

Finally, Dorothea Dix studied several jails asylums and poor houses in Indiana. Dix was a mental health advocate and a forerunner to the modern nurse. Through her studies of the hospitals and prisons she helped promote reform in these institutions. She came to Indiana to establish asylums for the mentally ill. But if she studied, as in went to school anywhere in Indiana, I could not find it.

I would like to find out more about the first patient's lives, but that was not the focus of the book.. Hopefully in the future, I will have the opportunity to write more about some of the patients and their lives before, during and after hospital life.

Please also note, any terms using the word "insane" are not to reflect my feelings toward people with mental health issues. First, wouldn't we all be considered people with mental health issues anyway? Several activities and conditions that are considered quite normal now were at one time taboo and considered a symptom of insanity- menopause, masturbation, hard academic study, infertility, phobias of snakes, spiders and other creepy crawlies. Anyone who has had therapy for a host of conditions could have been put into Central State Hospital. Second, I have nothing but respect and compassion for people with mental conditions that more than affect their everyday lives. I have seen people who struggle through getting the right combination of therapy and medication and who struggle with bad menstruation cycles and menopause. It isn't easy for them and when they truly manage their situations, they don't deserve the nasty comments and stigma attached to them. Just because you can't see the disease doesn't mean it doesn't exist. I used the word "insane" when it was part of the title of the hospital, to give readers a feel of what the thinking was like at the time. I moved to terms such as "mental health" and "mentally ill" when the hospital changed its name.

As for the book in general, I am sure people will disagree with the facts I've presented. I am hopeful in the future, more documentation comes to light so this volume can be updated with it. As with all history, it is a work in progress.

Acknowledgments

I would like to acknowledge the following people and organizations

- City of Indianapolis: For allowing me to legally document the hospital, its tunnels and grounds.
- Rick Bittle, Jason Young, and Sharon Miller for keeping me company on my documentation journey.
- My loving and historic minded husband, Michael: He's my best friend and my biggest supporter, despite my off-key singing. Thank you for the endless patience, support, meals, cleaning, tea, water, shoulders and ears, and "study breaks". "It's not the US yet. Still the colonies."
- Indiana Historical Society Library and Staff: Thank you for the speedy resources and mammoth photocopying.
- Indiana Medical History Museum: Thank you to Sarah M. Halter for fact checking and permissions.
- Indiana State Archives, especially Vicki Casteel, Alan January, and Michael Vetman: Thank you for all your help, especially when I was not particularly clear.
- Indiana State Library and staff: For its never ending supply of quick information and attention to detail.
- Paula Dunn: my editor: Without her, this book wouldn't be half as good. Thank you, thank you, and thank you. Remember, hospitals don't speak…. And it is "assessed."
- Megan Oaks, for her love of history and her scanning talents.
- Dr. Charles Bonsett: Indiana, history, and the medical community would be poorer without his knowledge and kindness.
- Lebanon Library, Lebanon, Indiana: Especially Eric Spall and Jamey Hickson.
- A special thanks goes out to my musical muses: Night Ranger, Joel Hoekstra, Jack Blades, Brad Gillis, Kelly Keagy, Loverboy, Fifth Dimension, The Left Banke, Yes, The Grass Roots, Boston, Steely Dan, Three Dog Night, and so many others. The late nights and quick concerts helped me focus and absorb the heady information contained in this book.

Table of Contents

Chapter 1: Early Mental Health	1
Chapter 2: Hospital Life	11
Chapter 3: Patient Life	25
Chapter 4: The Hospital and Farm Colony	37
Chapter 5: Staffing	41
Chapter 6: Treatments and Research	61
Chapter 7: Investigations into the Hospital	73
Chapter 8: Investigations	85
Chapter 9: Pathology Department	95
Chapter 10: Buildings	109
Chapter 11: Final Decline and Closure	141
Chapter 12: Interviews	161
Chapter 13: Today	175
Chapter 14: Central State Hospital Cemetery	179
Chapter 15: Central State Leadership	183
Epilogue	193
Notes	194
Photo Credits	197
Bibliography	198
Index	214

One

EARLY MENTAL HEALTH

Before hospitals, the insane were left to family and to prisons. If a location was "lucky" enough to have a place for the insane, it was usually no more than a shack, a pen or a place where afflicted people could run in an enclosed area or be chained. Many times, these places were no better than hog wallows.

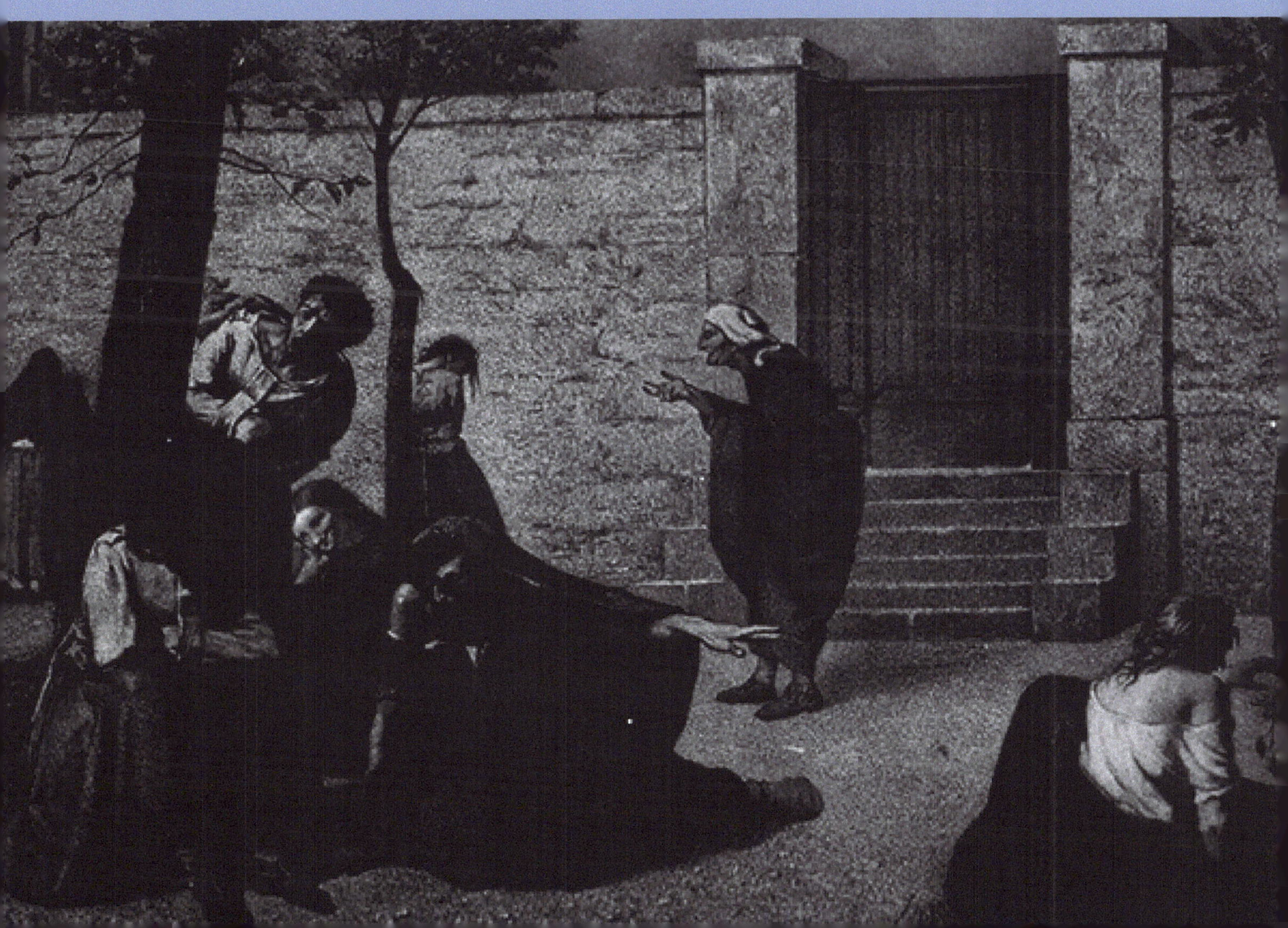

Early Society and the Insane

As society progressed, people believed prisons were a logical choice for anyone with behavior deviating from social norms. These were places of punishment, which is what society believed these people needed. Society didn't understand mental health and confinement put the rest of the population at ease. The buildings were made to do just this- to scare inmates and put them (and anyone viewing them) in awe. Later, hospitals would be modeled on prisons in architecture and structure making it easy to segregate the insane from society.

Prisons were strong, usually brick or stone structures, with an administrative regulatory atmosphere that separated the people inside from the rest of society. Routines were defined by blocks of time, with punctuality a must. Many prisons (and later hospitals) had bells to signal changes in the routine. Early prisons and hospitals were dedicated to work and solitude, labor and isolation. These mechanisms were designed to transform prisoners or the insane with the idea that they would leave the institution different people, not only by behavior but by personality. Prisons and hospitals were orderly, but by the 1850s (and much more pronounced in the 1880s), were corrupt and brutal- and also overcrowded. With few exceptions early hospitals housed the common people- the lower class. The upper classes were cared for at home, with private nurses and doctors.

As prisons were built to confine deviants and to transform their personalities for reintroduction to society, it is no surprise that early mental hospitals did the same- segregate the patients to transform (i.e. cure) them.

By the 1820s, penitentiaries were being built and two types of incarceration existed. In the Auburn, New York setting, the inmates slept separately and labored together during the day. In the Pennsylvania system started by Quakers, each inmate was kept in near silence and isolation, talking only with a handful of guards and other prison officials during their time in the penitentiary. Quakers believed this solitude gave the inmates time to ponder and repent. Any social deviants, including the insane, could be placed in these large institutions, whether they were criminals or not. Insanity in Colonial times was looked upon as no different than any other affliction- a lost leg, a missing arm. The insane simply melded with the rest of the people in society who could not fend for themselves and became the poor. The poor were cared for by the people in the Colonies. However, there was a differentiation by "moral character" within the poor population. The code was if someone was lazy and poor, they were not helped. If someone couldn't walk, couldn't work and was poor, they were cared for. Many times insane people were treated at home by skilled and unskilled doctors and laypeople. Pest houses were used in extreme cases of severe disease outbreak.
Religion played a huge role, especially in the Protestant church. Religious people believed that divine intervention had created some men rich and some poor. To help the poor was an opportunity for men to do good. Everything was based on doing good to attain entry into heaven.

Any deviant behavior was dealt with harshly. Flogging, whipping and even execution was common. People began to believe what their churches said about the gravity of every bad action. They believed they were meant to sin and to try to not sin was the best they could do. People supported each other, through punishment and charity. Strangers were a different matter, though- he might be the reason for disorderly conduct, and therefore outsiders were not trusted, nor helped.

By the mid-1700s workhouses and almshouses enforced strict codes for reward and punishment. These solutions were supposed to be for the benefit of the poor, but were nothing more than workhouses for the poor. In Philadelphia, almshouses were designed by the local government to be a benefit to the community because they were being constructed to care for the poor at a smaller cost than previous attempts. The insane were put in with the poor.

If insane people became too wieldy to care for, they were sent to the almshouse or a workhouse if they were destitute. Many workhouses looked like and functioned as industrial factories. Early almshouses housing the insane looked just like typical houses in the area complete with a garden in the front or back. They functioned like a large household and the people in them were like a family.

Hospital Formation

Religious beliefs shifted over time. People began to believe humans were inherently good and society tried to find other ways to curb poverty and crime. Society thought that a person turned to crime because of inadequacies in the family and therefore, the criminal spread crime throughout the area. This included insane people who committed crimes.

The first formal hospital opened in 1753 in Philadelphia. Six of its first patients were mentally ill. Dr. Benjamin Rush, who is largely referred to as "the father of modern psychiatry", worked at the hospital. His methodology included bloodletting and treating patients with toxic substances such as the mercury based calomel. He believed that psychiatric disorders originated from "hypertension in the brain's blood vessels". Bloodletting was thought to ease the tension and calm patients down. So it did, but mainly because patients were weakened by the loss of blood.

Rush also used a treatment called "The Tranquilizer". This was a chair built to "cure madness. It binds and confines every part of the body. By preventing the muscles from acting, it reduced the force and frequency of the pulse and by the position of the head and feet favors the application of cold ice water to the former and warm water to the latter."

Twenty years later, a second hospital opened in Williamsburg, Virginia. It was dedicated solely to mentally ill patients. This hospital differed from later institutions as it was smaller and kept to individualized care. It was modeled after Dr. Philippe Pinel's theories on moral therapy (a precursor to cognitive behavioral therapy). Pinel, was the psychiatrist in charge of the first Parisian asylums. He published articles on findings and theories about the relationship between emotion, social conditions and insanity.

Pinel believed that mental illness was curable. Therapies included good living conditions and basic behavior modification to encourage order. Moral treatments also include exercise, regular exposure to religion, training and activities for hygiene, and patient interests, such as woodworking, writing, music or art. Other methods of treatment were also used, including cold baths and drugs like morphine.

All that would change, however, with growing populations, additional identification of believed type and number of mental illnesses, and unfortunately, a somewhat unchecked ability for anyone with time and money to dispose of an unwanted relative. This need prompted large, state-funded facilities. These facilities were chronically overcrowded. As with any state endeavor, growth and change was low, with expansion occurring for the next 50 years. In America, over 100 Asylums were built, 60 of them before 1890. In Indiana, anytime money was requested for large scale projects, it usually didn't come in one lump sum and the stages of the project sometimes outlived the usefulness of the original idea.

After Dr. Philippe Pinel (1745-1826), who headed the Parisian asylums, asserted that kind and gentle treatment would help cure insanity, more doctors began to explore this new approach to treating the insane. Early efforts to diagnose insanity began with Isaac Ray's (1807-1881) A Treatise on the Medical Jurisprudence of Insanity. The belief was that anyone, including the rich, could become insane. They could be insane in certain areas but completely sane

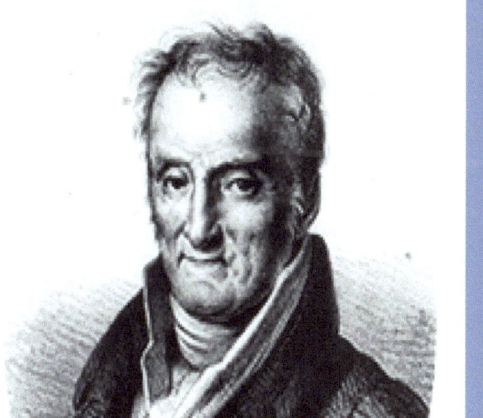

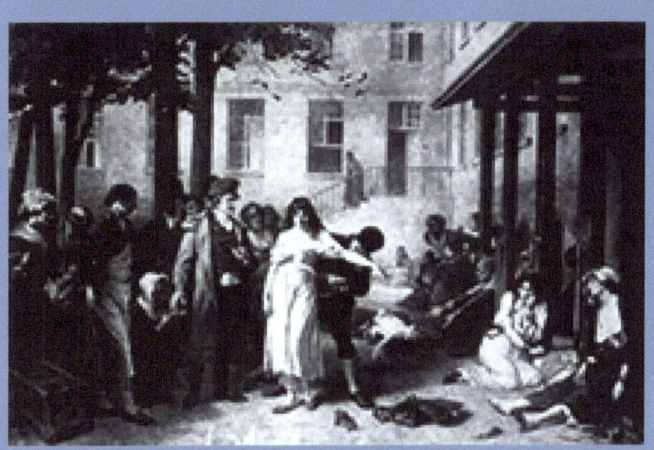

Left: Dr. Phillippe Pinel.

Below: "Dr. Pinel in the courtyard of the Salpêriere"

and capable of rational thought in others. If easygoing people became tense or angry all the time, or if religious churchgoers became radical freethinkers, they could be insane. In either case, they could be completely sane when they spoke about the weather, their childhood or a host of topics. Only by investigating a person's whole life and persona could a diagnosis be made. Pinel advocated researching and getting to know the patients, making extensive notes and then coming to an informed conclusion.

Although Dr. Rush condoned treatments which were somewhat questionable, he did not subscribe to coercion and restraint, physical punishment, and chains or cells. Instead, he placed patients in a normal hospital setting. This was the beginning of moral therapy.

Rush believed that to be doing something helped them feel useful and took their minds away from themselves. This was the start of what would become occupational, activity, music, art, and vocational therapy, He also was the first doctor to treat alcoholism as a mental disease versus a sin. He weaned people from alcohol using less potent substances.

These early efforts from doctors such as Pinel and Rush also included theories that insanity originated with social organization. This could mean "wrong" political thoughts, intellectual practices, economic practices, or "grave errors" such as school and family training. In essence, the insane couldn't help their behaviors. So how could doctors cure this insanity?

Doctors also thought insanity was hereditary. They believed it came from the mother more than the father and that intermarrying was also a cause. Some of the causes for insanity were errors in education. This could be studying too hard, not studying hard enough, studying and not maintaining a physically fit body, or reading romance novels. Doctors also believed that children were less likely to be insane; the use of tobacco, alcohol and narcotics also caused insanity; and in most cases, wanting a lot of sleep was a "precursor" to insanity.

Doctors thought by creating a place of social order and routine, where external influences could be curbed, insanity could be cured and so the asylum was the first resort. They already had a model in the prison structure for the type of place in which to create this almost Utopian existence. Prisons had the remoteness and structure needed for their inmates. These features were necessary to block bad influences.

Additionally, the terminology for the very early asylums included using "inmate" for patients, "cells" for rooms, "keepers" for attendants, and "asylum" for hospital. At Central State Hospital for the Insane, there is a heading in the

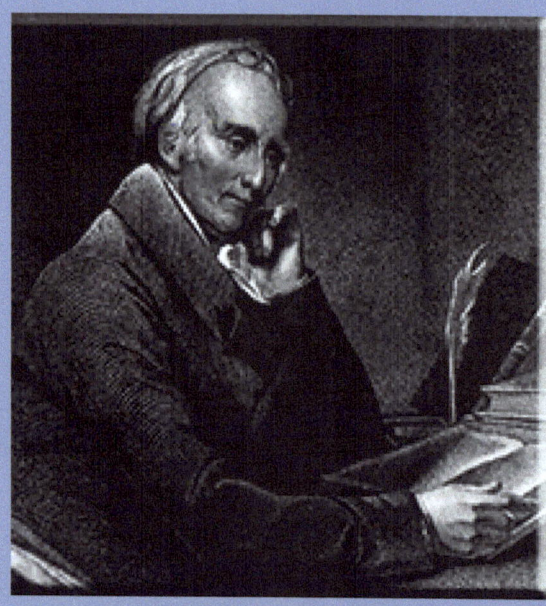

Above: Dr. Benjamin Rush, who is considered the father of modern psychiatry.

Right: An example of "The Tranquilizer," which Rush favored.

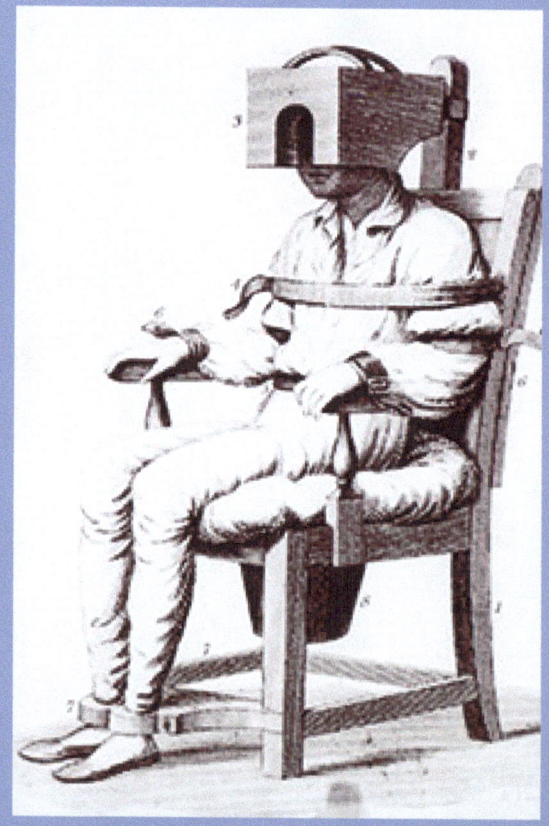

1861 yearly report that states "Health of Inmates", but under that heading, the term "patients" was used. Some rooms in the original building were called "cells" in one yearly report. Even as late as the early 1900s, "inmates" was still used to refer to patients.

In addition to truly wanting to help the insane, doctors were often ambitious in their estimation of the ability to "cure" insanity. The cure was really believed to be in the institution itself. Remove the patient from the society and the wrongness of their lives, make the hospital a separate society away from the rest of the area, and control and discipline the patient in a gentle and kind way. In short, the idea was to bring quiet and order to a member of a disorganized society.

This was an issue, however, because as much as doctors wanted this treatment for the patients, they also had to look at long term goals for themselves and the institution. To disallow the public access and information about the hospital activities would defeat the goal, but to allow too much public and family access could disrupt the patients. As a result, the doctors did try to create a "correct" atmosphere around the patients. Early on, visitors were not really welcome on the wards. Doctors felt it caused harm to the patients. However, they did want a public understanding of insanity, rejoiced when organizations and people thought of the patients' welfare. Controlled public tours were one way the hospital tried to educate the public but keep patients away from direct contact with outside influences.

INDIANA PRIOR TO MENTAL HOSPITALS

"Nothing great is lightly won; Nothing won is lost;
Every good deed is nobly done will repay the cost.
Leave to Heaven, in humble trust, all you will do;
But if you succeed, you must paddle your own canoe."
~Sarah T. Bolton, Indiana poetess

In Indiana, things were no better. Countless cases relayed by doctors of the deplorable conditions and the outrageous "care" for the insane.
- A widow wanted to commit her son because he forced the family into submission because of his rages.

WHERE WAS THE FIRST INDIANAPOLIS "CRAZY HOUSE"?

Before Central State Hospital was formed, the original "crazy house" was a log cabin at the corner of New Jersey and Ohio Streets. In 1827 the General Assembly set aside Square 22 for use as the state hospital and lunatic asylum. A log cabin was already on the site and was used as a "crazy house".

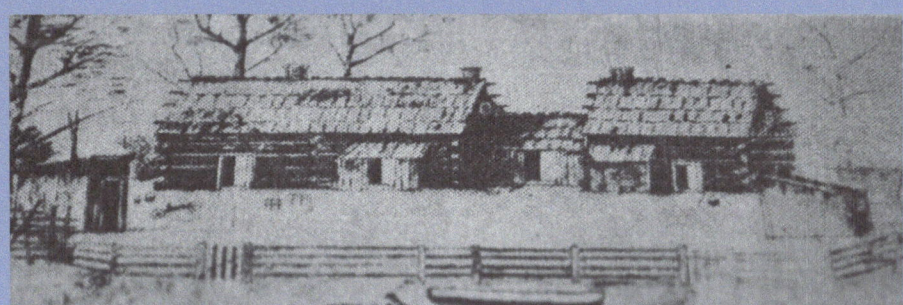

There are some newspaper articles which state a log cabin near the White River and Washington Street was where the first camp for the insane was. They were put into this area and fed, but received no other care. The author was unable to verify this information. It seems more likely that these were the Bolton Farm buildings. The Boltons had built a house and a separate building as a tavern on the property on the hill across from the old Employees Building (also known as the Administration Building)

- A man took his daughter to a poor house hoping she would get help. She did and years later, he was in the same poor house because he could not get into an asylum himself.
- A man came to Indianapolis after traveling all over Ohio, Indiana and Kentucky trying to find a place to admit himself.
- An insane old woman was kept in a log pen outside.
- Another insane woman was confined to a smokehouse, her cries upsetting those around her.

In 1832 the legislature received a memorial and a favorable report urging the building of the hospital and in 1841 a society was formed consisting of John Evans, MD, Isaac Fisher, MD, Edward Hannigan, and Caleb Jones, MD. They believed "the State of Indiana should take care of the mute, the blind, and the insane." During this time, Dr. Evans began publishing articles about the insane and the county institutions that housed them, such as poor houses. On December 7, 1841 Governor Samuel Bigger asked for action. He stated to the State legislature that when Indianapolis was made the capital that a "lunatic asylum" had been provide for in the form of an empty lot. Nothing had been done in Indiana with that property although other states had already established asylums for their insane. Bigger called upon the state to establish an institution where "they may be placed and submitted to proper medical treatment."

This message and the memorial of Drs. John Evans and Isaac Fisher were presented to the Committee on Education. On January 3, 1842, Dr. James Richee, the Chairman of the Committee on Education took up this cause with the committee, which resulted in a joint resolution: "…That it be made the duty of the Governor to hold a correspondence with the superintendent of the lunatic asylums of our sister states with the view to ascertain the most approved plan for the construction of an asylum, and the manner of conducting it, and any other information he may think necessary; which plans and information he shall communicate to the next General Assembly, with such recommendation on the subject of the immediate undertaking of the erection and establishment of an Indiana Lunatic Asylum as he may think proper."

The resolution was passed and approved by the governor on January 31, 1842. However, Governor Bigger did not mention this in the next meeting of the legislation. On December 27, 1842, the second memorial from Drs. John Evans and Isaac Fisher was presented and forwarded to the Committee on Finance.

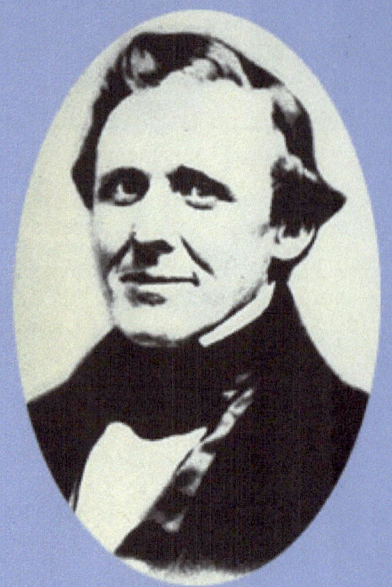

Above: Dr. John Evans, one of the founders of the hospital and the namesake of Evanston, Illinois. He was Governor of the Territory of Colorado until he was found to have had a hand in covering up the Sand Creek Massacre in which hundreds of Cheyenne were killed and dismembered and their bodies disrespected by the soldiers.

Below: Dorothea Dix, educator, reformer, and one of the first women to help transform nursing into a profession.

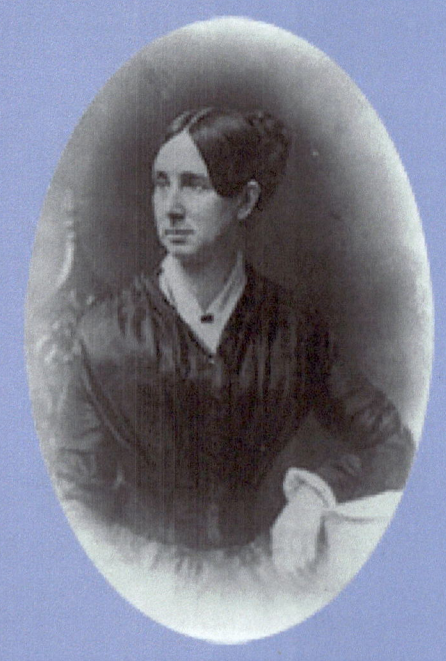

Just a few days later on January 3, 1843, the Committee on Finance stated that the topic would need to be postponed due to the "embarrassed condition" of state finances. Over the next two years, this subject would be presented to the legislature, the committees on Education and Finance. On December 19, 1843, through the memorial of Dr. James Matthews, the Committee of Education moved to discharge the subject of an asylum from any further discussion. This move was not approved. In fact, Mr. Buell of Warren, Indiana asked Dr. Matthews to report how much it would cost, the time to complete it, and all other pertinent information with regard to opening the asylum. Dr. Evans asked for a tax of one cent on every $100 to raise funds for the institution. This was agreed upon by the Committee on Education.

What is interesting to note is that Governor Bigger did not seem too awfully interested in the movement toward an insane hospital. Some speculation was put forward that this is why he was defeated for re-election in 1843. Whatever the case, Bigger's successor Governor Whitcomb was very interested, not only in a lunatic asylum, but also in a school for the education of the blind. He called upon the state and its people to extend its "warmest sympathy, and their relief to the extent of our ability…"

On Jan 15, 1844 the General Assembly approved an act that provided the erection of a state lunatic asylum. An amendment sponsored by Senator U.S. Connett, a physician, specifying "that one cent on the one hundred dollars be levied as a fund with which to erect a lunatic asylum."

> *'Then at least forty of our unfortunate fellow citizens who are suffering from insanity, who are now unable to obtain hospital care and consequently are without the proper treatment for their cure or comfort, may have a retreat from the cold and unfeeling treatment they too often met with from those not acquainted with their condition- a home where they can be surrounded with all the necessary comforts of life and kind attendants and friends to wipe away the tear of sorrow and give to the troubled and desponding heart, by kind words and every possible diversion, the cheering influences of hope and contentment – a hospital where they may have an anodyne for every pain and a remedy for every curable malady- where they may find a physician whose care for their welfare will be constant and unremitted, and who, in consequence of the entire devotion of his time and attention to the subject of their peculiar disease, will be able to direct every known means for their restoration."*

DORTHEA LYNDE DIX

One woman campaigned for change. Before nursing was a profession, Dorothea Lynde Dix was an educator, reformer and humanitarian. She is also well known for her "nursing corps" during the Civil War. These women and men were the precursor to the nursing profession as we know it today.

At 39 years old, Dorothea left her post as a veteran 24-year career school teacher and began her new career to fight for reformation in prisons and asylums across the globe. In 1841 when she began teaching at the Cambridge House of Corrections, she saw the same issues that were present in early mental health facilities throughout the world. The mentally ill were kept with criminals and were chained, left to starve and freeze, sometimes without clothing. They were abused, by the people who cared for them and by other inmates.

In 1843 Dix petitioned Massachusetts to reform the inhumane conditions for the mentally ill. In 1845, she wrote "Remarks on Prisons and Prison Discipline in the United States" which outlined her reforms for both prisons and mental hospitals. She was radical in her beliefs for the time. It was widely believed that the insane could not be cured and that putting them away was the best thing for them. However Dix proved by bettering the conditions around the insane, they could be helped. After all, some of the "insane" were really people who were depressed, or were suffering from post-traumatic stress syndrome (PTSD), pre-menstrual syndrome (PMS) and sexually transmitted diseases (STDs). One such case cited by her was "a young woman who was for years 'a raging maniac' chained in a cage and whipped to control her acts and words. She was helped by a husband and wife who agreed to take care of her in their home and slowly she recovered her senses."

Dorothea Dix visited the Indiana General assembly in 1845 and advocated for a state hospital for the insane. All of the recommendations for the building of the asylums were wrapped into Bill 182, run through the political machine and became law on January 13, 1845 and a Board of Commissioners for the hospital was formed. This Board of Commissioners was appointed, and responsible for approving and overseeing the budgets for the hospital. They were answerable to the State of Indiana and to its citizens for the running of the hospital.

For decades afterwards, Dix worked tirelessly to help better the conditions of the insane in countries around the world. In the U.S. alone, she helped establish 32 hospitals in 11 states, including Central State Hospital (then known as The Indiana Hospital for the Insane). She also helped established 15 schools for the "feeble minded", and a school for the blind. By 1880, she had helped establish training programs in new and existing hospitals. Between this work and her work during the Civil War, Dix established the groundwork for the nursing profession, and many other health care occupations. She advocated training personnel and not leaving them to their own devices.

The Bolton Farm

Sarah Tittle Barrett was born December 18, 1814 in Newport, Kentucky to Jonathan B. and Esther (Pendleton) Barrett. The family moved around and finally settled in Vernon, Indiana near Six Mile Creek. Sarah's parents farmed for food, flax and wool. Eventually the family became well off. They had nearly 100 cleared and fenced acres, a grist mill, and a larger house than the log cabin they began with. Still, Sarah's father wanted better for his children and sold his farm, moving the family to Madison, Indiana. This move would change Sarah's life forever.

Despite the fact that Sarah was almost illiterate when they made this move, she flourished with her new educational opportunities in Madison and became a writer. The Madison Banner published a poem with the caveat that she was "not yet 14 years old". She continued to be a contributor to the Madison and Cincinnati newspapers for many years.

Sarah's writing led her to Nathaniel Bolton, her husband. Nathaniel Bolton was born in Chillicothe, Ohio on July 25, 1803. He had no formal education but had skills to become a printer. When he and his stepfather George Smith, who was also a printer, moved to Indianapolis, they founded the first Indianapolis newspaper, The Gazette. Later Nathaniel also published The Democrat.

The couple married on October 15, 1831, traveling from Madison to Indianapolis on horseback. They lived at the Smith farm, which had originally been built by Nathaniel's stepfather, in Mount Jackson, Indiana, which is now part of Indianapolis. When Nathaniel's stepfather died, the Boltons made an inn by adding another log structure, and a frame building to the property. One of the rooms was used for social gatherings for the people who lived nearby. The Nathaniel Bolton Tavern was a place of community for the citizens of Indianapolis and members of the legislature. This may explain why later in life Bolton became the State Librarian, a clerk to a Congressional committee, and Consul to Switzerland.

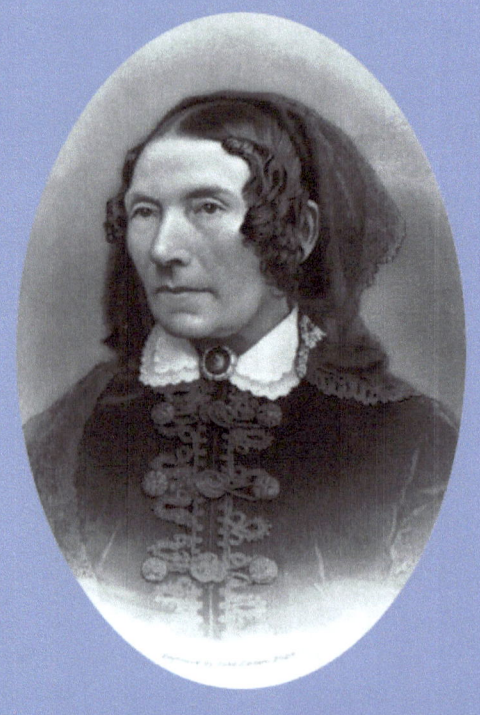

Left: Sarah T. Bolton, the "pioneer poet" of Indiana.

The tavern was situated in the central eastern portion of the property. The family had two children, a boy, James, and a girl, Ada. When James was born, Nathaniel planted a row of trees from the National Road (Washington Street) to the tavern. It was determined that the trees were about 20 year old specimens when they were planted. Many of the beautiful 200 year old trees stood until renovation of the land began in 2013.

During the era of the tavern, Nathaniel co-signed several loans and was obligated to repay some of them. Sarah worked very hard. She did the cooking, cleaning and farm chores. She also made butter, cheese and tended the children. Still, she found time to be an active part of the tavern, entertaining guests. She also found some time to write for special occasions, such as for dignitaries and friends.

It is interesting that a place so full of life, learning and community would be selected as the site for an "insane hospital". It was selected because it was four miles outside of Indianapolis, and on high ground. It may have also been chosen because of Nathaniel Bolton's political ties through his tavern's business.

Although some accounts say Sarah didn't want to sell the land to the state, the couple sold the farm to the State of Indiana on August 29, 1845 at $53 per acre ($8480; about $262,000 in 2014 money) and moved to Indianapolis, which had almost made its way westward to their farm. After the move, Sarah had much more time for writing. She and Nathaniel spent the next 12 years traveling for his jobs until his death in 1857. Afterwards, Sarah moved to Elmcroft (now part of Irvington). In 1858 her daughter died, leaving a grandson to raise. In her later life, Sarah moved to Beech Bank, which is now the Sarah T. Bolton Park.

CREATING A PLAN FOR THE HOSPITAL

On Jan 19, 1846 the legislature passed an act to provide for the erection of a suitable building for the use of the Indiana Hospital for the Insane." Construction began on May 5, 1846. The institution was originally constructed for 100-150 patients from all over the state.

The Bolton land was suitably cleared for the first building. Some sources state that patients were housed in the old Bolton home and tavern, but this seems to be incorrect. The house and the tavern were no longer in use by the time the first patient entered the hospital. The first building to be built on the property for hospital use was the Department for Men (see also Chapter 10 Buildings).

In 1847, in the Third Annual Report of the Commissioners and Superintendent of the Hospital for the Insane to the General Assembly of the State of Indiana, weather delays and contractor issues held up the building process for almost a year. During January, the water was so high, the Eagle Creek bridges were washed out and the fords were impassable due to high, rushing water.

The builders were unable to produce enough building materials because of the high water. The bricklayer, Mr. Clark was unable to keep a staff on hand to keep building at a quick pace and he was forced to relinquish the contract. A new contractor had to be found. Slate, expected to be delivered, was delayed in New Orleans.

Bradly and Karns did much of the carpentry work. Mr. J Willis and Mr. John Elder were the architects. Morrison and Turner supplied the brick. Mr. S.P. Ingersoll was the foreman of the masons. C. and J. Cox put up the copper gutters, R.R. Underhill completed the castings, and A. Haugh made flue openings.

Types of materials used on the original building included brick, slate ($8.50/square), tin, copper ($.025/pound-$0.15/gutter +75 cents for mitre joints, and 25 cents extra for elbows), plasters, iron nails, wood and iron trusses. Points of contention seemed to be whether slate or tin should be used on the roof and whether the dome should be made of copper. Slate was chosen for the roof because it was "cheap and more durable" than tin. Additionally, lime and hydraulic cement, stone, sand, hewn timbers, castings, and various sundries were needed. Labor, carpenters, casting work, repairs, printing and advertising, hardware and nails, and salaries made up other costs.

From the beginning, the hospital begged for more money. Lots on the original Square 22 "hospital block" were put up for sale, presumably to raise money. In 1847 there was a $10,400 deficit that would be raised through taxes, money from the treasury, or "in such manner as the Legislature may please to direct." The hospital staff stated that other states, such as Ohio, found it necessary to expand quickly after opening. The applications the hospital received so far from people in Indiana indicated this would be needed for this hospital as well. In the short term, they proposed changing the attic to patient rooms. "The rooms thus afforded are well suited for the accommodation of such patients as it will be found necessary to keep remote from the more frequented portions of the Institutions; or when more than the ordinary precautions are necessary to secure patients from running away."

Even though the hospital commissioners and the state legislature were aware that what they were building was too little for the accommodation of all the insane in Indiana, provision had been made for a second asylum in Indiana, yet to be built. Additionally, using Kentucky, Illinois, New Jersey, Massachusetts, and Ohio as examples, the hospital staff showed that Indiana was building something far better than in the other states because we could accommodate more patients.

More than two years after purchase, the hospital still wasn't open and the farm was in bad repair in 1847. The hospital commissioners had the fences repaired and prepared the current land and more land for farming. Part of the Bolton farmland continued to be farmed. The first farming lots were on the east side of the property. Several farmers (Harris and Morley, Patrick Adams, Z.R. Clark) rented the property and cultivated oats, corn, and fruits. Corn and oats were ground by the farmers at between $1.50 and $2.00 an acre. They also took care of livestock.

The hospital experienced more construction delays due to legislation indecision. One big issue was the heating system. The money had not been given by the Indiana State Treasury and the Board didn't want to incur this cost, so they got a loan to pay Mr. Reynolds, who put in the heating and air ventilation.

OPENING THE DOORS

The hospital took longer to build than was expected, so the hospital did not have all of the space it needed nor were all the facilities up and running. When the doors opened, the hospital was already overcrowded. It had 50 patients already admitted and en route to the hospital. Almost the same number were going to be admitted within a month. When the patients arrived, the staff was underpaid and under trained.

On November 7, 1848 the hospital opened. The first patients arrived from November 21 to November 23, 1848.

Patient Number	Name	County	Admission Date
1	Lacy Rich	Wayne	11/21/1848
2	Abigail VanBuskirk	Tipton	11/21/1848
3	Lucinda Brown	Marion	11/21/1848
4	Mary Whiteridge	Jefferson	11/21/1848
5	Rasina (Rosina) Wyatt	Jefferson	11/21/1848
6	Florintine Weide	Jefferson	11/21/1848
7	Melia Sheppard	Johnson	11/22/1848
8	Amelia Green	Marion	11/22/1848
9	Miss Nancy Little	Fayette	11/23/1848

Opening an institution to help the mentally ill is different than teaching the caregivers how the people should be treated. Most attendants, who spent the majority of the day with patients, had no medical training and received no real training from the hospital upon employment. They brought the only knowledge they had from society about the care and treatment of patients to their work. Attendants were used to treating patients the way they had been treated in the poor houses, streets and prisons. It would take years to change that way of thinking. By then, the institution had outgrown its purpose.

TWO

HOSPITAL LIFE

Central State Hospital was one of the first 15 public psychiatric hospitals in the United States. It was considered a leader in research and initiated many improvements that were adopted by other hospitals in, and out, of state.

Originally, the hospital was modeled after other hospitals that were considered successful in Ohio's Columbus Hospital for the Insane, New York's New York State Lunatic Asylum at Utica, the Kentucky hospital known under many names such as Fayette Hospital, Massachusetts' Worcester State Hospital, and the Kentucky Lunatic Asylum.

After Central State Hospital for the Insane was built, other hospitals were modeled after it, including Danvers State Hospital (also known as State Lunatic Hospital at Danvers in Danvers, Massachusetts), Athens Lunatic Asylum (also known as The Ridges in Athens, Ohio), Illinois Asylum for the Incurable Insane (also known as Bartonville State Hospital in Bartonville, Illinois).

Central State Hospital for the Insane was always a teaching hospital which drew many visiting physicians from other hospitals and schools. Treatments used in other hospitals were sometimes used at Central State when enough efficacy was proved through scientific research and demonstrations.

Practices in the hospital included Pinel's model of keeping patient records and getting to know the background of the patient to understand the reasons and type of insanity. Subscribing to Pinel, patients were to be treated with respect and care. As the hospital progressed, improvements were made to buildings and processes. Doctors and administrators found that prescription, admission, letter and account books were called for to keep track of patient records and the money entrusted to the hospital. With these new additions, the patients' treatment could be recorded from admission to treatment (prescription), and all correspondence could be tracked. "Upon arrival of patients in the Hospital, we have used every means in our power to learn their past history, parentage, education, religion and habits of life and all the causes which led to their insanity as well as to discover their precise physical and mental condition with a view to administer the proper remedial treatment."

By the end of the 1880s, Central State Hospital for the Insane was larger than the people it was to protect and treat. Due to neglect, corruption and a lack of money and trained personnel, Central State Hospital for the Insane was becoming synonymous with filth, abuse, starvation, and beatings. The constant political wrangling continued to harm the hospital and its goals. Early state government ran on political appointments, and so did the Indiana Hospital for the Insane. The superintendent was appointed and the superintendent could appoint and hire other staff, some of whom were politically charged as the hospital relied on political favor for funding.

Later, two world wars would take their toll as well. Despite advances in mental health diagnosis and treatment, the hospital declined. The hospital was old and retrofitting it to modern standards did little to curb the decay. Continued lack of funding, lack of money for personnel, and lack of trained personnel or effective training programs helped the hospital deteriorate into a crumbling warehouse for patients with no other place to go.

Early Hospital Life

From 1848 to 1888 the Indiana Hospital for the Insane was the only institution which provided treatment and care to patients in Indiana. From day one, this hospital was ill equipped to handle the influx of patients. When it opened, it was not prepared for the amount of people who came to them. Even though upgrades and additions for beds were made throughout its tenure, it could not handle the number of patients as Indiana's population grew.

County poor houses took overflow patients much to the patient's disservice. In 1865 the state enacted a law that provided the incurable and curable were treated equally. Patients were admitted based on a county quota because there was no room to take in everyone. This was ineffectual, because no one could predict the influx of people who needed care.

Many patients slept on thin mattresses on the floor. A consistent pattern of explaining how many patients had to be turned away because of lack of bed capacity became the norm. In the 34th annual report of the trustees and superintendent of the Indiana Hospital for the insane for the year ending October 31, 1882, Dr. Joseph G. Rogers, Superintendent, stated,

> *"What shall be done for those who still remain uncared for? .... The department of men is at all times crowded to its extreme capacity. The completion of the women's department will not obviate the necessity for the discharging or rejecting, annually, a large number of insane men who should be under asylum care. More than a thousand insane persons are necessarily scattered over the State outside of the hospital. Of their existence the great and good-hearted public is ignorant and how they are kept and treated it knows nothing. Those who are in a position to know feel that this helpless class should be under the watchful eyes, as well as the ministering hand of the State.*
>
> *"Indiana, with her vast resources and thriving population of two millions, should stand abreast, at least relatively of her sister States in the maintenance of her public charities; but she has not. Her people so ordered thirty years ago, in the State Constitution in which the care of the insane is made obligatory on the part of the legislature. Yet it has only been partially done."*

He went on to state how other states including Ohio, Illinois, Kentucky, Michigan, Wisconsin, Iowa, Missouri, Kansas, Nebraska and California were able to house and care for their insane with far more insane people in them.

> *"This should be felt to be an individual obligation by every member of the next General Assembly for in every constituency are to be found families who are obliged to keep an insane skeleton in the closet and who would appreciate such relief move than any other good which could come to them."*

Patient Success

Among the successes mentioned:
- A woman who had illness, several family issues and who suffered anxiety and loss of sleep went to Central State Hospital, overwhelmed with gloom. She was given proper medical treatment and her mind calmed. When she was given light employment, amusements and lots of exercise in the fresh air (walking and carriage riding) for four months, she was restored and returned home.
- A farmer was placed in jail for religious excitement due to Mormonism. He was sleepless, noisy, violent, and raving. Through solitude, baths, medicines and diet, he calmed and his restraints were removed. With exercise and labor, he was cured in three months.
- A young woman was admitted for two months. She was maniacal and gave herself "bleeding injuries." The woman was incoherent, approaching dementia, lost her memory, and had no emotion and no interest in anything. With the use of "remedies" she was restored.

Surgery, Deaths and Disease

Surgery

Part of the myth of any mental institution is that secret surgeries are performed on a regular basis. The yearly reports of Central State are full of types of surgeries performed and outcomes, even when not favorable. One case of a man with paraphimosis (1) failed when he died of a heart attack during surgery.

Other examples of surgeries include:
- The doctors treated a case of ergotism (usually occurring from eating grain tainted with the fungus, Claviceps purpurea). The boy was successfully treated and was able to keep most of his limbs. However, necrosis caused part of his leg to be amputated. After the amputation, he fully recovered.
- A man came to the hospital who had been hit in the skull. He had a small depression the "size of birdshot." Since the quarrel that had given him the injury, he had been suicidal and despondent. At first, a trephine was used but that caused a lot of blood loss. Then the doctors maneuvered and eventually pulled out the bone pieces that were pressed into his brain. When the man awoke, he said he "felt like a new man." He left the hospital on the sixth day and went back to his new life.
- Surgeries were also done based on doctor and superintendent decisions (see the case of June Highsaw in the closure chapter). While Highsaw was most certainly not the only case such as this, the surgeries, while not secret, were part of patient history and not public record.

Deaths

The death rate at the hospital was 7% in 1848, which was less than Ohio (8%) or Massachusetts (10%). As the years went on, the death rate fluctuated between 2-10%, except in years where maintenance was allowed to lapse. For example in 1853, the death rate soared to almost 15% when 14 deaths occurred among 500 patients, many due to poor ventilation in the building.

Some patients arrived ill and succumbed to the illness. In 1872 the hospital reported a decrease in patient death. It was attributed to the county poor homes which had not "poured their human debris into the Hospital." What was meant by this is that by the time many patients made it to the hospital, they were not only mentally ill, they were also sick beyond repair. By county poor homes not giving the hospital their sick and dying, the patient deaths decreased.

Other patients contracted illness at the hospital and it had its share of flu, pneumonia, and other diseases. However, there were never any large scale epidemics.

Accidental deaths happened, such as a patient who was "engaged in police duty" in a vehicle near the hospital and crushed by the engine belt of the car.

Occasionally, patients would kill other patients. In 1886 a quiet man was sleeping on a bench in the Grove when another more violent patient picked up a slat from the fence and struck him with it, killing him instantly. Staff said the two men never quarreled, but the violent man stated, "He was my enemy. I had to kill him."

In 1896 a patient hit another with a chair, which irreparably fractured his skull, killing him. On the morning of July 9, 1919 Thomas Edwards, a patient, attacked Mrs. Mary L. Kelley, a forewoman of the laundry and Fred Pfister, another patient, with a pipe iron. They both died. The attack seemed to be without warning or provocation.

Other deaths due to understaffing also occurred. May 16, 1904 a patient died of scalding in a bath. The male attendant had been by himself from Tuesday to Saturday for the most part, aside from times when he was sleeping and when the night watchmen took over. The attendant had a patient working with him to bath another patient. The patient due for bathing had been stripped. The attendant stepped out to remove soiled clothing as was the rule, thereby breaking the rule of leaving two patients in the bathing area. The attendant stated he knew he was breaking one rule, but upholding another and that "if I had help on the ward, it would not have been necessary to have left the bathroom." When the attendant returned, the water was on, the patent to be bathed was in the tub, and the other patient was standing beside the tubs. The attendant asked his helper why he'd turned on the water, but got no response. The attendant asked for someone from Ward A, which was nearby, to call a doctor. Dr. Watters stated it couldn't have been too long for the patient to be in the water because "the flesh was not coked." The attendant was subsequently discharged from the hospital, although Dr. Watters (2) didn't think the attendant had done anything wrong.
In the 1980s and 1990s up to 18 cases were found to be due to understaffing and negligence.

Suicides

Suicides were not uncommon but they were not out of control. It was always less than 1% of the patients who committed suicide with usually two to ten patients per year who killed themselves.

The first two suicides happened in 1852. One man killed himself with a handkerchief around his throat. Over the years, patients hanged themselves, killed other patients and died by a variety of self-induced means, sometimes unintentional. In one case, a man had been smuggling meat back to his room, and at 12:30am one evening, he died by "meat choking" when he tried to eat it. Two patients died by suffocation. The most common methods of suicide were hanging, followed by drowning (usually in a bathtub, or if they had ground privileges, Eagle Creek) and then slitting wrists or other area of the body. Sometimes patients would find a chemical, such disinfectant, and drink it.

Suicides rose in the 1880-1909 period. In 1901 John Stiffani died from a severe scalding while bathing. Another man hung himself by taking the leather straps from his restraints and tying them to the bed, forming a noose and dropping his head into it.

One particularly gruesome attempted suicide involved a woman who had been addicted to opium before she was admitted to the hospital. She gave herself a stomach wound and pulled out four feet of intestine. The wound was closed with a suture, the hernia mass was carbolized and returned to the body cavity, and the external wound closed by sutures. She survived.

Civil War and the Return of Dorthea Dix

During the Civil War (1861-1865), the hospital administration noted that other states were improving and growing their hospitals and thought that for the sake of humanity that Central State Hospital for the Insane should be expanded to care for the sick, meaning insane people who were also sick with a physical ailment such as heart problems or a chronic condition. The hospital experienced tremendous overcrowding due to the "rebellion" (Civil War) when so many fathers, brothers, and sons were at the front (3).

After the Civil War, the hospital tried to make due with less. They did not receive appropriations for new buildings or much of the repair work. Because of this, space that would have been used for patient rooms and treatment were taken away from the patients. However, when Dorthea Dix revisited in the early part of 1867 and made numerous suggestions for improvements, including more buildings, repairs and improvements for patients, the hospital received more money for expansion for a short time.

Because of Dix' visit, the north wing of the original building was completed. The hospital also received a carpenter's house. The grounds were brought back up to their pre-war beauty and the hospital began growing Concord grapes (Hartford Prolific). Dix gave a Mason and Hamlin's five octave cabinet organ (4) to the new chapel in the north wing.

New Hospitals and Other Institutions

Three new hospitals did form eventually: Evansville (1890), Logansport (1888) and Richmond (1890). The Richmond and Logansport hospitals were almost not built because Mr. David S. Gooding (Hancock County) of the Indiana House of Representatives Ways and Means Committee believed the State had been "misled" in the necessity for three new hospitals. These hospitals were forbidden to discharge patients until "their physical and mental condition justifies it." However, the policy did not apply to Central State Hospital.

Logansport (Longcliff)

It opened July 1, 1888. It was nicknamed Longcliff because it was built near a cliff (a rock formation) overlooking the Wabash River. Instead of the Kirkbride plan, which was falling out of favor, it was built on the cottage plan, providing a homier atmosphere. Built on 281 acres, 160 were purchased from the Andrew Shanklin family, and the 121 were donated by Cass County residents.

Evansville (Woodmere)

It sat on 160 acres three miles east of Evansville and opened on Oct 30, 1890. Woodmere was its nickname, suggesting a peaceful retreat. It was originally built on the Kirkbride plan.

Richmond (East Haven)

Plans began in 1878 and construction in 1884. Because of the issues between the state and planning, the hospital buildings were used by the Indiana School for Feebleminded Youth. When they transferred out, the buildings were left in disrepair and were vacant for a time. More updates needed to be made to them and on July 29, 1890 the hospital opened. It sat on a little over 300 acres of land. It was also built on the cottage plan.

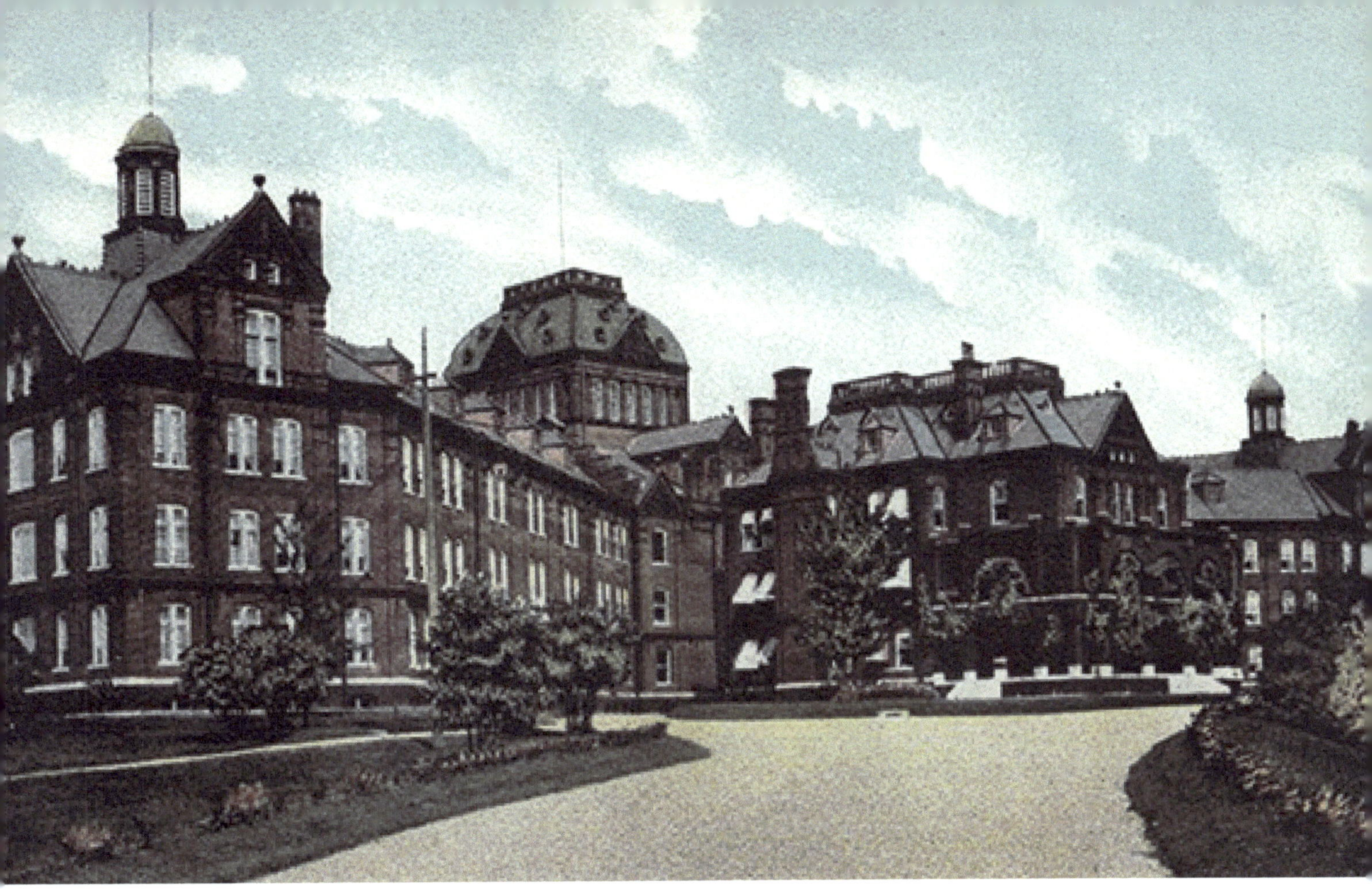

Above: Evansville State Hospital
Below: Logansport State Hospital

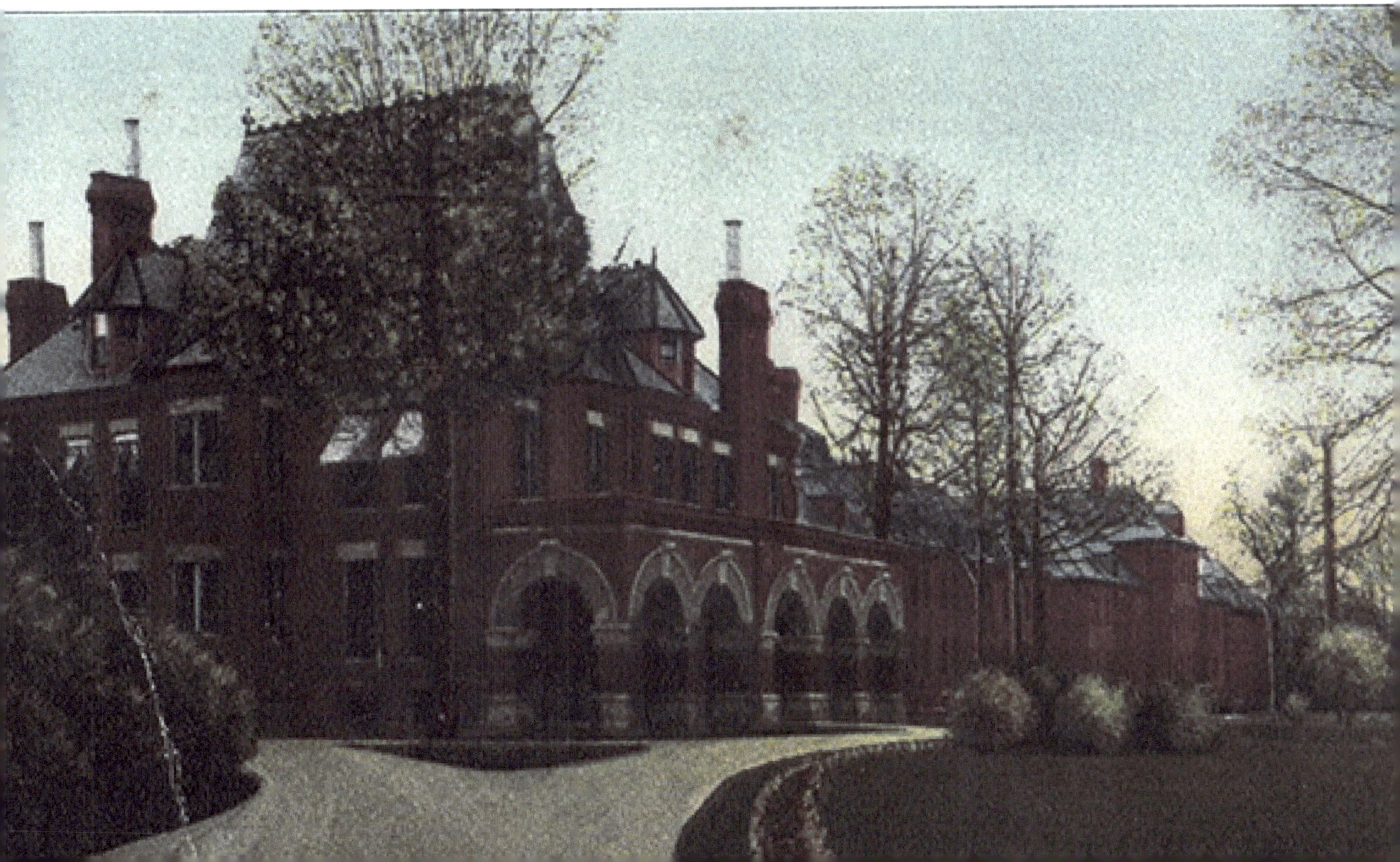

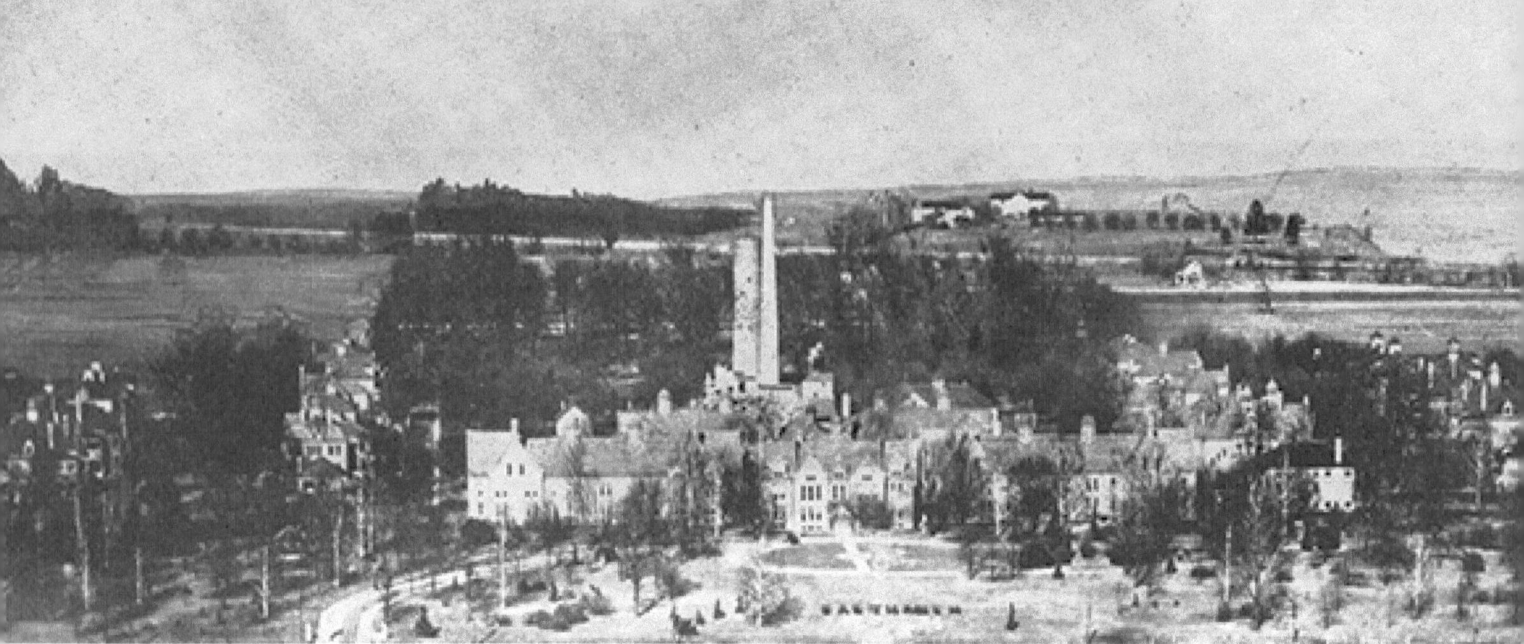

Above: Richmond State Hospital

Additionally, several other institutions opened.
- In the early 1900s, Marion County opened its own facility, The Asylum for the Incurably Insane (located at the county poor farm) for 200 patients. The hospital was overcrowded by 400 patients. Despite 300 new beds being bought, 200 of these patients were "not in as fortunate care as the rest of the population due to lack of space." They slept on thin mattresses in the floor in halls, or wherever space was available.
- In 1905 the Madison State Hospital (the Southeastern Indiana Hospital for the Insane) was started. It sat on a 400 foot bluff known as "The Hill." It cost over $1,200,000 to build. It used the utilitarian cottage plan as its basis. Originally, it contained 1,265 acres and sat next to Clifty Falls State Park.
- The Indiana Village for Epileptics was finished in 1907.
- In 1909 the hospital for Insane Criminals was established at the Indiana State Prison in Michigan City.

By the time these facilities were built, they did not alleviate crowded conditions, nor did they change the perception that mentally ill people were "skeletons in the closet." Perhaps this still had something to do with the word "inmates" still being used in Central State Hospital's annual reports as it was a prison throwback word as late as 1898!

By 1900 the cycle of overcrowding, repairs and lack of money was still prevalent. However, new innovations were added to the hospital. A telephone system switchboard was installed to replace the old speaking tube method of communication. With the new telephone system all departments were connected and quick communication was now possible.

Fire Protection

By 1867, fire insurance became important. Many old buildings were made of wood that combusted easily. The Sanborn Company created maps to assess fire insurance liability in case these buildings burned. The maps were not limited to the wooden buildings; all buildings on the property were assessed, including Central State Hospital. As a result of the Sanborn maps bringing the hospital's attention to potential risks, the hospital asked that the State make a contingency that they would have their buildings rebuilt in case of fire.

Fire prevention became paramount in Indiana, especially when an Illinois insane asylum lost 19 patients because of lack of fire protection and evacuation planning. The hospital suggested to the State of Indiana that the hospital should also have fire insurance to cover over $3,000,000 worth of assets at the hospital. It is unknown if the State did purchase insurance for the hospital.

The hospital was lucky. It never had a fire with loss of life. Many of the fires were small with little property damage. Below is a sampling of the types of fires which the hospital buildings sustained damage:
- Between 1884 and 1885 there were 3 fires (no locations mentioned) $60,000 damage.
  - In 1904 a fire burned in the third ward of the Department for Women.
  - February 13, 1906 a fire burned the basement of the Department for Men.

- In 1926 the hospital had four fires: laundry for $4000, two others at the laundry at 'small losses', and one in the Department for Men at "no loss".
- In 1935 the Men's Recreation Hall sustained $200 damage from a fire due to antiquated wiring.

Hospital Projects

Although the hospital administration asked for many things, it always took multiple times of asking and many years to complete. They asked for the Men's Department building to be complete and it was completed 22 years after the hospital opened. The Women's Department took nearly that long. In 1894 the administration asked that the Men's Department be torn down and a new building built. This did not happen until 1931 when the Men's Cottages were built.

Other projects that were not funded by the state included:
- A natatorium and bath house
- Tuberculosis department
- Building for convalescents, contagious disease and acute cases (although a Sick Hospital was built)
- The Sick Hospital was outdated, being built in 1899 and needed updating or a new building should be built.
- Buildings for the untidy (i.e. patients who could not bathe or groom themselves on the most basic level)
- Training school for employees
- Pavilions for "outdoor patients" (which could have been convalescing tuberculosis patients).
- Support for hydrotherapeutics (Although hydrotherapeutics existed in a rudimentary form, a full area wasn't built and equipped until much later than the early 1900s.)
- A freestanding separate chapel

During the 1880s, in addition to regular maintenance which was hit or miss depending on money, several major improvements occurred, outside The Department of Women:
- The fence on the National Road (Washington Street) and a gate at Vermont Street were installed. In making the hospital more home-like, the administrations requested the block of lots to the south west of the hospital be bought and destroyed. They believed that the hospital farm was open and vulnerable to anyone who wanted to come in and "pillage" it for food. Fletcher recommended that the houses be condemned and an iron fence placed around the entire hospital. It took some time to get the fence and when it was installed, it gave little to no protection to the farmland.
- A new railroad spur was put on the grounds by the Indianapolis Decatur & Springfield Railroad to the north. It passed to the rear of the men and women's buildings and went to the coal yards, wood ricks and stores, saving the hospital from having to haul coal and other supplies from beyond Eagle Creek.
- A well was also dug and a pump house installed for the Department of Women. Water mains for the hospital's own water system (and city water) were installed.
- Wire screens were placed on the windows of the Department for Men to keep pests out.
- Roads and walks were regraded, leveled and graveled.
- Fire drills were perfected.
- The street car tracks were removed from the hospital.

Name Change

Originally the hospital was named simply the Hospital for the Insane. Within a few years, the name changed to the Indiana Hospital for the Insane. March 11, 1889, the hospital's was changed to Central State Hospital for the Insane. March 3, 1927 it became Central State Hospital.

World War I

World War I was not kind to the hospital. The hospital still lacked space. Its medical staff was called to war by the Army Medical Corps. The men who manned the wards were drafted into the military. Nurses worked for the Red Cross. The attendants and domestics were able to get larger salaries outside of the hospital and left their work. Dr. Dodds stated in the annual report of the Northern Indiana Hospital for the Insane ending September 30, 1920 "The state hospitals…. If not for the faithful, loyal, well-trained men and women who remained at their posts, some of these hospitals should have had to close their doors." Moreover practically no increase was made in the appropriations and there was not sufficient money to meet the increased cost in subsistence and repairs.

The gardens and fields provided ample food, so the patients noticed no difference to their diet during this time. Shortly after the war, the State Board of Charities, who had helped get more land for farming, saw fruition of some of its goals. For example the trees were now bearing fruit which alleviated some of the food costs. Small eating areas in some of the existing buildings or additions were made for infirm patients.

The diagnosis of shell shock or post-traumatic stress disorder (PTSD) came out of WWI. With so many resources in the Army Medical Corps, group action, techniques and study made diagnosis quicker and treatment stronger. Additionally, some of the improvements to medical techniques and equipment helped foster neurosurgery as a specialty medicine.

Although the yearly reports indicate occupational therapy continued to be refined and was considered an integral part of a patient's treatment, the U.S. Public Health Service disagreed, especially with regard to veterans. Henry Ladd Stickney, a supervisor, visited the hospital and was displeased. He wrote a report to the State Board of Indiana Charities, which supervised the well-being of people within state institutions.

Stickney took issue with the bad condition of the men's wards. He also did not believe there was real vocational or occupational therapy available at the hospital other than working around the grounds and buildings. The organization believed for most of the time that veterans had little to occupy their minds.

Additionally, Stickney believed that hydrotherapy should have been a part of the therapy rotation. There seemed to be no attempt to provide this to patients.

Because of these issues, he recommended that without changes, War Risk Insurance claimants should be moved to a private facility, or to a different state or governmental facility that could better serve their needs.

The stock market crash of 1929 changed the hospital. Funds were even more limited. Repairs, except for the most critical, went undone. Because of the State provision in the constitution that prohibited Indiana from bonding itself for indebtedness, the hospital could not enter the Public Works Administration program early on in 1934. This program, when finally entered, allowed some minor repair work to occur: roads, sidewalks, drives.

However, not all was bleak. During the 1929-1940 period, because of the lack of jobs, more qualified people were applying for jobs. Central State had waiting lists for any job that was posted and the vacancies would be filled within 24 hours. The down side was that needed training programs were unable to be created due to perpetual lack of funds and some patient care did suffer.

The hospital believed that public education was key to the public's support of the hospital. The more the public knew and understood, the more they appreciated and were proud of what the hospital was accomplishing. Much needed repairs were completed and the Department for Men was dismantled making way for the Men's Cottages to be built, which allowed for more modern housing and treatment for patients.

In 1930 hospital officials stated that in 82 years, 33,623 patients had been admitted and 23,388 were discharged, and 8,487 died. Of those people, in addition to the chronic mentally ill, they found the public were sending older people to the hospital, which was not right in most cases because nothing was wrong. To alleviate crowding, patients from Jasper, Newton, Benton, White and Carroll counties were being sent to Logansport.

By the end of the 1930s, outpatients were sent to IU School of Medicine for consultation and surgery. They were considered well enough to be treated by someone outside the Central State Hospital system.

World War II

In 1939 as Europe began World War II industry in general, especially manufacturing, began to pick up. The lower paid but higher qualified state employees gained during the post-WWI years, were leaving to go to these jobs, leaving the hospitals inadequately staffed and with under-trained staff. Still, with the perpetual lack of funds, no money existed to put decent training in place or offer more money to the staff they had or could hire.

The Men's Department program was interrupted by the "national emergency" of the bombing of Pearl Harbor and the announcement of the U.S. entering WWII. This action had a devastating impact on Central State Hospital. Materials, especially anything metal or industrial related, were very difficult to get. Even more personnel left, and the men especially, could not be replaced. There was no time to train any of the people the hospital could hire.

The war's toll on the hospital resulted in damaged patient care and dilapidated building conditions. One example at the Logansport State Hospital shows that a doctor had no one to man the wards one evening. The night supervisor took her keys and gave one to the best patient on each ward with instructions that if fire broke out, the patient was to unlock the doors and let the other patients out. The patients rose amazingly to this task on several nights.

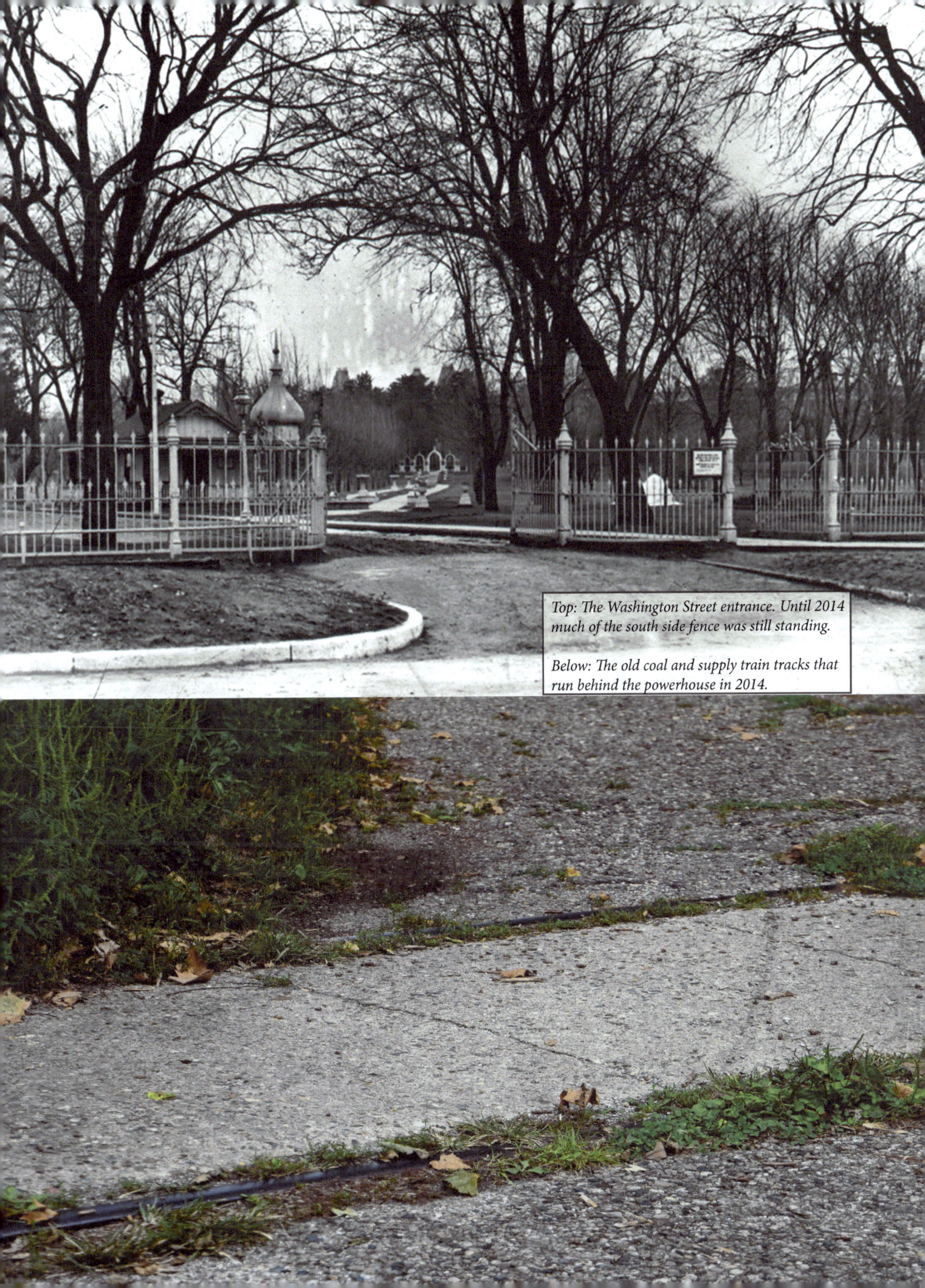

Top: The Washington Street entrance. Until 2014 much of the south side fence was still standing.

Below: The old coal and supply train tracks that run behind the powerhouse in 2014.

The patients ran the hospital during the war becoming "trustees" who would perform attendant duties, check on other patients and perform watch rounds.

Additionally, the hospital did not offer social services during the war. The librarian helped find patients places to stay after they were released due to housing shortages.

Central State Hospital did its bit for the war effort. It organized under the Civilian Defense for blackouts and air-raids with assignments of personnel to duties and stations. Hospital staff was given courses in first aid, training of air raid wardens, and instruction in chemical warfare by the Office of Civilian Defense and the Indianapolis Fire Department. Personnel bought war bonds through payroll deduction. The hospital pulled together to collect scrap metal, discarded rubber, tin cans and waste paper.

In February of 1943 Central State Hospital was taxed further by a fire at Evansville's State Hospital. The fire destroyed most of the hospital and patients had to be sent around the state. Central State Hospital received patients from Vanderburgh, Greene, Sullivan and Knox Counties. Because of the influx of patients, employees were forced to sleep on the third floor of the Women's Department.

Also, psychiatry took an odd turn. Nazism and its atrocities were becoming known. Germany was losing its grip as the standard for medical education. In the eyes of the academics, many ideas were explored in psychiatry which were "bizarre and impractical. These theories contained many fanciful suggestions ….. they were the fruits of visionary minds, they lacked scientific soundness and were without value to the patient."

A reorganization of duties occurred during WWII. The hospital shared dual control with the Division of Mental Health in the State Department of Public Welfare. As the Public Welfare Department had become very hands off, Central State Hospital was largely left to its own devices and truly became a place onto itself. In 1945 "An Act Concerning Mental Cases" was passed that allowed for one central authority over mental hospitals. However, because of the staff shortage, the act could not be carried out immediately. In this bill, a teaching hospital was proposed to be erected. This hospital was built on the grounds of Indiana University School of Medicine in Indianapolis and was named Larue D. Carter Memorial Hospital.

Post World War II

After the war when materials became available, another inadequate program for rehabilitation and repair was launched. Over $287,300.00 in improvements and repairs were needed, weren't fully realized. Hiring and keeping personnel continued to be a problem. The Superintendent warned that unsatisfactory conditions due to a lack of doctors and turnover of attendants were "likely to continue without adequate pay for all." Consequently, women were now working on the men's wards due to staffing shortages. Only five full time registered nurses (RNs) worked at the hospital, although there were openings for 16. The hospital also had seven full time and four part time part time social workers.

The hospital moved into a new age. More treatments were available and seemed to have a better effect. Drugs were being developed to help the mentally ill. Psychotherapy was now widely used. Occupational therapy continued to be refined and was considered an integral part of a patient's treatment. Family was becoming more involved. When a patient was released, the hospital asked that the family provide a six month update with the patient's condition.

An interest in efficiency began, and new ways to complete tasks appeared. A new procedure to streamline patient care was implemented. New patients were put in the Admission Ward and checked for fever and disease. In the second week, blood and spinal fluids were examined and the doctor ordered a urine analysis, blood counts, x-ray and other tests. Once the tests were back, the doctor spoke with staff about patient care going forward including: insulin therapy, electric shock and malaria treatment. Patients stayed on the Admission Ward for six months. If they were not ready to go home, they were assigned a ward.

Additionally the hospital introduced new record keeping. An inventory of drugs was kept to control their use and distribution. Ward diaries were instituted for anything out of the ordinary and changes to population. Narcotic control books were used to pinpoint any excessive drug use. Ward cards used in Cottage 4A and 4B, and Cottage 3B helped doctors who make rounds.

Nursing policies were being standardized and reporting as well. By this time all restraints for men except Cottage 7 were gone. In Cottage 7, 26 men were in seclusion and 27 in restraints. 1By 1957 nurses from DePauw came to the hospital and were given temporary accreditation after being surveyed by the Indiana State Board of Nurses Registration and Nursing Education. Central State was unique in the state and country for using college students to help fill some gaps. The nurses had four weeks of clinical education and testing, then went to the hospital to apply. After this the nurses were given six months to go to the accrediting agency and completed eight weeks of psychiatric nursing courses.

The public was treated to a variety of news coverage during this time. Emphasis was placed on the aging hospital and the treatment of patients. A variety of scandals appeared in newspapers.

On March 6, 1949, Richard Lewis, a reporter, wrote about his visit to the hospital with Indiana State Representatives. "In the catacomb like recesses, " Lewis wrote, "we saw the living dead." The infirmary inhabitants were "aged and feeble" and "skeletonic." They lay under "thin, dirty blankets" and "babble." The walls of the infirmary wards were "alive with roaches…a rat scuttled across the broken concrete floor, leaving his droppings in a shallow chuckhole."

Some people on the tour compared the smell to that of Dachau concentration camp. Lewis, who had been to Dachau, pointed out the difference- that being that the inmates of Dachau were liberated. These people would not be, until death.

The women's building, which had bars on the windows, looked like a prison to Lewis. Plaster fell from walls, plumbing didn't work and some wards had one bath for 50 patients. There were two psychiatrists for the entire facility and one of them was the medical director. Normally ten to 12 RNs would be on staff at a facility this size. There were two positions at Central State Hospital, with one nurse on staff and the other was not replaced for almost a year. No surgeon was on staff. One research director was employed. "Only the tiniest spark of psychiatric work can be done here."

In 1953 Governor George N. Craig was appalled by "Old Main" (Department for Women). "I doubt there is a cheap boarding house in even the remotest area of any of our larger cities which is comparable to conditions I found there." Sixty people were using one tub. The hospital employee pool was sadly lacking:

The hospital had	The hospital was short, according to hospital requested funding	American Psychological Association (APA) Standards
240 attendants	12	needed 112 more
12-13 doctors	--	needed 24 more
7 nurses	31	needed 158 more
2 psychiatrists	--	unknown

Patient Donation

Jewel MacComber Christie died as a patient of Central State Hospital in 1936. She and her son set up a fund which helped purchase electromyographic, encephalographic, and electro-cardiographic equipment. The initial donation was $17600. Jewel Christie sustained a fall, began using drugs and got addicted. She was eventually admitted to Central State Hospital when she was found wandering the streets of Anderson, dazed (5).

Dr. Williams, stated he had money for 25 more nurses "if I can get them." Administration said that they were having problems attracting staff at the pay rates they had. The governor ordered state health and personnel officials to work out an employee procurement process for state institutions. His plan included using 30 inmates of Indiana penal institutions to provide carpentry skills and general clean up. An orchard sprayer and 500 gallons of Dichlorodiphenyl-trichloroethane (DDT) were provided to kill insects until new screens could be provided for windows. Other factory and state farm work at the State Farm and Reformatory stopped and manufacturing the screens became the priority. Patients were eating on the floor so penal plants also were to manufacture 800 heavy duty chairs, 500 tables, 500 storage units. The National Guard supplied old beds and the Indiana Board of Health supplied an X-ray machine that was not in use.

Also, it was alleged that patients were still involved in housekeeping despite the 1966 Federal labor law prohibiting them from working even as part of therapy. Court cases were still being fought in the early 2000s trying to get back pay for patients who were performing work.

A scandal involved the twenty year old adopted daughter of a prominent family. The girl tried to get out from the inside but a "no visitors" order was given. Her foster parent testified she was of unsound mind. Attorney John Raikos helped free her before she was given electro shock treatments. The judge, George A Henry, said that a full report of the girl's condition was never provided and therefore, she was free and declared of sound mind. Then he told the foster family that they equated care in dollars and cents and not love.

Staffing continued to be slow and not many attendants or nurses stayed for a long time. According to Miss Martha Rogers, Director of Psychiatric Nursing "Most attendants are assigned to these areas for short periods and then transferred to less physically demanding and more pleasant duties elsewhere."

Money, Maintenance and the Cost of Care

Money

Of course, no institution is ever going to get all the money for all the projects they need, but the State of Indiana had a pattern with regard to the hospital. On April 3, 1857 the General Assembly told the Board of Commissioners for the hospital that no money had been appropriated. Staff was let go and the 303 patients were released. On April 21, 1857 the Board of Commissioners created guidelines stating that the counties must pay for the hospital expenses, but it didn't work well as very few counties could afford this. Finally, by October 5, 1857 the hospital was told money could be received from the treasury to support the hospital until the General Assembly met again.

Again in 1863 the Legislature didn't make an appropriation. The Superintendent said the omission was "less than inexcusable". All of the patients were returned to their county poor homes, family and friends. Somehow, the farm survived with an additional 15 acres of clover field turned into a vegetable field by staff who had nowhere else to go or live. The old garden was reseeded to grass.

Late in 1863 money was given to the hospital to reopen and continue operation. No back pay seems to have been appropriated. Because of the monetary issues, the hospital asked the state to amend the law stating that clothing expenses should be charged to the county where the person resided to $40 per patient.
Sometimes vendors were made to wait for money. For example, in 1861 the hospital had to defer the coal payment because they had no money. In 1864, Calvin Fletcher Jr. co-owner of Western Commercial Nurseries, provided shade and evergreen trees for $359.35 and said he "would wait on the money till the legislature appropriated the money to be paid for them."

Maintenance

Maintenance was always an issue at the hospital. The bids were posted three times in the newspapers and then a contractor was selected. Sometimes, the building materials were not what they were supposed to be. By the time the Department for Men was completed, several small outbuildings had been built. The old wing of the Department for Men needed repairs.

Between 1873 and 1879, the hospital buildings received little maintenance. They were overcrowded, and in bad repair. It was hard to provide care for the insane under those circumstances. Patients were still in "the Basement" of the Men's Department and employees were now six people to a room to make more room for patients. In 1875 no maintenance budget was provided and in 1877 and 1879 the hospital received only about 25% of what it requested.

In the 12 years after the hospital opened, it was clear the administrative wheels were not moving fast enough

for the influx of patients. The hospital was in a constant state of being reactive to issues and not proactive. Maintenance was often neglected.
- Twelve years after the hospital opened, the hospital also needed repairs to the roof for leaks.
- They also asked for gas lighting because the oil lighting put out "noxious carbon" and presented a fire hazard.
- The administration also stated "in damp weather when the atmosphere is light the stench from the water closets is intolerable. The air is impure and can account for some of the deaths."
- The wooden floors needed to be re-laid and covered in lead.
- A previously minor plastering that was repaired. By the time the money was appropriated, the plaster was so damaged from rain water and leaking water closets that it had to be torn out and completely redone.
- The old boiler was crumbling to pieces and couldn't be sold.

COST OF CARE

The initial startup costs for the hospital were calculated at less than $400 per bed (compared with other institutions that were $500 per bed. Even with this lower per bed cost, the money given by the Indiana State Legislature, and the money made by the farm, and loans, wasn't enough to help finish the hospital buildings.

Between 1853 and 1854 the cost of running the hospital jumped. For example, the cost of building and labor went up as did the cost for foodstuffs. The hospital used two less barrels of flour but the cost went from $1,074.87 to $2,093.77. To defray meat costs in the long run, the hospital grazed cattle on 60 acres of land.

Doctors estimated that people who were caught and cured early on took about 21 weeks to cure at a cost of $64.32 each. The incurable were on average sick for 13.5 years before admission. If they had been in the system for those years it would have cost Indiana $1,418.56 per case. The incurables were still being cared for in hospitals and jails, county poor homes and in "private pen or out-building". Doctors estimated 80% of these cases, if they had been caught early, could have been cured.

Eventually, the center of the hospital's Department for Men was in danger of collapsing and taking the rest of the building with it. Because of the lack of attention given to the original problem, it would cost almost $100,000 to fix the problem and therefore only the immediate repairs necessary were performed. The hospital continued its reactive versus proactive approach.

Still, the superintendent wrote in 1874 that he believed the hospital truly provided "comfort and cure" and wished the State would be as generous as the citizens had been with their support. The Superintendent went on to say that buildings "should not be built by parts, but constructed as a whole from foundations to roof without intermission, as a matter of economy and utility." This was never to be.

The Department of Women, the second major building on the hospital grounds, opened in 1874, but was not completed until 1886. By that time, repairs were needed to the older sections and the Kirkbride plan was obsolete. They also found that the new bathrooms, sinks and water closets were needed to make the building home-like.

When the hospital had a $26,000 surplus, the hospital administration wanted to use the money to furnish the Women's Department, which never had been fully furnished. The hospital was told to return the money to the State Treasury. Oddly enough, the State Treasury reappropriated the money. The next year, only $15,000 for repairs was requested, knowing it wasn't going to be enough for everything. The hospital received $12,000.

During the 1880s, the hospital also asked in an effort to save money that
- Any out of state patients had to be paid for by the state they came from
- Any patient with sufficient means would provide their own clothing and expenses.
- Female insane who could not be brought in by their immediate relatives should be taken to a skilled female attendant and only the expense of the transfer be charged (this would save 50%).

OVERCROWDING

In the year after Central State Hospital for the Insane opened, it seemed to run smoothly, despite overcrowding. However, a $10,000 deficit was incurred in 1848, and by 1851 that figure grew to $18,000 (over $530,000 in 2014 money). It increased to $22,000 in 1852 with half the debt being discharged by the end of the year. It increased again from $11,000 to $12,000 between 1852-1855, when it was finally discharged.

The chronic shortage of space, staff, and coin was catching up to the hospital. By 1851 the hospital was more than overcrowded, staff slept four to a room or sometimes in patient rooms and there seemed to be no end. The administration asked for $35,000 for two new wings off the main building, stating it would take three years to complete them. The south wing was opened in 1853. Due to a lack of appropriations and other delays, the north wing was opened in 1870, 19 years after the space was needed.

Overcrowding was out of control. In order to accommodate patients and the overcrowding, patients had to be put in the basement. These basement rooms were for the worst of the worst patients.

- Known as "the Basement", these "low, narrow, dark, damp, unventilated, difficult to warm prison-like and foreboding" areas were "unfit for the habitation of human beings, leaving out all consideration of cure." The cells were located under the front wards.
- Patients slept on straw mattresses which were destroyed almost immediately. They were also not allowed to eat at "common tables with the rest of the population."
- Gloves, muffs, wristlets and straps were employed daily.
- Patients in the front wards had to listen to the noise associated with the most difficult patients. It disturbed the less unfortunate patients in sleep and daily routine and destroyed some of the benefits the hospital could bring their conditions.

After WWI, Central State and other institutions played catch up on repairs for years. Reorganization of departments, extensive repairs, painting, plumbing, paper hanging, new floors, ceilings, walls, roofs, gutters, downspouts, walks, roads and lawns were all neglected during wartime. Additionally, replacement of some articles was necessary due to being worn out, broken and an inability to be repaired: bedding, carpets, rug, shades, furniture, dishes, instruments, farm and garden implements, wagons, harnesses.

While Superintendent Bahr was in office, he was in charge of a colony that was located at Fort Benjamin Harrison ("Fort Ben") in 1948. At the time, there was a waiting list. Three hundred senile and 'deteriorated' cases went there living in three barracks with refurbished kitchens.

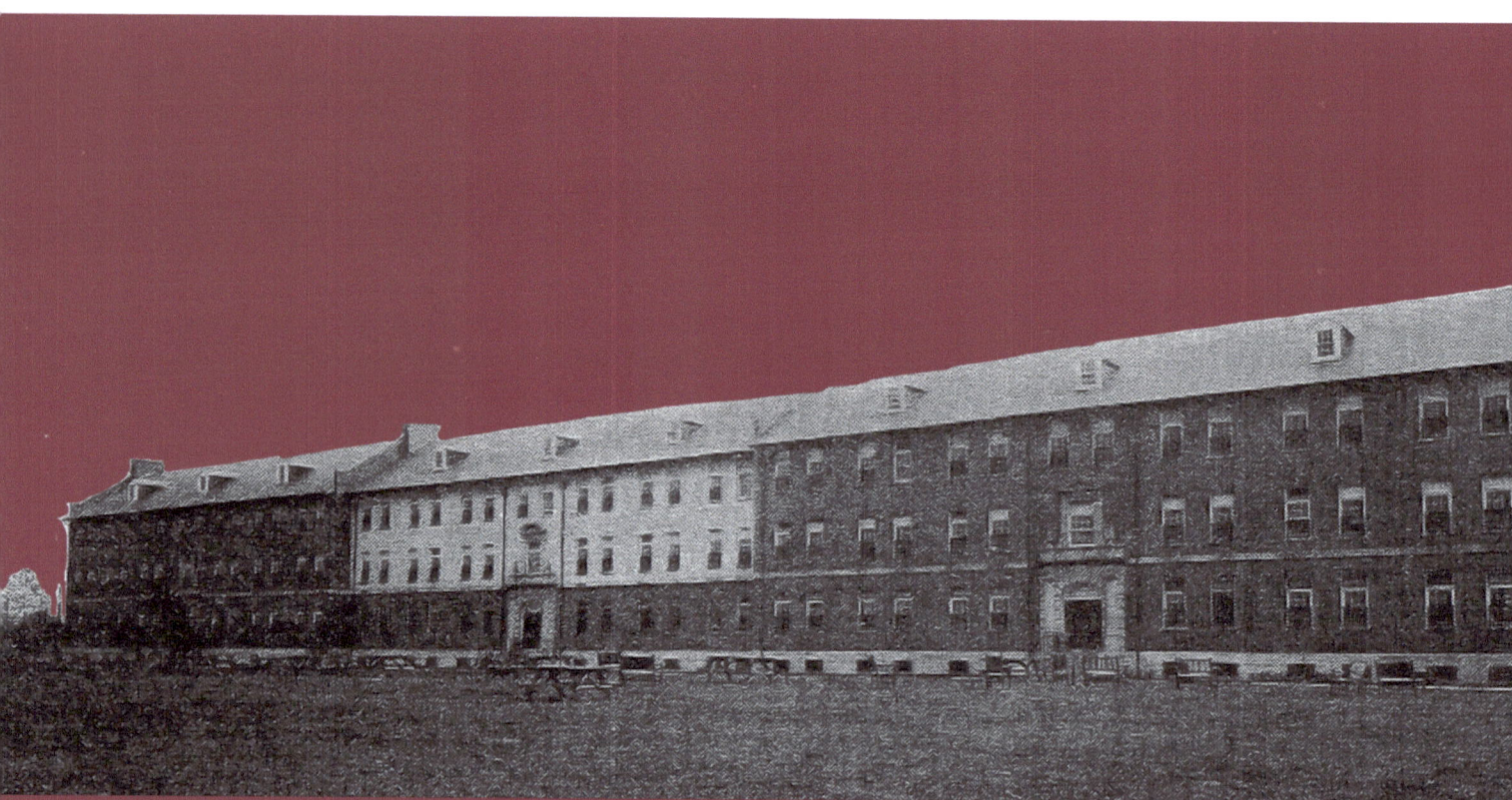

Three Barracks Building at the Fort Benjamin Harrison Colony.

Three

PATIENT LIFE

Patients came from all walks of life - farmers, laborers, merchants, blacksmiths, physicians, coopers, gunsmiths, daugerrean artists, dentists, tinners, house workers, school girls, teachers, tailoresses, mantua makers, milliners and paper makers and those with no occupations.

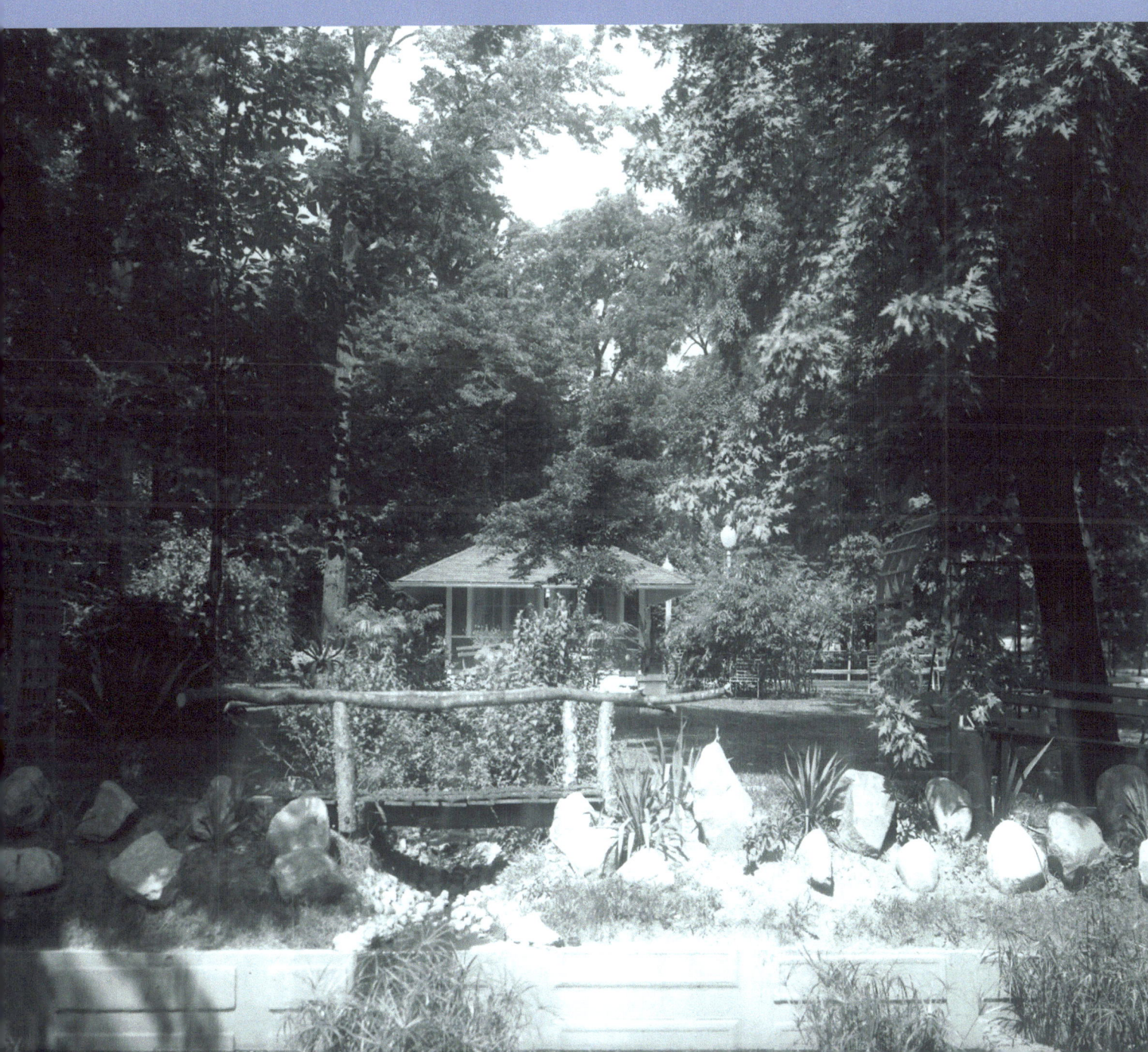

At the beginning of the hospitals, patients were classified into two types of insanity- criminals and all the others. Criminally insane people could have many different classifications but since they were apt to harm others, they were kept in prisons. All of the other insane fell into a variety of classifications based on their type of insanity.

During the early days, the hospital was locked. This was to ensure the patients would not wander off, or hurt themselves or others. Still, it was not uncommon for patients to "elope" (escape). Most were patients who were given ground privileges and left. Many times they would be returned or come back of their own accord. Anyone who didn't return was marked as "discharged unimproved."

The staff was penalized highly for any missing patients. Punishment ranged from fines, to demotion, to working extra hours, to dismissal without references. Security consisted of attendants and other staff keeping the peace until the early 1900s when a police force was formed specifically for the hospital.

Patients who were too sick, or unable to function within groups, such as angry, violent and suicidal patients, spent much of their time on the wards or later in padded cells to keep them and others from harm. Seclusion rooms were also used for patients who made a lot of noise at night and disturbed other patients. Sometimes these rooms were used as a reward for patients and afforded them a little privacy. Other times, they were used as a restful respite for agitated but non-violent patients.

Segregation of male and females was normal until after about 1900 when they were in the same building, but in different wards. Patients had little to no privacy and even less personal space. A patient could expect a highly regimented and scheduled day with little variation and with staff always looking on.

It was common in the infancy of the hospital for the patients to work at the hospital. The reason was twofold. First, it was part of "moral therapy" and it seemed to calm and focus the patients, if not help them. Additionally, there was never enough money or staff for everything that needed to be done.

Bonding between patients occurred but rivalries also existed as in any group situation.

Women

Mental healthcare for women and men varied somewhat. Some patients were admitted for short periods. Women seemed to come in more from the stress and exhaustion of everyday lives. Who can blame them? Cooking, cleaning, childcare, social norms and options were very different than they are today. Some women had lost their major breadwinner through accidents, divorce, abandonment or the Civil War. Many times, once they had de-stressed, they went home. They were also put in asylums as a result of giving birth to illegitimate children, problematic miscarriages (note that this is not the stress of having a miscarriage, but the simple fact that a woman may have had several), rape, the then undiagnosed post-natal depression, lack of wanting sex, or wanting sex too much.

In one case, a woman had just finished college, had no job and was living with her brother. Instead of supporting her emotionally, the brother told his sister what she'd done was a waste and wrote a doctor for advice about his sister's "erratic" behavior. The doctor advised the brother to have his sister admitted. Whether this was because he thought the woman was insane or to protect her from her sexist brother, is unknown.

Aside from employment for the hospital, in Victorian times, women didn't do manual labor that was considered "men's work" at the time. It was all based on the Victorian ideals of gender roles and femininity. The women stayed inside in the early times of the hospital making sheets, bedspreads, comforters, pillow cases, under bed ticks, window curtains, dresses, double mattresses, table clothes, pantaloons, pillows, and doing the mending, ironing, washing and other housework.

The domestic department was one of the areas that needed the most help. Sometimes patients had no family or friends. Even if they did, family and friends were not always forthcoming with the clothing they needed. Plus, with the large quantity of people at the hospital, a large number of bedding, linens, and decorative textiles were needed.

To give you an idea of how industrious the staff and patients were, in the 1853, the domestic department reported that it made 182 dresses, 10 skirts, 25 chemises, 30 coats, 22 vests, 59 pantaloons, 13 drawers, 10 night dresses, 302 sheets, 105 pillow cases, 39 bed ticks, 4 bed quilts, 26 table cloths, 53 shirts, 187 towels, 9 sacks, 27 curtains, 53 comfortables (1), 50 pounds of carpet rags (2).

Women would also make fancy items for sale. For example, in 1850 the fancy items (unspecified as to what they really were) brought the hospital $40 in income.

In the 1860s, clothing allowances for women were " two strong gowns, two flannel petticoats, two pairs of woolen stockings, one pair of shoes, two handkerchiefs, at least two chemises and a large warm shawl or cloak, two night gowns, and two quilted skirts". Women's clothing consisted of dresses made of cheviots, oil prints and gingham, undergarments of half bleached muslin and cotton flannel, seamless hosiery. Clothing for men included woolen jeans, material for coats, pants and vests; cheviot for shirts (3), and cotton flannel for undergarments.

Men

While women may have had spouses or other family to care for them, many men did not. After the Civil War and later after the World Wars, more men were admitted to the asylums for conditions that are now collectively called symptoms of Post-Traumatic Stress Syndrome (PTSD), which can affect anyone after a traumatic event. Because of the overwhelming alcoholism and delusions that often came with it, which were enough to be admitted, doctors had a difficulty distinguishing between PTSD and psychosis. Generally, fewer men were in the hospital in the beginning than women. Escape was far more common with men. Some researchers claim because of the fewer number of men that the wards were less likely to break out into unstable conditions. The men's daily schedule was the same as that of women but instead of the indoor duties, they worked outdoors. A commonality among men and women was that they worked together in the kitchens and bake houses. They also cleaned their own wards. Mens' wards generally had more structure and discipline, given that many of the men were in the military. Men were allowed to join sports teams and a band. Farming, gardening, workshops and engineering were also suitable for stable patients.

Routine and Structure

In 1851 you could be admitted to Central State Hospital for no less than 39 reasons. Typically in the early years, patients would be declared insane by a family member and/or doctor and sheriff. Once at the hospital, the patients were evaluated and sent to live on appropriate wards. First there was a distinction by ward between quiet and tidy patients, quiet but untidy patients and loud and untidy patients.

As patients progressed in their treatment, they were put on the appropriate wards. Sometimes, the chronic stayed in their same wards for years.

The routine became rising between for breakfast between 4:30-5:30 a.m. for attendants and shortly after that for patients. Breakfast consisted of coffee, tea or cocoa, and oatmeal or sometimes bread. Then it was off to their tasks for good and mobile patients. The others would have to wait to be taken outside.

Lunch came at 12:30p.m. and would have been food from the farm: some sort of meat, vegetables, milk and

Miss Case 8101

One unfortunate case that shows how desperately the mentally ill needed options came in 1952. A patient known as Miss Case 8101 had already spent 63 years in the institution and was the one person who spent the longest time in any Indiana institution. She was admitted January 17, 1889, when Benjamin Harrison was president and the Eiffel Tower was about to be unveiled. When Miss Case 8101 arrived, a chestnut horse brought the 19 year old young woman up the curved drive to her new home. Her original file was lost and there were only a few notations since 1926, one of which was from her sister saying what to do when Miss Case 8101 died. It was assumed Miss Case 8101 was brought in during a time when people were admitted for being 'queer' or "not right".

Miss Case 8101 was an average child in a middle-class Irish family and spent a lot of time alone, writing letters to people her parents did not know. She was shy and didn't care for people, fearing their criticism. When she was ten years old, her father died due to a complete financial loss (5). Her mother provided for the family and Miss Case 8101 finished eighth grade. Shortly afterwards, the family moved to Kansas City and Miss Case 8101's nervousness became more pronounced. The doctors said she needed familiarity so they moved back to Indianapolis, but it didn't help. Miss Case 8101 came to Central State Hospital with extreme disturbances and religious hallucinations. Later, she seemed to mellow into a "pleasant, chatty woman." It was believed that if she'd been able to have electro convulsive therapy treatment, she might have fared better, "but the knowledge came too late."

CENTRAL STATE HOSPITAL

DEPARTMENT FOR MEN

Clothing Requisition, 1st Class

(CAPABLE OF ATTENTION TO DRESS)

2 Coats, woolen.

1 Vest, woolen.

2 Pair Pants, woolen.

1 Overcoat, woolen.

1 Hat or Cap, woven in one piece.

4 Shirts, white muslin.

4 Undershirts, cotton flannel.

4 Drawers, cotton flannel.

6 Handkerchiefs.

6 Pairs Half Hose, Balbriggan.

1 Pair Shoes, light and comfortable.

1 Pair Slippers, full calf.

1 Pair Suspenders.

> Early clothing lists for patients who are able to dress themselves.
>
> Patients who were unable to attend to their dress were dressed by attendants.
>
> Sometimes the family provided garments, other times the hospital provided them.

N. B.—The above articles MUST BE NEW, or as good as new. Partly worn clothing is useless to the insane patient. Pack in a cheap calico bag. Trunks and valises will not be received.

RECEIVED, with the patient, the above Schedule of Clothing, new and in good condition.

....*Supervisor.*

....19.......

CENTRAL STATE HOSPITAL

DEPARTMENT FOR WOMEN

Clothing Requisition, 1st Class

(CAPABLE OF ATTENTION TO DRESS)

3 Dresses, gingham, or oil print, plain.

1 Best Dress, cotton, wool or silk, neat.

4 Drawers, Wamsutta muslin, plain.

4 Chemise, Wamsutta muslin, plain.

3 Night Gowns, Wamsutta muslin, plain.

2 Underskirts, striped cotton, plain.

2 Underskirts, mixed flannel, plain.

6 Handkerchiefs.

6 Pairs Hose, good Balbriggan, plain.

1 Pair Shoes, light and comfortable.

1 Hat, Hood or Bonnet, plain.

1 Shawl or Cloak.

3 Under Vests.

N. B.—The above articles MUST BE NEW, or as good as new. Partly worn clothing is useless to the insane patient. Pack in a cheap calico bag. Trunks and valises will not be received.

RECEIVED, with the patient, the above Schedule of Clothing, new and in good condition.

....*Supervisor*.

....19........

bread. Patients were then back at their jobs, or taken outside when the weather permitted. There were always staff shortages in the women's wards and to ease the burden, sometimes patients were given paraldehyde (4). Dinner, or tea as they called it, was at 6pm and the food was much the same as lunch. Bedtime began around 8 or 9 o'clock. Patients slept on beds, but when space and equipment was hard to come by, they also had to sleep on cotton or feather ticks, (thin mattresses) that were placed on the floor.

The grounds were beautiful, but the maintenance department replaced the wood fence by the Department for Women' with barbed wire. The hospital wanted better control over how people were committed. The hospital's process contained too many loopholes and records mentioned parents dropping off deformed children, or angry family members dropping off wives, husbands, etc.

The way patients were admitted changed throughout the hospital's life. Originally, people could apply for admission either for themselves or family and friends. Later, admission was petitioned by a sheriff, judge, local doctor or a combination of these who would sign paperwork. Once the hospital staff received the paperwork, a determination for admission would be made. Later, doctors would work directly with patients and family to have them admitted.

The biggest change to patient life in the 1880s was the use of restraints. They were abolished by Superintendent William B. Fletcher in 1885 but reinstituted in part by Superintendent George F. Edenharter when he took over the position.

Also during this time, women now had access to women doctors, most notably Dr. Sarah Stockton, who graduated from the Women's Medical College of Philadelphia. Her dissertation explored mental illness and its treatment.

Race Issues

Many people believe that African American's were denied treatment at Central State. The question of admitting colored people to the institution came up in 1855 and again in 1856. The Superintendent thought they should be admitted but that it would be "absolutely necessary to build rooms isolated and purposely for them." This does not prove they were admitted in 1856 and certainly shows they had not been admitted before 1856. No records exist of any separate "colored" area, although their treatment on the wards could have easily been segregated by the staff.

From the records, we know:

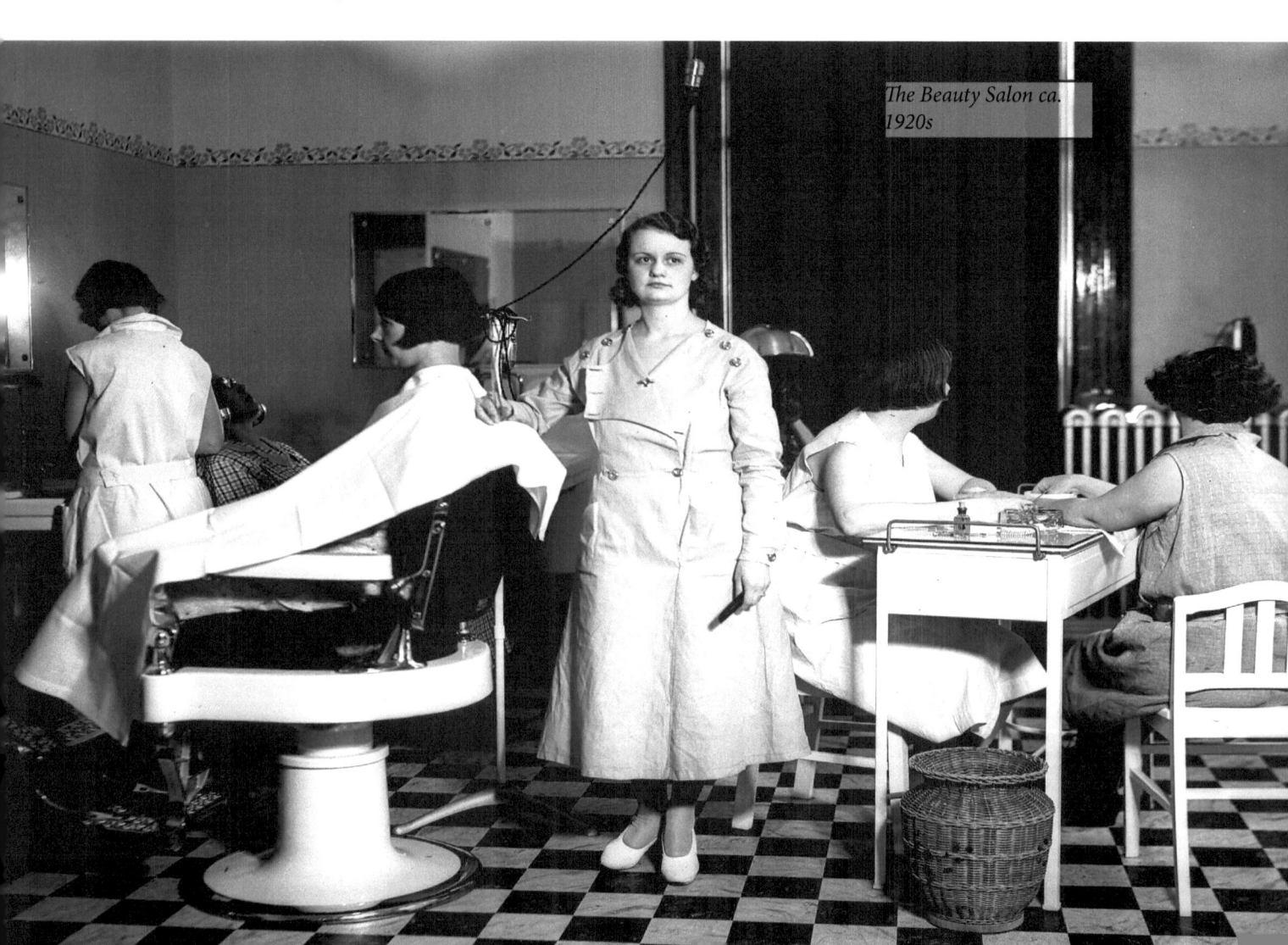

The Beauty Salon ca. 1920s

- The earliest record found of a black patient was Charles Cox. He was admitted in 1887 by his mother June Cox because he drank, was violent and had delusions that he could turn people and places into snakes.
- The earliest distinction of "colored" patients in the yearly reports was in 1890 there were a total of 9 colored men and 6 colored women admitted during that year.
- The earliest known burial at the hospital of an African American patient is Robert Alexander who was buried in Section 2 of the hospital cemetery on July 11, 1905. (See Chapter 7 Cemetery).
- By 1944 the yearly report stated, there was "no restriction for admission based on age, color or sex."
- Other information concerning African-Americans in the hospital includes:
- A newspaper account from January 17, 1900 states that John Turner "a young colored man" assaulted and killed his wife in 1899. A witness testified that John had a grandfather who was a patient in Central State and who died in 1899 at the hospital.
- On February 14, 1901 the Indianapolis Journal reported that Levi Kent (also known as Levi Glenn, "who was a Negro", died of tuberculosis and that he'd been at the hospital since 1899.
- On February 27, 1901 the Indianapolis Journal reported that the former Central State patient and "black man", George Ward, was lynched, being hanged from a bridge over the Wabash River in Terre Haute and burned.
- On June 3, 1902: Wilis Perry, "colored", was taken to the hospital because he was suffering from dementia.

Diet

The kitchens also benefited from the patients. The workers and patients prepared and cooked food, and they cleaned kitchens and dining rooms. They were also employed to take trays of food to other patients.

Patients unable to eat with the rest of the population ate in their rooms. Later, separate kitchens were built for men and women's wards and trays were brought from the kitchen through dumb-waiters and through tunnels to the wards. The hospital began to use a "sick diet" for patients who were on diet restrictions and required specific foods. In the 1950s a free standing kitchen/dining room used by patients and staff was built.

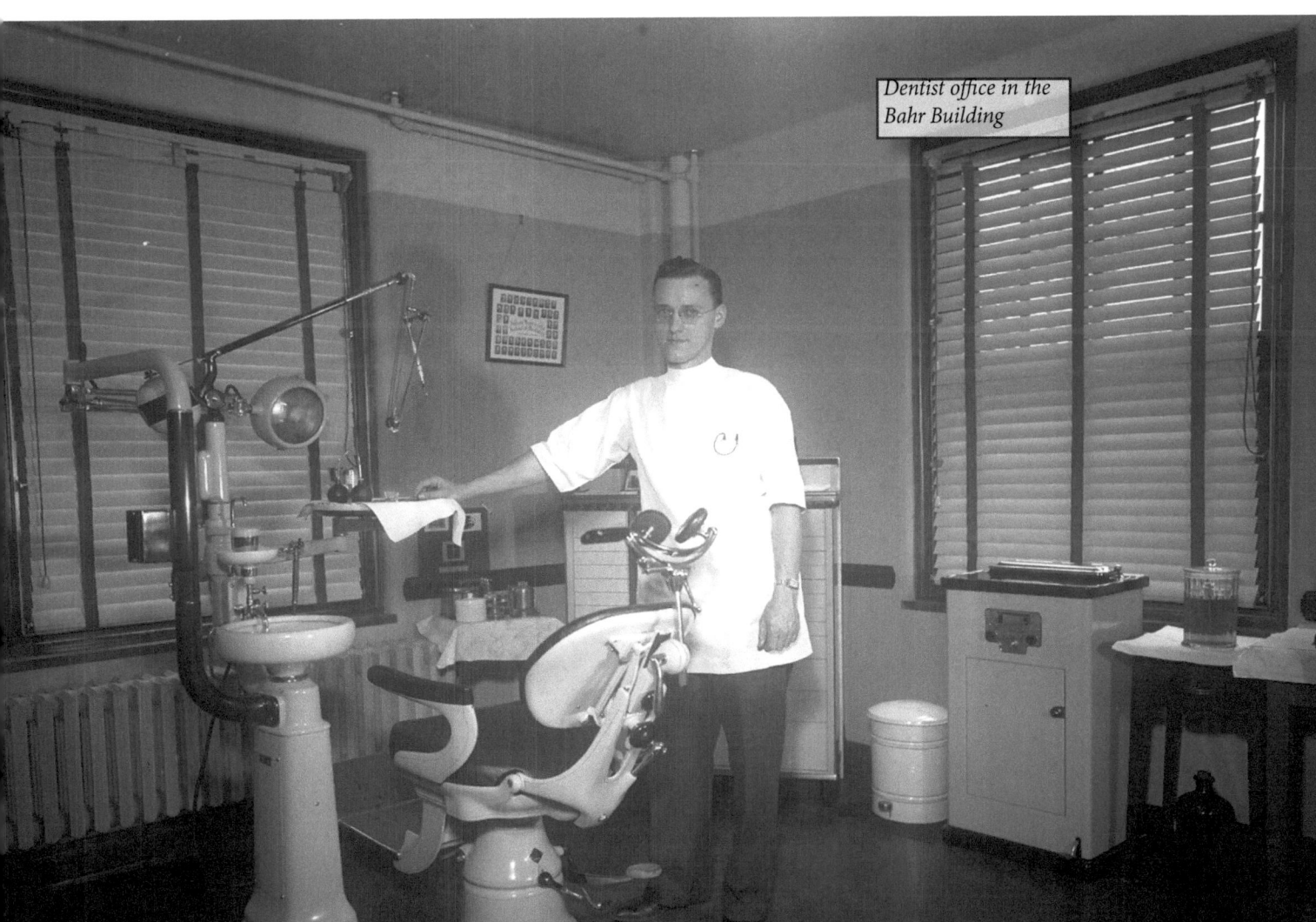

Dentist office in the Bahr Building

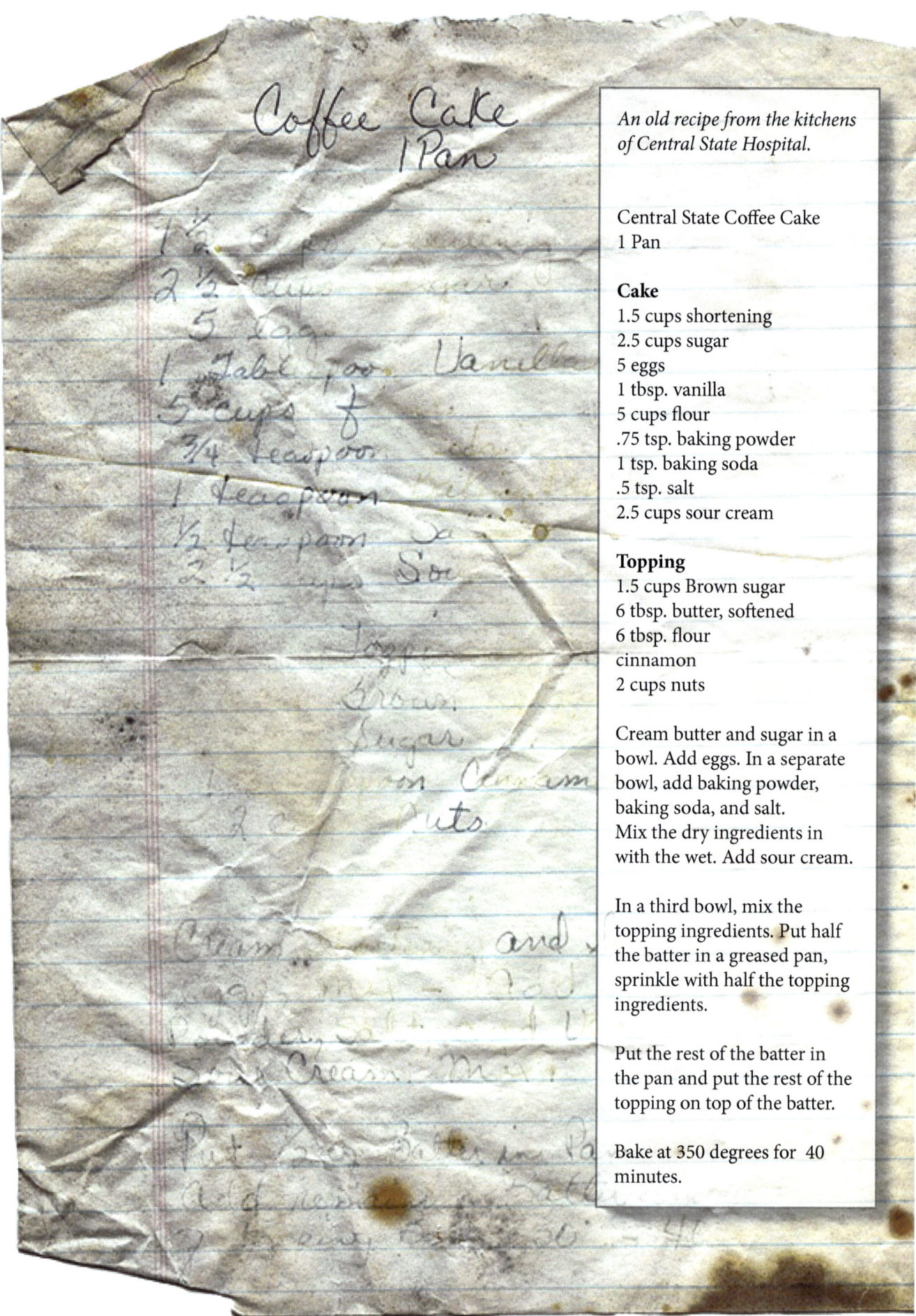

An old recipe from the kitchens of Central State Hospital.

Central State Coffee Cake
1 Pan

Cake
1.5 cups shortening
2.5 cups sugar
5 eggs
1 tbsp. vanilla
5 cups flour
.75 tsp. baking powder
1 tsp. baking soda
.5 tsp. salt
2.5 cups sour cream

Topping
1.5 cups Brown sugar
6 tbsp. butter, softened
6 tbsp. flour
cinnamon
2 cups nuts

Cream butter and sugar in a bowl. Add eggs. In a separate bowl, add baking powder, baking soda, and salt.
Mix the dry ingredients in with the wet. Add sour cream.

In a third bowl, mix the topping ingredients. Put half the batter in a greased pan, sprinkle with half the topping ingredients.

Put the rest of the batter in the pan and put the rest of the topping on top of the batter.

Bake at 350 degrees for 40 minutes.

The patients seemed to eat well, although there were allegations of mismanagement of food funds and substandard food served. On Thanksgiving Day 1885, 1800 pounds of turkey, three barrels of cranberries, 200 gallons of oysters and a large supply of the "necessary accessories" were served to the patients.

According the 1886 yearly report, milk was "used freely, each patient having as much as he wished". Additionally, 1,120 quarts of strawberries from the farm were consumed, two (train) car loads of watermelons, apples, grapes, oranges and bananas were also eaten.

Beef, bread and potatoes were the basis of the diet, as were other items from the farm and outside vendors. Early in the hospital's life, a typical day meals would consist of:
- **Breakfast:** meat, hash, bread and butter, coffee, tea, milk,
- **Dinner (lunch):** boiled potatoes, roast fresh pork, sweet potatoes, cabbage, pickles, and ginger cake.
- **Supper:** peaches, bread and butter, tea.
- Feeble people on a special diet had choices off a special diet menu which contained milk, cream, tea, coffee, chocolate, beef, tea, beef essence (5), eggs, oysters, poultry, bread and fresh meats.

By 1959 a typical menu was:
- **Breakfast:** beef stew, hot rolls, pickles, fruit Jell-O, beverages; cornmeal bacon oranges, coffee or milk buttered toast; French toast, oatmeal, scrambled and fried eggs
- **Dinner (notice it was still not called lunch):** ham steak, roast pork, baked chicken, fish sticks, corned beef brisket and roast beef
- **Supper:** includes sausage and creamed macaroni, braunschweiger and beans, vegetable soup and cornbread, salmon salad, bologna and creamed beef on toast.
- Substitutions were made when there was a lack of a product or lack of help to prepare it.

By 1961 a typical menu was:
- **Breakfast:** Fruit juice, cold cereal, hot cakes, butter and syrup, coffee and milk
- **Dinner (notice it was still not called lunch):** Baked ham, browned potatoes, green beans, bread and butter, orange Jello cubes, beverage
- **Supper:** Chili, crackers, lettuce and oil/vinegar dressing, bread and butter, apricot upside down cake, beverage

The old dining rooms were used as dormitories. The new dining rooms were used for the patients, who were served by "trustees" (patients who were well enough to be trusted to do important tasks). The reason for the new dining rooms is because there were over 40 meals a week that had to be transported to buildings, distributed to wards and then put onto plates. Before the new dining rooms, the food was not hot or cold when appropriate. Additionally, hungry patients were angry, and attendants hurried to get food out, making portioning mistakes.

In the late 1940s, the cannery provided 40000 gallons of vegetables. Improvements in food included the use of a variety of methods other than boiling meats and using more seasonings. Hot foods and cold foods remained hot or cold based on better containment and transportation systems. Men and women ate together at the farm colony. Special diets were now more accommodated.

Therapy and Activities
(See Treatment Chapter)

Work and recreation was central to life within the hospital. Patients were also encouraged to participate in pleasurable activities. Early occupational, art, writing and music therapy commenced (although it would be called "moral therapy" for many years).

Artisans and tradesmen were employed to teach patients skills. The result of their work was used to benefit not only the patient, but the institution. Men learned to farm (including butchering and livestock) and learned the carpentry and machine trade to help with the everyday running of the hospital. Women washed, cooked, sewed and cleaned. Artwork and writing was used in decorations around the institutions. Sometimes women would serve as secretaries.

Even shoe repair and maintenance employed patients on site. At some institutions, patients were paid for this work. At Central State Hospital it was considered part of their treatment and legal until 1966 when the Fair Labor Standards Act (FLSA) ruled that mental patients should be paid minimum wage. The hospital administration calculated how much each patient would earn if they were in mainstream society and translated this figure as a savings for the hospital.

The social activities of the hospital progressed with those of society as a whole, and interaction with outsiders was encouraged much later, helping to rehabilitate them. Sports teams were organized amongst men and inter-hospital rivalries formed. Walking within the grounds and woodlands was the most widely used form of exercise available.

Both men and women had access to a library on site at the hospital. Many of the books were donated by advocate for the insane, Dorthea Dix, the original matron, other workers, well-to-do people, and others. Additionally, newspapers and other publications were donated by several organizations, including:

- Family Visitor (Indianapolis)
- Indiana State Sentinel (Indianapolis)
- Indiana State Journal (Indianapolis)
- Christian Messenger (Indianapolis)
- Decatur Clarion (Greensburg)
- Wayne County Whig (Centerville)
- Richmond Palladium (Richmond)
- Democratic Pharos (Logansport)
- Indiana American (Brookville)
- New Albany Ledger (New Albany)
- Greenfield Spectator (Greenfield)
- Wabash Weekly Gazette (Wabashtown, now Wabash)
- Fort Wayne Times (Fort Wayne)
- Madison Weekly Courier (Madison)
- St Joseph Valley Register (South Bend)

During the 1880-1950 time period, Central State Hospital still had a very regimented day. Still, during free time, many professional and amateur organization from outside the hospital came to entertain the patients, including the Masonic Dramatic Club of Indianapolis, the orchestra and choir of the Institute for the Blind, Haverly's Georgia Minstrels, Miller's orchestra. Other recreation included using the moving picture machine and stereopticon.

In the 1880s, with the idea that family and friends cheered the patients and did them good, visitors were on the rise. Patients were also encouraged to go on "furloughs" or leaves where they could start integrating back into life outside the hospital. They attended the annual state fair. Additionally, patients had activities at the hospital including a bowling alley, pool tables, a pipe organ and stage scenery for the patients. The hospital also hosted an annual field day and Fourth of July pageant, parties and a weekly Thursday dance as well as Halloween, New Years and Christmas parties.

Superintendent Max Bahr instituted giving Christmas gifts and this continued after his death. Organizations including hospital Indiana and State Mental Health associations ask for donations of new and used items to help make Christmas special for the patients. Everyone received a gift that was personally addressed to them.

The hospital was also conscientious of religion and education. Reverent L. Harrison of Indianapolis began giving services on a regular basis. These services were done inside the Department for Men, the Department for Women, and out in the groves when weather permitted.

Patient classes were not given until March 1885. At that time, a school was set up in the Department for Women, although men and women attended. They attended classes two and a half days a week. Classes focused on vocal music and gymnastics, as well as math, geography, languages, reading, writing, and grammar. Additionally, knitting, crocheting and embroidery were offered. Many patients created items that were used at the hospital. Initially, about 175 people participated in classes.

Another part of education was letter writing. Below are examples of some of the letters:

C.S.: "I used to be unhappy here, not that I was treated badly, but that I was losing my school. I am content to stay, for I am learning as much as I could in any other school. I am in fractions."

L.M.: "I am going to school now and I think that is helping me, for now I won't get any further behind. I think if I stay here this winter I shall have learned something."

W.C.: "I believe I told you I was in school. We have music twice a day. I enjoy it very much. I attend church and Sunday school every Sabbath. So you see the State understands her business."

A.B.: "They talk of sending me home, but I don't care much about it. I am treated so well here *and am learning so much. I am studying reading, writing, arithmetic, grammar, geography and music. But Dutch is the best of all. I will write you a German letter before long."*

S.K.: *"I will write a few lines to let you know I am feeling better than I ever did in all my life. Indeed, I feel more like a man than I ever did before. I think I am improving very fast in my studies. My loving teachers, you do not know how much I love them. Our Superintendent comes over every Sunday morning to Sunday school. In the afternoon we go to church, we boys sing in the choir. Dr. Thomas comes in our school often to see how we are getting along."*

Over 60% of the patients volunteered to work during the 1880s, which was considered a good form of early occupational therapy. Dr. Fletcher believed occupations, good food and outdoor exercise can go a long way in helping mentally ill. Men made and repaired brooms and reupholstered furniture and painted. In 1886 their labor was valued at $3,500 in savings for the state.

The 1950s held new promises for the mentally ill. For people in mental hospitals with syphilis, penicillin was available to help them beat the disease and leave the hospital. Additionally, psychotropic drugs were available to help schizophrenia and other chronic conditions for patients.

During this time, more emphasis was placed on drugs and psychotherapy with other types of occupational, art, music and recreational therapy given as needed and warranted. Even the Women's Press Club would go to the hospital in the 1950s and lecture on topics in the news.

To get patients to do what was needed for their care, the hospital instated a points system for privileges. Certain activities were worth certain points. Accruing points meant that when therapy was attended and drugs taken, you could store points for trips off the grounds or being able to have a part time job.

As part of a more relaxed atmosphere, patients could send and receive uncensored mail, use pay telephones or manage limited amounts of money. They could also have visitors from 10a.m. to 8 p.m. every day of the week- a far cry from the restrictions of the early hospital years.

Recreational therapy included volleyball, basketball, lounging, games, a nature corner which included parakeets, fish, and plant life; movies, dances, stage productions, softball, basketball, badminton, touch football, games, dances, holiday programs, off-ground excursions, hobby clubs, and a newspaper published by patients. The Grove, a beautiful shaded area located in the middle of the property, was used in summer with basketball hoops, shelter and small hard surface area. Miss Rogers, a staff member, helped fix up the basement of Cottage 2, known as the "hole of Calcutta," for use as a playhouse and a place where patients could listen to music, play games and socialize. But the hospital had no money so with the patients help, a pool table was re-covered with old Army blankets, as felt was too expensive to buy. Games and a stereo were added.

In the 1970s, patients had access to many traditional programs as well as off-site programs. In the southeast corner of the Men's building basement (room 383), Mr. Lou Reagle was in charge of these therapies. Activities Therapy consisted of four departments: Music, Recreation, Occupational and Vocational Industrial Therapy (VIT). Access to the departments was through an Activities Therapy (AT) form through an AT representative. In the 1970s, communications was a huge issue. The AT personnel were trying to get prescriptions with goals versus activities. Additionally, if a patient regressed, a new referral was needed. If the patient progressed, new goals were needed. As Mr. Reagle wrote, "The AT program may be exacerbating his problem because a factor was not indicated about the patient."

Typical programs offered at the hospital included "Activities of Daily Living", "Dance Class" and "Community Orientation". Additionally, the hospital was trying to "select" patients that would benefit from off-site programs as well. A transition was in place, requiring each area of AT to have an off-site component. For example, the "Activities in Daily Living" class would have patients going to the supermarket to buy their own food. This was all in preparation for them to be equipped to leave the hospital.

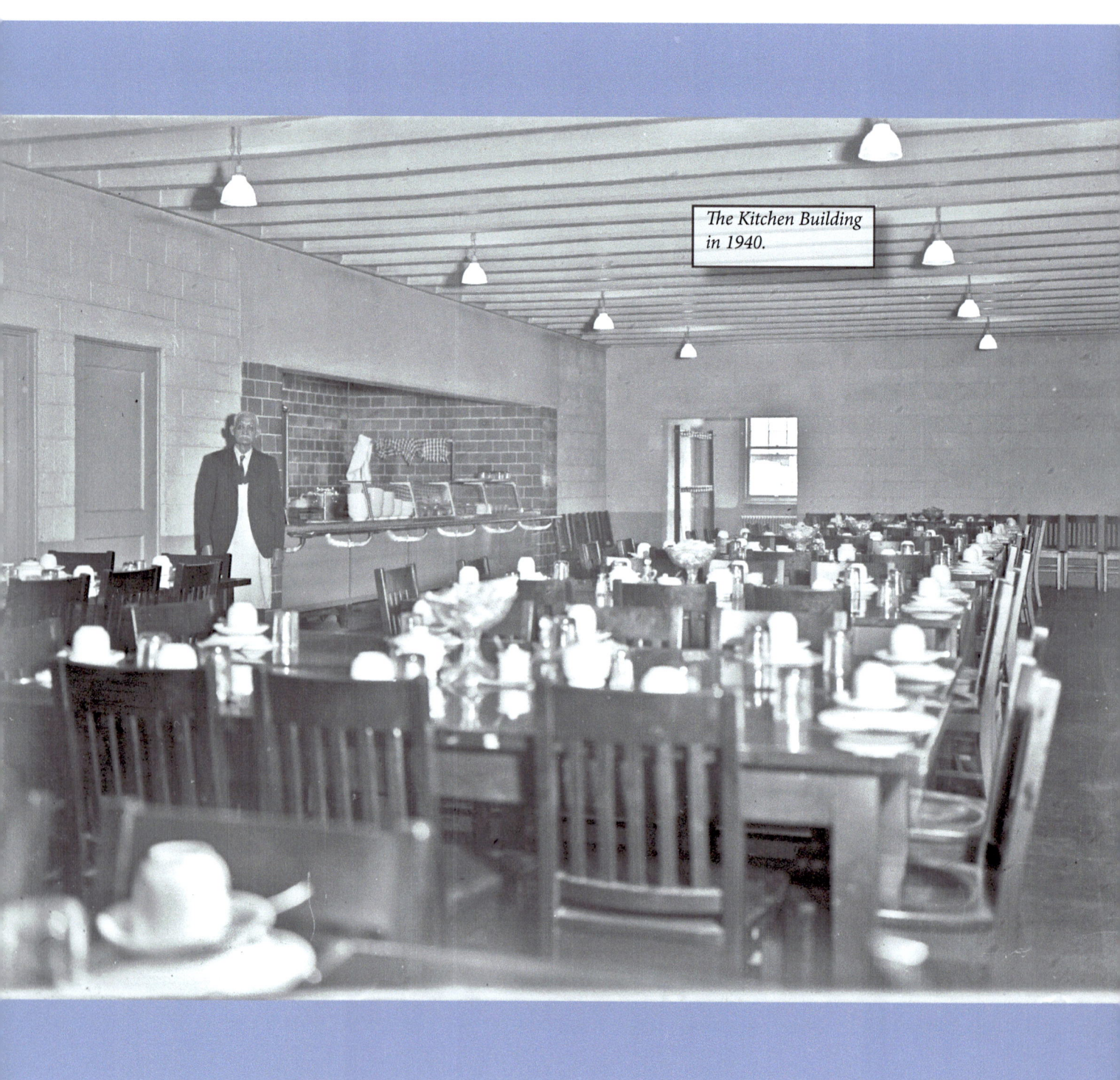

The Kitchen Building in 1940.

FOUR

THE HOSPITAL and FARM COLONY

The farm helped defray costs from 1848 to 1968. Farm land extended from Vermont Street to Washington Street and about half way from Warman Street to Tibbs Avenue The north side was farmed; the south side was pasture for livestock in the 1800s. The south west side of the property also contained a farm field.

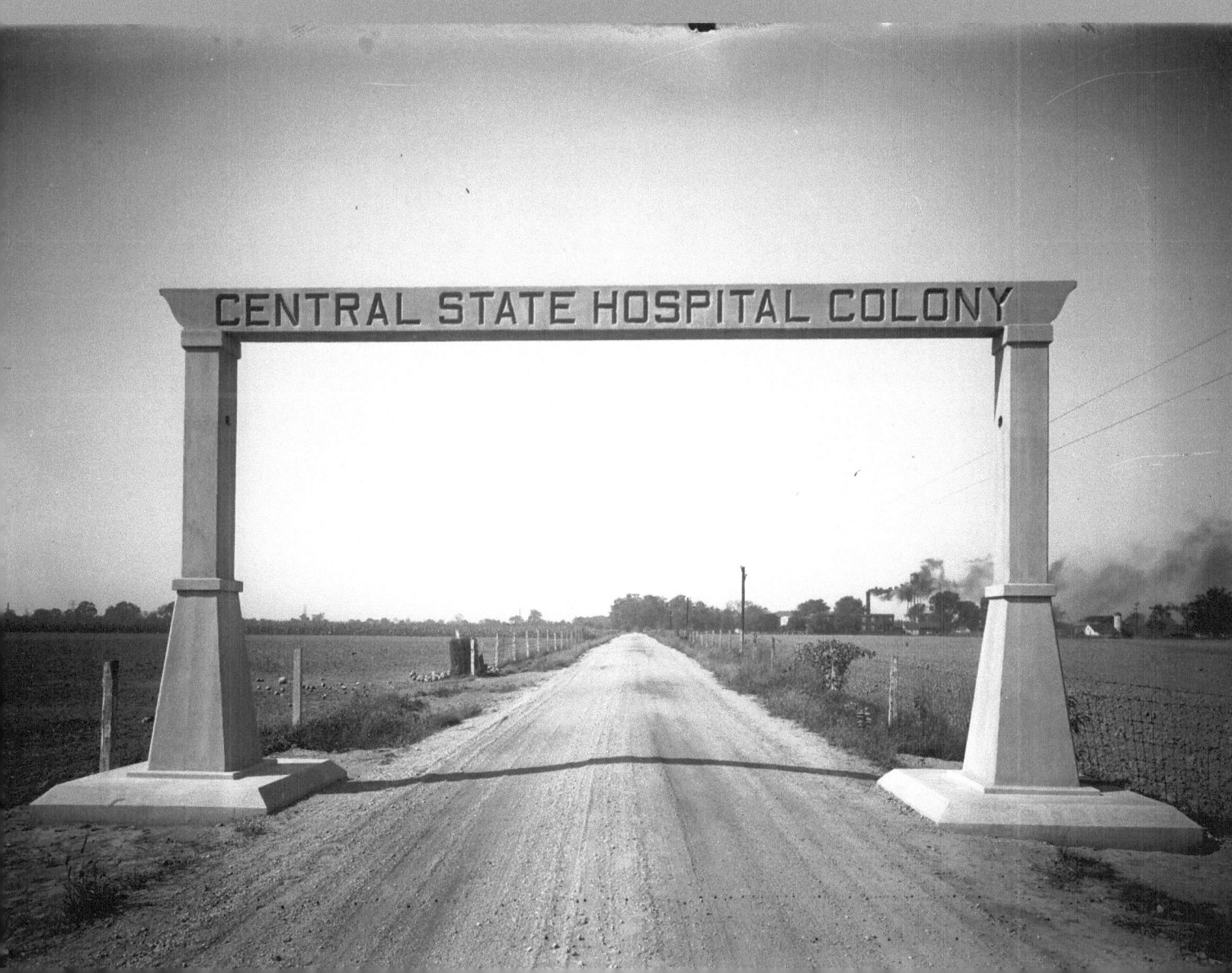

The Hospital Farm

Central State Hospital was responsible for two farms- one on the hospital grounds and the Farm Colony that was taken over in 1938 from the Marion County Poor Farm.

In addition to the farms, Central State also had greenhouses, located east of the Administration Building. In 1885 Superintendent George F. Edenharter asked for money to build them because "These houses furnish the most effective medicine in the form of flowers for a great number of our patients." These greenhouses were used to grow seedlings for the farm and Farm Colony, and for the numerous flowerbeds around the hospital grounds and patient rooms.

Also, for a time in the 1880s, land was rented in the neighborhood for a kitchen garden, which consisted of mostly herbs and other more delicate plants such as lettuce, spinach and other leafing greens.

Many years, minor droughts hindered production of crops. In 1870 the potatoes had to be bought for the winter supply because the "Colorado bug" destroyed the entire crop. Several years, early frosts also damaged crop production.

However, the farms were usually productive, providing an abundance of crops for use at the hospital and other state run institutions. The hospital sold much of what it produced to increase the money it had available to it to run the hospital.

Central State Hospital Farm and Colony

The farm was where the Bahr Building was later built on the east side of the campus. The asylum farm was by far the biggest employer of men and some female patients. The farm grew good fruits and vegetables for the hospital kitchens.

To do farm work, there was a horse barn, a farm and garden barn, which housed a variety of wagons and tools: two horse wagons, one one-horse cart, one ox cart, one two horse spring wagon, one one-horse spring wagon, one large coal wagon used for heavy hauling; one large family carriage; one rockaway; one open top buggy, three wheelbarrows, two sleighs and one large ox sled.

Over the years the following crops were cultivated: Corn, Irish potatoes, sweet potatoes, oats, turnips, onions, parsnips, beets, tomatoes, carrots, beans, peas, pork, hay, cabbage, strawberries, lettuce, celery, shocks corn-fodder, milk, radishes, green onions, dry onions, leeks, green beans, dry beans, pickles, pumpkins, eggplants, watermelons, carrots, parsley, spinach, asparagus, early beans, grapes, muskmelons, early cabbage, drum-head cabbage, veal, straw, blue grass seed, pickle cabbage, rhubarb, butter beans, shorts and bran, cauliflower, lima beans, green apples, kale, oyster plant, celery plant, red peppers, hay, oats, wood, and cucumbers.

Also 20 to 60 acres were dedicated to pasturing livestock- oxen, bulls, calves, pigs, and mules. Horses were also bought and stabled for the use of the hospital. The doctor's horses were also stabled and fed in the barn.

During the 1880s, a lot of construction took place. 2,000 yards of solid roads and pathways were created, including the iconic Main Driveway that people remember that went from Washington Street north past Kirkbride Way and west to the Department for Women. Seedlings were raised to become plants for the grounds and the greenhouses were able to produce beautiful flowers and plants for the hospital wards. It also produced and incredible amount of bedding plants. For examples, in 1925 it produced 5.000 geraniums, 12,000 petunias, 6000 achyranthes (which inhibited arthritis and acute edema), 9,000 alternantheras (used possibly as an analgesic), 4000 canna, 1,000 begonias, 4000 pansies to name a few. Potted plants for the wards totaled over 9,000. Over 5,400 bouquets of cut flowers such as zinnia, larkspur, stevia, and gladiolas, made their way into the buildings.

A new kitchen garden was made available in the 1880s and worked farm space on the McCaslin farm that was 2 miles from the hospital. Grass was planted as well as fountains installed.

Central State Farm Colony

In 1938, the hospital took over the Marion County Poor Farm and changed it to the Central State Farm Colony. The colony was located on Tibbs Avenue near 23rd Street. About 300 patients lived and worked at the Farm Colony. They were not paid; it was considered therapy. Types of crops raised were sweet potatoes, tomatoes, cabbage, green beans, cauliflower, field corn (for livestock), corn and popcorn. Most of these were used at the hospital, although strawberries were often traded to other state institutions for other crops.

Even when farming was no longer considered therapy, patients still worked at the farm. Bill Parish, the last Farm Colony Manager said farming as a therapy still worked, "Anytime you keep a patient busy, it's better than sitting all the time." He felt the closing of the farm was "very sad and heartbreaking."

Patients did receive a trade off working at the Farm Colony. Some patients lived at the colony under minimal

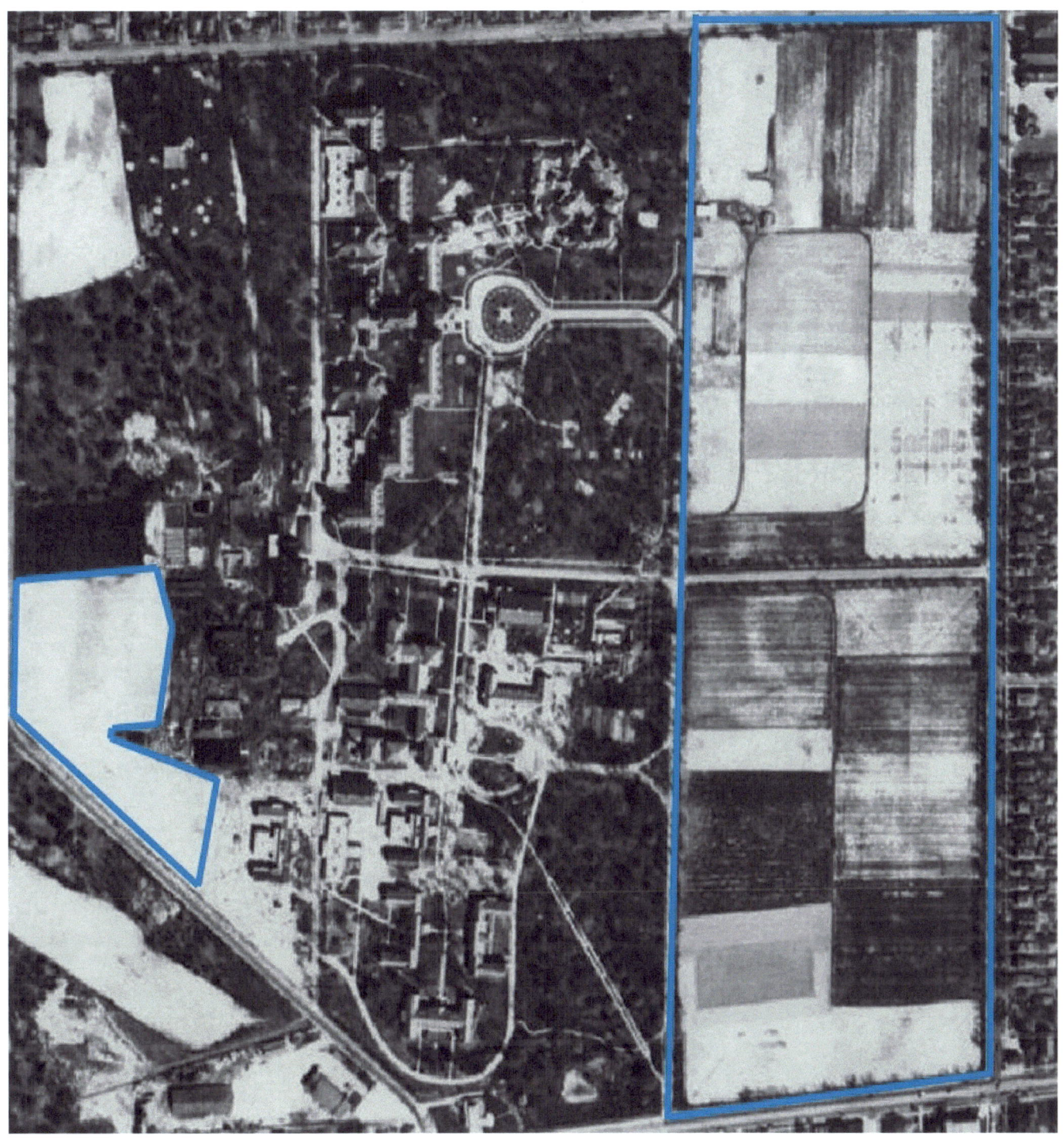

Top 1937 aerial view of Central State Hospital. The blue outlined areas indicate where the hospital farmed on site. Notice tthat the original Men's Building has almost been completely razed to make way for the cottages in the center bottom of the picture.

supervision. Only the most stable patients were sent to work there. The atmosphere was relaxed and somewhat less regulated than the hospital farm or property. Locked doors were almost non-existent. During the Indianapolis 500, the patients and staff would climb the water tower and watch the race since the west side of the farm butted up to the race track property.

Colony buildings in 1939:

- Two story building with several wings
- Frame building
- Administration building
- Boiler room
- Brick barn
- Granary
- Tool shed

By the 1940s, with cheaper ways to produce food, most state farm land was closed and sold. This was not the case in Indiana. The hospital kept the farmlands at the hospital running until 1968 when it was converted to other uses, such as Bahr Park. The Farm Colony land was phased out by 1968 and the land transferred to the Marion County Commissioners and eventually was sold. The closure was due to fewer vegetables being needed at the hospital, and labor laws changing, making patient labor illegal. The hospital didn't have the money to pay people to work on the farm. They were under hiring freezes on non-essential positions more on than off during the 1970s-1990s. The Farm Colony ceased in 1968 and the buildings were demolished between 1972 and 1978.

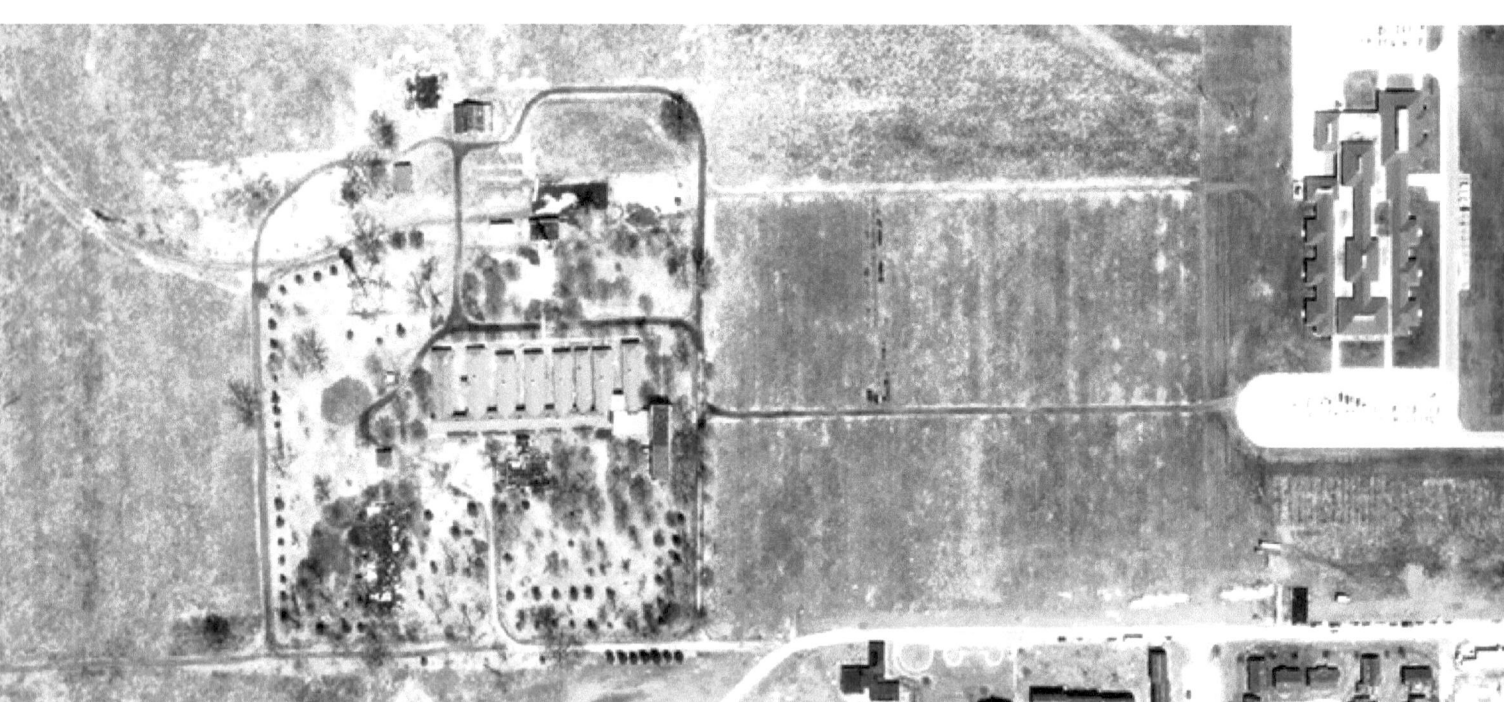

Bottom; 1972 aerial view of the Farm Colony.

FIVE

STAFFING THE HOSPITAL

The staff of the hospital from the top down did not have ample free time. They lived on the grounds of the hospital. They ate at the hospital and they slept at the hospital. Whenever the hospital was short staffed, administration knew where to find staff needed because they were on the grounds.

In the early days of the hospital, most staff had one day off. They worked 10-24 hour shifts, depending on the needs of the hospital. Staff weren't paid hourly. They were paid by the week, month or year. If an attendant was paid $20 a month, it didn't matter if the attendant put in 160 hours that month or 260 hours.

Staff lived and breathed the hospital, with only an afternoon or a whole day off every week or sometimes every two weeks if they were lucky. Staff had to ask for vacation time and were sometimes denied. Fraternization between male and female staff members was forbidden, punishable by termination.

Because of overcrowding and lack of space, sometimes the floor staff (e.g. attendants and domestic staff) were forced to live four to six to a room. Sometimes, they had to sleep in the same room (1) as the patients. In the 1930s, 100 employees were sleeping in the Department for Men, with 50 employees sleeping in the same rooms with patients. When the patients were quiet, it was not a bad experience, but if the patients were loud and restless, it didn't make for restful sleep. The staff were most likely living sleep deprived existences. It was a hard, gritty and emotionally draining existence.

As the hospital grew, staff no longer lived at the hospital for the most part and were hired via human resource departments. Hours were shortened and vacations became routine.

Still, in times of trouble, the hospital sometimes continued to take over the lives of staff by canceling vacations, and by understaffing and overtime.

One interesting side note, in 1901, newspapers mention Statehouse and Courthouse teams playing baseball "on the diamond" at the hospital. The exact location of this diamond is unknown at present.

Early Staffing

Staffing the hospital was largely done by comparing other hospitals and using the Kirkbride methodology (2). The hospital administration would visit other hospitals or read about the way they ran their hospitals in journals. Sometimes, the administration would also go to conferences and network to find out more about how other hospitals were run and staffed.

Dr. Thomas Kirkbride was a leader in mental health during the 1800s. He was born on July 31, 1809 to Quaker parents. He attended the University of Pennsylvania Medical School, graduating in 1832. He became the superintendent of the Pennsylvania Hospital for the Insane by 1840. By 1844 he helped found the Association of Medical Superintendents of American Institutions for the Insane (AMSAII) and was its president from 1862 to 1870. As part of his attempt to improve medical care for the insane, he developed the Kirkbride Plan and wrote about it in his work, "On the Construction, Organization and General Arrangements of Hospitals for the Insane with Some Remarks on Insanity and Its Treatment" (1854, revised 1880). Of seventy five guidelines for creating and building a hospital, Central State Hospital was compliant on at least 60 of the recommendations. Because of time and records, compliance on 10 of the recommendations is not known.

Kirkbride recommended hiring the following people to staff the hospital.
- Board of Commissioners
- Board of Trustees
- Physician in Chief (Superintendent)
- Two Assistant Physicians
- Steward and Matron
- Chaplain
- Consulting physicians
- Others: drivers, entertainers, etc.
- Two night watchers (Central State Hospital had no night clocks but two inside night watchmen and 13 outside night watchmen)
- Two supervisors
- Two teachers or two companions (did not employ, had volunteers); one for women and one for men
- 32 Attendants (16 for men; 16 for women)
- Two special attendants (one for men and one for women)
- Two seamstresses
- One farmer and three farmhands
- One gardener and three assistant gardeners
- One jobber/teamster
- One carpenter
- One engineer and machinist
- Two firemen (At the height of Central State specific firemen, the hospital had room for 35 firemen!)
- One baker and one assistant baker
- One carriage driver
- One gatekeeper
- One cook and three assistant cooks
- Four female domestics
- Two dairy maids (Central State had one)
- Three washerwomen
- Four ironers

In addition to a Board of Commissioners, Board of Trustees, Superintendent and physicians, the hospital started out with the staff below. As you can see, it was not as complete as Kirkbride recommended.
Six attendants ($20/month)
- Two head attendants; ($10.53/month)
- One fireman ($20/month)
- One laborer ($15/month)
- One teamster ($12/month)
- One house assistant ($12/month)

- One washer man ($12/month)
- One washerwoman ($10.53/month)
- One cook ($20/month)
- One assistant cook ($7.58/month)
- One tailoresses ($8.67/month)
- One ironer ($8.67/month)
- One chamber maid ($7.58/month)

Each person received board which included a place to sleep and meals. In the first year of the hospital the monthly cost of staff outside of the doctors and builders was $262.70 ($7743.97 in 2014 money) or $3,152.40/year ($92,927.59 in 2014 money).

Board of Commissioners/ Board of Trustees

Kirkbride recommended that a Board of Commissioners form to plan, build and open a hospital. It should be no more than 12 people serving a term of one year. The people appointed should have public confidence and be a man of business, liberality, intelligence, and benevolence who were willing to faithfully attend to the duties of the station above all political or personal influence.

The Board was to visit the hospital regularly to attest to its running, and appoint the supervisor, but maintain a distance (i.e. no personal relationships with staff or anyone affiliated with the hospital).

The Board of Trustees was to help run and advocate to the legislature for the maintenance of the hospital.

Thomas Kirkbride

Kirkbride's early experiences with the mentally ill were influenced by York Retreat (Lamal Hill, York, England). Its leader Samuel Tuke, a Quaker reformer, used the moral treatment for the people at his retreat, as did the Association of Medical Superintendents of American Institutions for the Insane (AMSAII), of which Kirkbride was the head for a time. Kirkbride's work attracted supporters who believed Kirkbride was advancing treatment for the insane. Kirkbride also attracted peers who thought his work was unneeded and hindered progress in treatment for the insane. In Kirkbride's work with patients, the overwhelming majority seemed to respect him, although one patient did try to kill him. Kirkbride believed fervently that the insane had much to offer and could be cured. In fact, after his first wife died, Kirkbride married a former patient. Kirkbride was a proponent of abolishing as many mechanical restraints as possible from insane asylums. He died of pneumonia on December 16, 1883 at his home on the grounds of the Pennsylvania Hospital for the Insane.

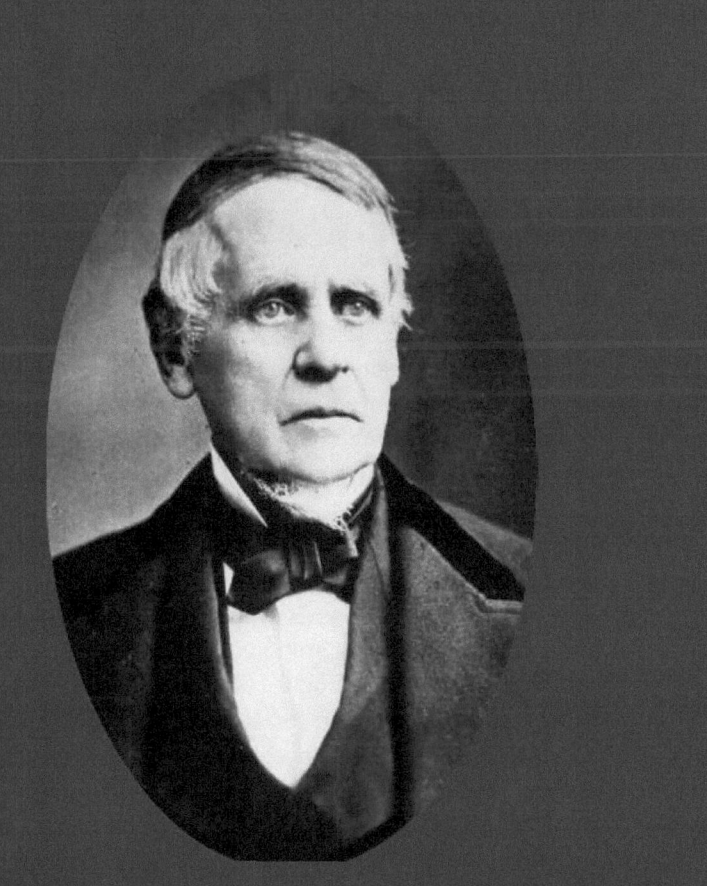

Superintendent

The Board of Charities or the Board of Commissioners appointed a "Physician-in-Chief" or Superintendent. The physician appointed as Superintendent should be "of high moral character and his skills should fit the position." The superintendent was responsible for appointing other key staff such as Assistant Physician, Steward and Matron. He hired and fired staff. The superintendent was responsible not only for who was hired and how they performed but also the running of the hospital.

The Superintendent's family lived in a suite of rooms in various buildings over the years. Eventually this practice stopped and people commuted to work (3).

Notable Superintendents

The most influential superintendents during the 1880s-1920s were Dr. William B. Fletcher (1883-1887), Dr. George F. Edenharter (1893-1923), and Dr. Max Bahr (1923-1952).

Dr. William B. Fletcher (1883-1887) was affiliated with two institutions. First in 1869 he helped form the Medical College of Indiana. He was also a professor of mental disease at the Central College of Physicians and Surgeons. He was seen as a man of reform, serving on committees dealing with reformatory and benevolent institutions, temperance and public health. He introduced bills to help public health, safety, prisons and common schools. He also supported employing female doctors for the women's department at the Indiana Hospital for the Insane (including Dr. Sarah Stockton) and opposed the repeal of the act that created the State Board of Health. Dr. Fletcher oversaw the building of the Department for Women (also known as Seven Steeples). He also supported providing less "stupefying drugs" to the patients and as a result, hydrate of chloral and bromide of potassium usage was reduced by one-third.

Fletcher gave dignity to patients by stopping the secret burials and employed the hospital chaplain to conduct services. Because he felt "moral force" was stronger than restraints, he appointed a chaplain and offered weekly services and public burials. He abolished the "209 restraint chairs, 120 cribs, 101 camisoles, 108 restraint straps, 56 wristlets (hand-cuffs), 55 pairs of gloves (leather mittens), 11 pairs of anklets and 2 leather collars (collar restraints)." He had actually run the institution for several months without these items when he destroyed them in a huge bonfire, becoming known as the man who built "humanity's bonfire." This act received a lot of attention from the press including other hospitals and journals. Fletcher also started the practice of performing autopsies to

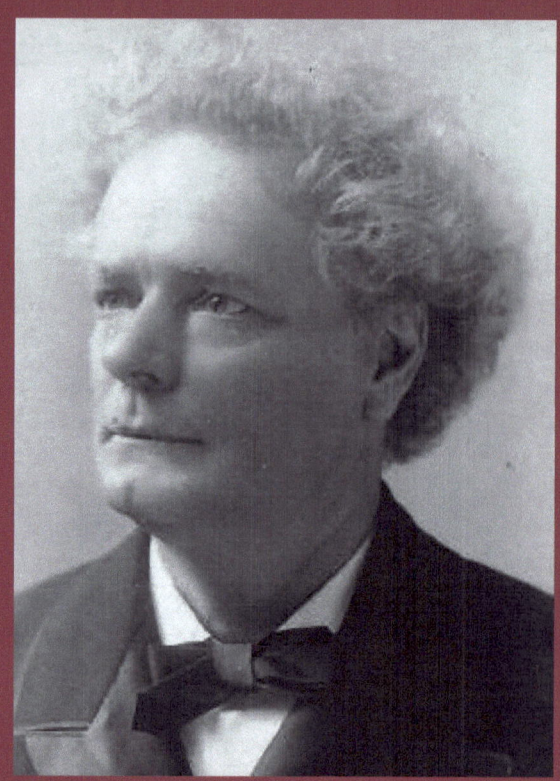

Dr. William B. Fletcher kept his reformist spirit despite the political agenda that came with the position. When he first became Superintendent, he reduced the medicinal whiskey, water and cod liver oil hospital usage from three gallons a day to one pint believing it was more "injurious than beneficial." He gave extra malt beer to patients who didn't have appetites. By 1887 he removed alcohol from the hospital entirely. He also provided a married man and woman to each ward to be in charge of attendants. (Young men were considered too "fiery" and apt to "strike blows.")

study the insane body.

The act of abolishing restraints, while well intended, unintentionally created havoc. Attendants were responsible for a large number of patients. There were no psychotic drugs for angry, violent or disturbed patients. Restraints had been seen as the answer. For people who said that restraints were necessary to prevent suicide, Fletcher pointed to like numbers with or without restraints and that noted one woman was able to strangle herself in a locked crib.

However, the staff adapted and sometimes patients who "disfigure themselves or pick their clothing to pieces… have had to wear mittens made of bed ticking." Occasionally patients were shut in their rooms. Overall though, Fletcher said, "The patients seem to be better without restraints. " Records show that in 1889 restraints were used one time, attesting to the fact that Central State Hospital was not a deliberately abusive organization where patients were tied and chained on a regular basis.

In 1886, Fletcher asked why they had to return a surplus of $26,000 to the State Treasury and why it could not be appropriated for the continued care of the over 1,700 patients. When he spoke out about the moral issues within the hospital, it cost him his job. But the price was worth it because many of the abuses were eliminated.

Dr. George F. Edenharter worked as the superintendent from 1893-1923. He brought back "mechanical restraints," (4) although they were out of style. He stated they were necessary citing "the bruises they sometimes caused lasted only several days while the potential harm from drugs used to quiet patients was incalculable" Still, he admitted strait jackets were used "more often when the institution was short on attendants" and they were "often left on longer periods of time than required."

Edenharter used restraints and said that "restraints" was misleading because different institutions regarded restrains and their levels differently. For example, many hospitals didn't consider applying hypodermics a restraint. At Central State Hospital, restraints were used sparingly, and at the request of the doctor only. These consisted mostly of locking a patient in a room. A camisole was also used. The sleeves were really long, so the patients couldn't grab anything. However, Edenharter said the camisole should come off as soon as the need was gone. "The habit of pumping drugs into patients in order to keep them quiet is reprehensible." Edenharter did not practice surgeries on the insane. Edenharter also saw that the hospital grew and expanded with the times. During his tenure, he saw old buildings replaced, new activity buildings built, and added new and additional equipment for operating rooms and the pathological labs, occupational therapy departments and malaria therapy of paresis program. He was by all accounts a "caring soul" who genuinely wanted to help the patients. He made regular visitation of the wards his priority.

The early 1900s saw a need for reform. At the same time, strides were made in the treatment of patients. As reform and innovation progressed, the Indiana Hospital for the Insane became known as Central State Hospital and earned respect as a teaching and research facility.

After Edenharter, Max Bahr served 54 years at Central State Hospital. Twenty nine years were spent as Superintendent. He saw the demolition of the Department for Men Building (the original hospital building) and construction of five new men's building. Mayer Hall and the Employees Building (also known as the Administration Building) were also built. He began the Occupational Therapy Department. He was known as a gentle, kind man who toured the wards often. When he died, he left money to be used for an ongoing program to purchase Christmas presents for patients.

Doctor's Duties

The doctors hired by the Superintendent were to be "of high moral character and his skills should fit the position." The doctors were to make rounds every day with the superintendent in the morning and in the evening alone. Doctors also lived on the hospital grounds, but later this practice ended. They were on call every evening and stayed on call for a week or more during the rotation.

They were expected to visit patients every day, two times a day (morning and afternoon). At CSH there is evidence that this was not always possible. Doctors' time was limited, which led to a sporadic and inconsistent completion of records. Expectations were never quite followed through with to the exacting scale they should have been.

Additionally, doctors were expected to report on research, and attend meetings and conventions related to medical causes. By the early 1920s, clinics were provided to patients for eyes and dentistry. Lectures for students and the public continued. Doctors gave talks at county historical societies and several articles appeared in literature.

Sarah Stockton

Dr. Sarah Stockton worked exclusively with the women in the hospital. She believed that some insanity and abnormal workings of the female organs were related. Many insane women had irregular periods. It was believed that because of the nervous energy and cerebral movement, the body used the menstrual blood as a power source for the body. If women had no periods or women who had reached menopause, were also susceptible to insanity.

Dr. Stockton had cases of giving tonics to uteri and vaginas when enlarged and prone to endometriosis that met with success. She admitted little was done surgically, pointing one year to four cases:
- Two of trachalorraphy which were successful
- One perineorrhaphy, which was successful
- One laparotomy, which resulted in peritonitis and the patient died.

TREASURER

The treasurer was a salaried position. His duties were to keep the books and pay the bills of the steward when proper documentation was presented.

STEWARD *(later Bookkeeper)*

The steward made all the purchases for the hospital including building materials. He was to promptly provide receipts and bills to the treasurer to ensure timely payment. He was also responsible for male domestics (5), the attendants for the male patients, and male patient comfort.

The steward also was responsible for other staff such as night watchmen, farmers and farmhands, gardeners and their assistants, jobbers, carpenters, engineers and machinists, firemen, bakers and their assistants, the carriage driver, and the gatekeeper.

MATRON

The matron was responsible for the domestic running of the hospital, meaning the laundress, washerwomen, seamstresses, female domestics and ironers. She was also responsible for the female patient attendants and the comfort of female patients.

She was also responsible for cooks, their assistants, and bakers and their assistants, and dairy maids.
Many times the matron was part of a married couple who shared the duties of matron and steward. Other times, she was the superintendent's wife.

ATTENDANTS

Attendants were the people patients saw the majority of the day. The superintendent hired these staff members.

The attendants were sometimes worked 24 hours a day, as in the early days. In the 1940s, the attendants were "prisoners" of their work. They had to live on campus, sometimes on wards and were on call 24/7 with a half day they could leave the campus. Carrie Lively talked about her work in 1899, "The first two weeks were a horror to me. At first I could not sleep because of some maniac yelling or someone moaning or suffering." Carrie was lucky. She and some of her coworkers had every other evening off. "The grounds were beautiful and we could go anywhere on the grounds we wished and we could sit on a swing with a friend or just rest and talked." Earlene Floyd, another attended said, "I love the patients. Just like a family, we help each other get through the day."

Kirkbride, in his book on hospitals for the insane, recommended people with the following characteristics be hired.
- Pleasant expression and mental cultivation
- Good temper
- Patience
- Coolness and courage
- Cheerfulness
- Good worker
- Sympathy
- Moral character
- Good health
- "and that indefinable something that can only be called tact"

Kirkbride also recommended that attendants be prepared for what their job entailed. He stressed that they needed to be "prepared for insults and charges when unfounded," and if they expected gratitude, they should quit. Moreover, they should expect sometimes to receive some verbal and physical abuse from patients. Because Kirkbride acknowledged the attendants had a "high stress job", he believed they should be given "ample recreation time and uninterrupted sleep."

Attendants and Assistants had a strict set of rules to follow. The following guidelines are from 1848:
1. Self-respect is paramount and this will be reflected in the department and duties executed.
2. Dress shall be neat and clean. Conduct will be impeccable.
3. Everyone will treat everyone with respect, a cheerful attitude, moral obligation
4. Duty to institution:
   - Engagements will be completed properly. Leaving the hospital requires a 30 day notice.
   - You will dedicate your time to the hospital without extra compensation. You will not sell services or goods to anyone, especially patients.
   - You will not leave the hospital without permission. You will return by 9p.m. or ask permission before hand.
   - You will maintain the neatness of the hospital at all times.
   - You will not give anyone your keys. Males will not enter female areas.
   - Doors must be locked at night. Lights are required by the Superintendent must be burning at all times. Leaving your post without permission is a violation of your duties.
5. Duties to patients:
   - Patients will be treated with respect and equality.
   - Each patient will be groomed in the morning and the beds aired.
   - Patients will be comforted when irritated, encouraged and cheered when melancholy and depressed. They will not be pushed, collared, or rudely handled. If any of this is witnessed, you will inform the Superintendent.
   - When patients curse or are abusive, attendants must be cool, and calm. Violence and blows towards the patents are never tolerated.
   - Patients will never be restrained.
   - One attendant will always be in the hall with the patients and will not leave without permission. You will keep the patients occupied, tidy and cared for at all times.
   - At meals, one or more attendants will be present to assist with the meals. You will ensure patients do not take silverware with them.
   - Nothing sharp will ever be given to a patient. No medication will ever be given to a patient unless it is prescribed. No letters or other articles may be given to patients without Superintendent approval. Clothes of suicidal patients and sharp objects will be removed from every room every night. You will always know where your patients are.
   - When patients leave, they are not allowed to do anything but be with you unless permission is obtained prior to leaving. Attendants are responsible for the well-being of the patients when they are out.
   - Medication is given 30 minutes before the meal. The cups used will have the patients names and will be returned within one hour of taking them, cleaned. You will not hold any conversations other than those about patients with the assistant physician or superintendent.
   - All damages to patients or materials are to be reported daily to the superintendent, matron or steward.
   - When a patient is acting or speaking inappropriately, you will gently redirect their conversation or actions. They may be placed in their rooms but if so, you will report this to the superintendent or assistant physician.
   - You will make the patients comfortable morning, noon and night.
   - Every patient will be assigned to an attendant. You are responsible for your patients and their care and well-being at all times.
   - Food is not allowed in the wards. Patients must be at every meal except in cases of illness, or high mental excitement unless permission has been obtained.

6. Duty on Sabbath:
    - Sunday is a day of rest and quiet at the hospital. No visitors are allowed.
    - All attendants who can be spared from their duties will attend services.
    - The superintendent will decide which patients attend services.
7. Miscellaneous rules:
    - No drinking on or off campus. No smoking on campus.
    - No one can be admitted to the wards except with the permission of the superintendent
    - Strangers must obey visiting hours.
8. Stated hours for meals:
    - Waking bell rung two to three minutes:
    - 4:30a.m. (June/July/August)
    - 5:00a.m. (March, April, September, October)
    - 5:30a.m. (November, December, January, February)
    - Breakfast served one and a half hours after the waking bell. (6, 6:30 and 7a.m.)
    - Dinner is at 12:30 p.m.
    - Tea at 6 p.m. (Tea was considered supper)
9. The hospital closes at 9:30 p.m. and everyone stays in their own apartments after that time.

Even with this strict code, abuses happened. Attendants were sometimes uneducated people, with no background in medicine. The hospital did not provide a robust training plan. In fact, in the beginning, attendants were brought in, given a tour and a talk with the Superintendent, and sent into the wards. They were put into the worst wards to condition them and as they proved themselves, were sent to better wards.

During the reformation years, because there was more emphasis placed on the comfort of the patient and the violent (regardless of gender) were considered soothed by a woman's voice, the female supervisor of attendants administered all medicines and performed bed and clothing inspections for several years until these duties were passed to attendants and nurses.

Throughout the years, there were not always enough attendants. Prior to about 1950, it was not uncommon for one attendant to cover three or four wards at night. As the population grew, a "Trustee", meaning a patient who was in good shape would watch over other patients. They were not paid or trained. In 1958, Bill Parish started at Central State as an attendant. "We had so many patients, it was all we could to keep patients fed and bathed."

This changed in the 1960s when the Federal government ruled that unpaid patient labor was illegal. In 1966 the Fair Labor Standards Act (FLSA) ruled that mental patients should be paid minimum wage but several cases were brought before the court in many states because the Department of Labor (DOL) would not enforce it. Years later, court cases were still being fought to get patients back pay with interest. Trustees were gone. This ruling made the case that more staff was needed. In the 1960s and 1970s funding increased from the State and more people were hired, including attendants. In 1993 the staff to patient ratio was two to one. This may be because fewer people were being admitted as the hospital was closing down.

As more became known about mental health and education conditions improved in Indiana, more educated people came to the hospital to work as attendants. Additionally, the hospital did more training. At the height of training, newly hired attendants, with or without, a medical or psychiatric background, attended a four week program of training that included clinical supervision. They could aspire to move from institutional trainee, to Attendant, to a Psychiatric Attendant I and on to Psychiatric Attendant II (6), the latter being reserved more for supervisors. In the 1980s, a Psychiatric Attendant III and IV were also added.

Attendants did not take guidance from nurses, but only "written orders from the doctor." The Administration believed that the attendant personnel were "over-achieving, especially when you consider the typical socio-economic background and educational preparation….We know the attendants, by and large, do a very credible job…."

Security

There were three night watchers in the department for women, and a total of 13 employed at the hospital. These night watchmen visited wards every 35 to 40 minutes. By the 1960s midnight staff did rounds of patients and the grounds every 15 minutes.

Nurses

After Kirkbride's methodology lost favor, other staff members were hired, most importantly, nurses. In the beginning, nurses worked long hours and lived on the hospital grounds. They were expected to wear uniforms and be unmarried. Later, as nursing progressed, they were allowed to wear uniforms that progressed from dresses, hosiery and hats to regular street clothes and later, scrubs.

In 1928 the hospital had 139 nurses and attendants for 1, 611 patients. In 1949 the staff to patient ratio was 6.3 to 1 and it was 4.2 to 1 in 1911, but there were eight patients to every attendant. Central State was consistently below national averages on patient staff ratios.

Martha Rogers, RN (Third Floor, Old Main Building) wrote in the 1970s, "The Nursing Department attempts to provide the best possible nursing care to patients via two basic subdivisions: Nursing Service and Nursing Education." Nursing Service was responsible for directing nurses' care for patients by "striving to give nursing care of the highest possible quality". Nursing education provided clinical instruction and experience necessary to nursing personnel to give skilled nursing care. Both divisions worked together to "promote and encourage nursing studies, program of in-service, promotion of good human relations, evaluation of nursing care quality and others.

In the 1947 annual report to the Governor, Superintendent Bahr recognized the fact that the staff was the first line to the patients. "The medical personnel requires professional and technical skill of high order and it demands attention and service given in an atmosphere of sympathy for the individual and understanding of the disease. While the building and medical facilities form the essential foundation on which the work must be built, the real heart of the problem lies in the quality of the service rendered by the staff. There must be sufficient number of attendants, sufficiently well trained and supervised to care of the patients to carry out the physician's orders and watch for symptoms which should be reported."

The Nursing Education Department was responsible for designing, planning and implementing the nursing education program. This included not only formal but informal learning. In-service programs scheduled every other month were attended by nursing personnel. These programs included new nursing procedures and techniques as well as general information. The Registered Nurse seminars were held bi-weekly. RNs and other personnel attended these sessions.

Nursing Service was different. Registered nurses and attendants were part of this department. The trainees received courses in basic attendant nursing including skills, growth and development, anxiety, conflict, ethics etc. It was an on-the-job four week course with continuous clinical supervision. It was an "opportunity for students to discuss beliefs and ideas about mental illness, with particular emphasis on dealing with misconceptions and fallacious infor-

Below: A view of how nurse's shoes changed. Left, a 1910s pair of shoes. Right, a 1970s pair of shoes.

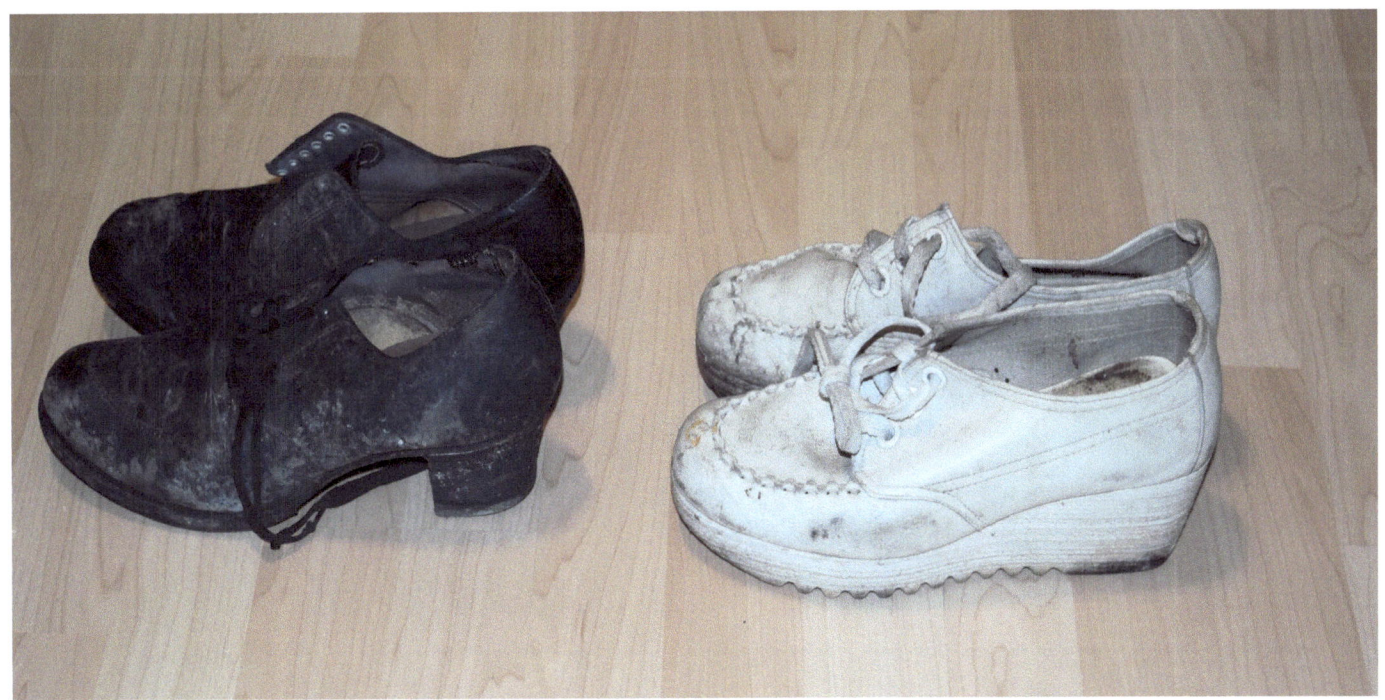

mation about mental illness." Once the course was completed, the attendant is assigned to a ward area and supervised practice of basic skills. After six months, if successful, the attendant is considered a permanent employment.

The biggest issue this department experienced in the 1970s was the salary scale for registered nurses. It was lower than pay in other agencies and made it difficult to build a robust nursing staff. There were only six nurses in 1972 at Central State Hospital.

Nursing service was responsible for planning and implementing nursing care for the patients, continuous training, supervision and evaluation of personnel, coordination with other departments, developing public relations, and selection and assignment of personnel.

In addition, the nurses were responsible for being consultants and resources for the patients, planning nursing units in new buildings, phasing out service in certain ward areas, opening new wards, and participation in surveys and departmental planning.

In 1968 the nurses began organizing the unit system, functioned on treatment teams and were involved in planning for the patient. Due to a smaller inpatient population and fewer wards, nurses and attendants were able to better use behavior modification techniques.

One of the most prescribed techniques was remotivation. About 40 Remotivationists collaborated regularly to share experiences, make plans and discuss issues relating to their situations. Remotivation was used for isolationist patients so that they could relate their experiences, become more social and realize what kind of contribution they could make. The Remotivationists recorded patient progress and reported regularly to treatment teams.

Nurses created "nursing care plans" for each patient that were reviewed quarterly. These plans were not kept in with the patent's record, but in a Kardex file at the ward level. They were generally thrown away and not recorded, once the patient left the hospital.

(See the chapter on Central State Leadership to see more about staffing at the hospital.)

STAFF ISSUES

Staff was hard to get and keep because of work and pay throughout the 146-year history of the hospital (7). For example, in the 1880s the hospital believed the salaries paid to the male attendants was too low ($20 per month) and that it should be $30 per month. The Superintendent made $2,000 per year and the hospital wanted it raised to $3,500 per year. A few years later it was raised to $3,000per year. In 1907 the female attendants made $18 to $22 per month

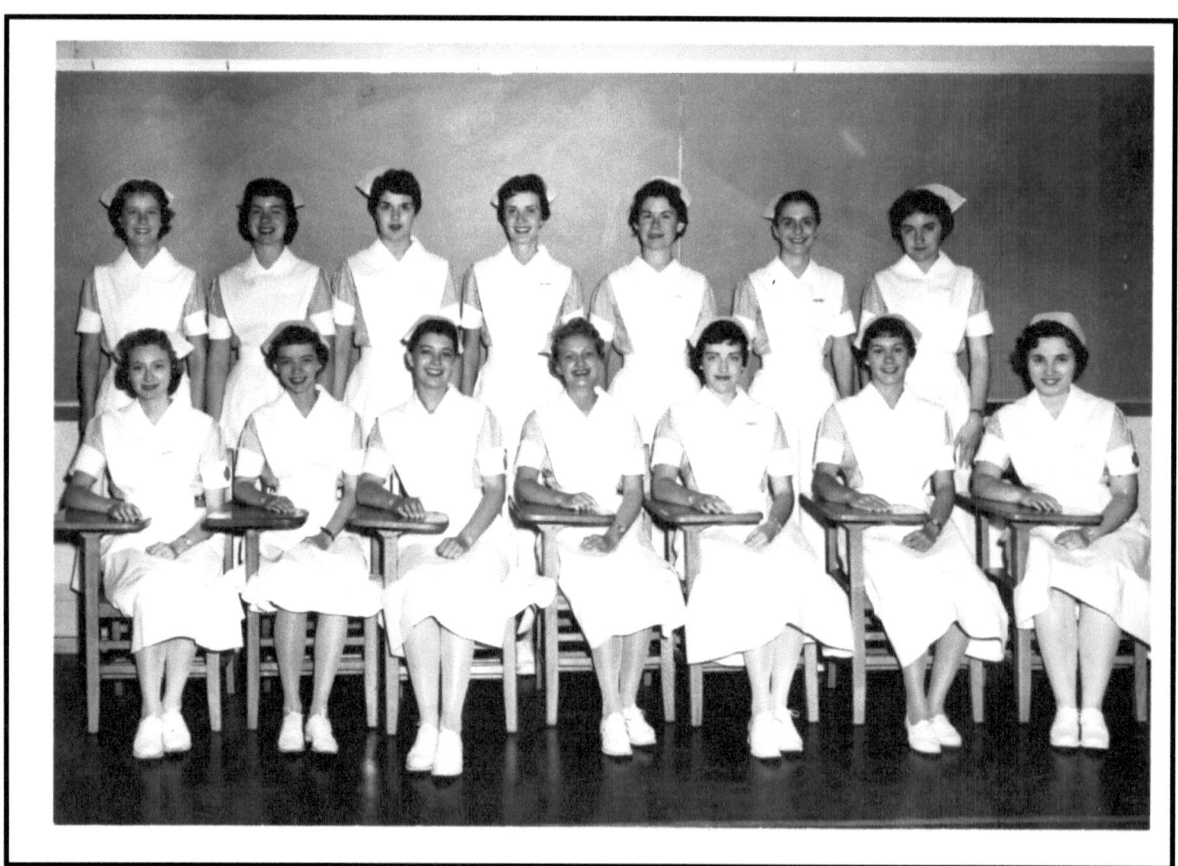

to start and then they could reach as high as $27 per month. Male attendants at the same made between $28 to $32 per month with a maximum of $39 per month.

Even in the last years before the hospital closed, it was difficult to hire staff, most notably nurses, because they could make $3,000-$5,000 more per year at a non-state run facility.

Thievery also occurred amongst the hospital staff who lived on the grounds. Several newspaper reports show that the employee quarters were pilfered by unknown people. Most likely, it was another employee, or an outside person, as any patients would have been caught with the items.

Even the doctors were not immune from complaints. In 1921, Dr. Sarah Stockton (8), 79, was accused by Otis Browning, a discharged supervisor, of not being fit for duty since 1919. He also wondered why Dr. Stockton was allowed to be a patient in the sick hospital and have everyone at her beck and call and still receive a salary. Otis was discharged because she refused to take coaching for her work and approach with coworkers. Otis accused Dr. Edenharter of liking Catholics more than anyone and playing favorites.

Educating staff was never handled properly at the hospital. In the beginning the staff had no medical background and little formal education in many cases. Training consisted of rules and regulations.

In the 1890s, more training was provided by assigning mentors to the staff members (mostly attendants) to get them acclimated to the wards. After WWI and more prominently after WWII, training grew to be a month to six weeks long. This additional training included a high level overview of how to deal with crisis in the wards and how to perform common tasks, such as bathing patients.

Finally in the 1960s, a two month program was developed. This training continued with previous information, as well as training on how to become different types of attendants. CNAs and nurses also attended this training. By 1970 more training was created outside of the basic new hire training. Given to the patients as well, over 50 seminars were held per year educating thousands of the hospital staff and patients. Topics include diabetes, sickle cell anemia and drug abuse education.

Housekeeping and kitchen staff also attended more training on sanitation and processes.

From the information available, the hospital did not seem to provide any type of hospital wide training for safety beyond the basics of what to do if a patient was out of control. For many staff members, this meant calling for security. For nurses and attendants, this meant taking the patient down to the floor and sedating them.

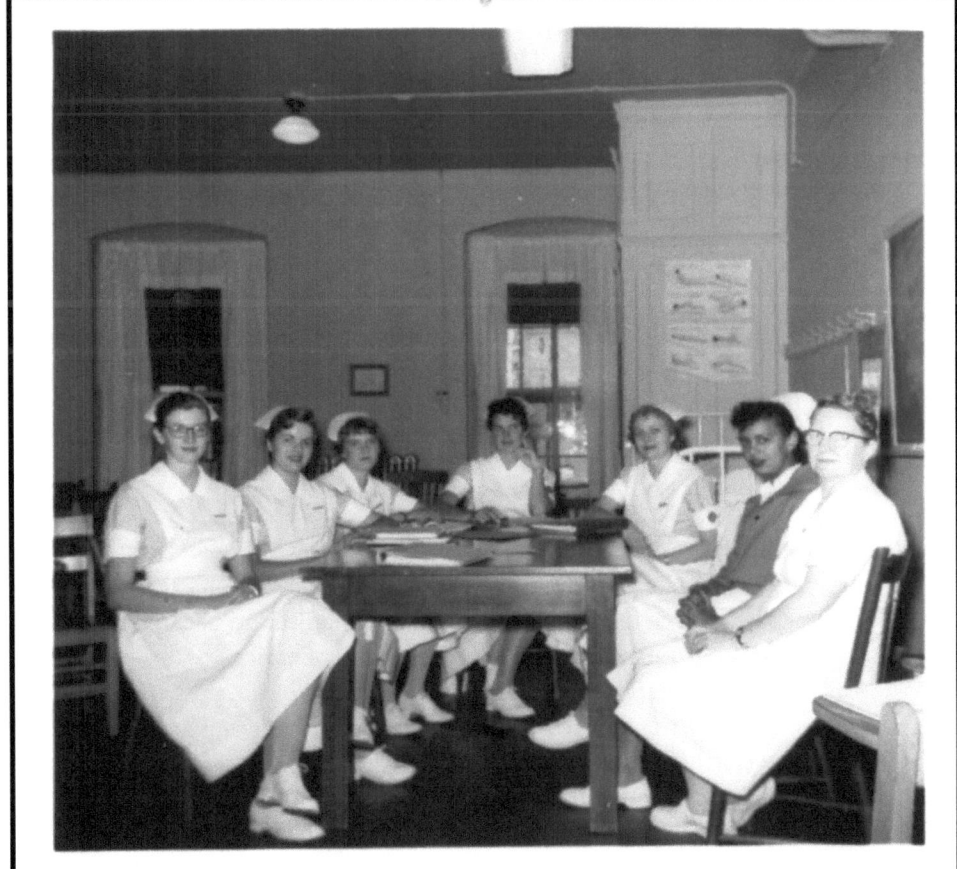

Opposite and right: Groups of DePauw University nurses. This program was one of the first to formalize modern nursing in Central State Hospital.

Evolution of Staff

Throughout the history of the hospital, staffing needs changed. More patients were being treated as outpatients. Because of dropping populations, wards were closed. Instead of individuals, departments were listed in the yearly reports. One of the largest changes was the direct admission of patients to treatment units, which eliminated the need for central admission services. This treatment on a unit allowed the hospital to form a team of people to take care of patients where all members of the staff were responsible for the care of the patient and not just carrying out orders from a physician.

Clinical Director

In the 1970s during a time of change, Donald W. Reed, MD the Clinical Director the Bahr Treatment Center (Front Corridor, South End) wrote,

> *"What does a unit do as a group? The unit sets up a team and all are involved in the care and management of patients. Everyone on the team should have the chance to say his piece…..It is the physician who is legally responsible for the patient care. Another professional may be unit leader but cannot abrogate the physician responsibility."*

Additionally, he stated, "Are there any efforts to standardize unit operations? No. I will intervene only if gross indications of failure appear. It works better if you are free to try new approaches you think will work." This was a disservice to standardization and best practices for what should have gone on in the hospital.

He agreed that "It is hard to get treatment approaches going when attendants change."

This is a bit contradictory to what the staff wrote about their departments in the 1970s. The staff declared that some had issues getting others to listen, getting forms completed, etc. However, with no standardization coming from the top down, the hospital was bound to continue to founder. Additionally, although there was an acknowledgment that changing attendants resulted in treatment approaches going awry, there was no suggestion for fixing this problem. Overall, there was a message of yes, we have problems, but we're ok with the status quo.

Below is a sampling of staffing in the 1970s.

Housekeeping
Where: Main Floor, Men's Building, east of the lobby, phone 318
Head: Mrs. Cordelia Lewis

In addition to 48 employees who had a minimum of two in-service training programs that consisted of instructions for maintaining proper sanitary conditions, 12 patients were on "industrial assignment" within the department. Patients were also included in the in service training programs and were always supervised.

The Housekeeping Department's goal was to
- Prevent the spread of disease by employing modern sanitation methods
- Provide a clean and attractive hospital environment
- Provide a therapeutic outlet for patients referred for industrial assignment through Vocational Industrial Therapy.
- Foster good hospital community relations.

Volunteer Department
Where: Main Floor, Old Main Building (9)
Head: Mrs. Rachel Bash

Early in Central State's history, this department had volunteers, although it was not an organized department or an official department of the hospital. In 1956 Glenna Bolstad became the first full time director of Volunteer Services. In 1976, the department was renamed Community Services.

The volunteer department accepted and disposed of donated items and conducted educational tours. However, their primary goal was to use the volunteers in the most efficient way possible. The Volunteer Director would assign the volunteers and they would be supervised by the department in which they worked. Volunteers were largely used in the hospital to assist with recreational activities, occupational therapy, library therapy, nursing care and clerical projects. For a time until the Admissions Ward was phased out, experienced Gold Ladies, being the best of the best volunteers, provided weekly programs for patients, including crafts, refreshment and recreation and their one-to-one contact alleviated some of the patients' initial fears.

Psychology Department
Where: Main Floor, Men's Building, West
Head: Dr. Werner Kuhn

Psychologists were interested in the science of human behavior. Assessing patients with tests was important throughout the patients stay at the hospital. Dr. Kuhn's philosophy was if you're going to test, make sure it is recorded and worth the time. He stated that psychologists would give recommendations in response to questions asked and that although psychologists were the most helpful in getting programs set up, the recommendations need not be adhered to. Group and individual therapies were offered with B.F. Skinner's work being one of the most prominent forms of psychology used. Kuhn also believed more research and tracking of the research should be done because he viewed it as knowledge.

Medical Records Department
Where: Center basement, Men's Building
Head: Mrs. Mary Sigler

The Medical Records Department made applications for Social Security, Veterans Administration (VA) and insurance benefits. Social Workers were expected to obtain a signed release so that Medical Records could determine benefits. Additionally, Medical Records needed to know when VA patients were in service, the branch and serial number of claims- in addition to all the other information required.

The department tried to have the medial record assembled by noon the day after a person was admitted. Dictation was sent out for transcription. Medical Records also had to make copies of lab reports for a patient's chart, the Bahr Treatment Center and the ward physician.

All cases of syphilis had to be reported to the Board of Health. Gonorrhea did not. Coding and diagnosis were imperative parts of the medial record.

If patients were going out for extended leaves, any "handicapped conditions" had to be reported, if the patient wanted them to be. The hospital was afraid if they oversaturated patients with handicaps, the patients would not find employment.

New paperwork was required to be filled out when a patient returned from family care or convalescent leave. All records were to be returned to Medical Records by 4:30 every day. No social history was released for any patient outside of the state and Marion County hospital system without express permission from the hospital.

Social Services Department
Where: Bahr Treatment Center Main Lobby
Head: Mrs. Rosa Harding; Mrs. Wiegman (chairman of the pre-admissions committee)

The major functions of the Social Services Department were to:
- Help patients and their families in their understanding of mental illness and help them make constructive use of hospital services.
- Help prevent unnecessary disintegration of the family
- Aid the treatment team in understanding patients in relation to their social, economic and emotional environment.
- Participate in education and training programs in the hospital and community.

Social workers screened potential patients. Mrs. Wiegman, who was the Chairman of the Pre-Admissions Committee, would make a determination on if the patient was right for Central State. Upon admission, the social workers helped patients obtained patients' medical and social histories, explained hospital policies to them, and helped them acclimate to the new environment. During the patient's stay, the social worker was the liaison between the patient and the community. The social worker was responsible for ensuring contracts with family and services were in place for the patient. The social worker would also conduct family therapy, and conversations with the patient and family to help determine if the patient was ready for release. If the patient could not return home upon release, the social worker helped devise an alternative plan.

In 1972, 72 patients were in family care. Mrs. Beverly, a social worker, was responsible for presenting reports to certify family care homes. Six patients were in a halfway house. They were employed and monitored in the evening by social workers.

The department also worked with IUPUI's Graduate School of Social Services. First and second year students came to the hospital to gain experience in the field. Mrs. Michau, a supervisor in the department, supervised them.

Drug Room
Where: Basement, Old Main Building
Head: Mr. Ralph Monteith

Early drugs at the hospital were vegetable compounds for the maintenance of physical health. After the advent of phenothiazine derivatives to control psychoses, more drugs than these compounds were used. Between 1962 and 1971 over 19,000 prescriptions were filled at the hospital, with the majority of these filled between 1969 and 1971. At first, keeping track of these prescriptions required little paperwork. With changes from the Bureau of Narcotics and Dangerous Drugs, the pharmacy had to keep better records, which increased its workload.

In the 1970s, pharmacists were on call over the weekend. Doctors could still get the keys from the Superintendent's Office to get whatever drugs they needed. A note was to be left. Later, this practice was abolished. Additionally, Monteith suggested any unused drugs be returned to the pharmacy.

Marking Room
Where: West End, Service Building
Head: Mrs. Norma Bond

The Marking Room ensured that patients had the clothing and other items they needed. It was divided into four parts: Hospital Supply, Home Supply, County Supply and Trust Fund. The biggest issue came from Home Supply as many patients' families forgot or didn't send clothes and other items needed. Bond stated, "It isn't the Clothing Room's fault that a patient does not have clothes. We can purchase what we need. We will pay for it somehow. Staff should call the Marking Room when a patient needs clothing."

Bond believed the patients should look "as good as possible." At this time, there was an issue that the clothes looked better in the Marking Room than on the patients. Clothes were not being ironed and cared for well enough, but the Marking Room only had ironing facilities and did not have permanent press equipment in the laundry room.

In 1971, 359 patients were on County Supply at a cost of $10,538 for the year. Over $18,000 was spent on clothing for trust fund patients. County items were issued right away, Trust Fund items were issued in just a few days and Home Supply was "luck." Donated clothing (which was sometime earmarked for specific patients) was distributed as well. Patients were sometimes allowed to choose clothing from the donated pile, although many times it was in too poor condition to be useful. Many donations were sent to Goodwill, the Salvation Army or Volunteers of America.

Bond stated ill-fitting clothes were sometimes due to relatives giving up on buying clothes or sending the wrong size. Sometimes patients would take other patient's clothing.
If clothing was sent in on bid from a supplier for the Hospital Supply and found unacceptable, it was shipped back to the owner.

Maintenance Department
Where: Powerhouse
Head: Mr. Bill Holgate

In 1972, 85 employees worked on the maintenance of Central State Hospital. They worked in the power house, on the grounds crew, and in plumbing, electrical and other trades. Approximately 20 patients also worked on the maintenance department, mostly as grounds crew members. Holgate stated, "It seemed to have been more important to get the patient to help the hospital than to teach him skills that he can use."(10). There was still a ban against hiring former patients (unless an "exceptionally well justified application" was specially approved.) so the hospital had to "rely heavily upon the patients to get the work out." (11)

Dental Section
Where: Bahr Treatment Center, Front Corridor, North End
Head: Dr. Jerry Follmar

New dental patients were examined each Thursday. Any issues with the teeth, mouth, throat or gums were documented. Proper brushing and hygiene was taught to patients. Forms recording this information were kept for each patient. Because the population was dropping, in the 1970s dentists were able to devote more time to each patient. They wanted the patients at Central State to have the "quality of dental work that others recognize as quality and admire." They performed every dental procedure except fixing a broken jaw.

At one time the patients brushes were kept at the office and they had to contact the office to get them. By the 1970s, the patients had their own brushes in their own rooms.

Even after a patient left the hospital, the dental office tried to follow up with the patient- in two months if memory was an issue for the patient and five to six months if it wasn't. Dentists received extra money for replacing dentures and used the plastic type because the others were prone to breaking.
However, dentists refused to treat patients who did not comply with hospital rules for "decent grooming." If appointments, which were coordinated with the wards were missed, dental privileges were withheld.

Information Desk
Where: Main Lobby, Men's Building
Head: Mrs. Virginia Saxe

The information desk did more than just give instructions. It was also a "clearing house". It took orders from the doctors for the patients and granted leave to patients. People working the desk were responsible for security in the sense of screening all relatives and friends coming to visit. They dispensed medications to the relatives for patients going on leave. When medication returned with a patient, it was sent to the pharmacy and its return date and number was recorded.

The Information Desk also worked very closely with Social Services. They kept a ward book which indicated where each patient was located. They assisted other departments such as Recreation, with this information as well. However, sometimes when patients would leave or come back from a pass, the desk would not receive accurate information and the patients could not be found.

All ward visits were recorded at the Information Desk. Social Services and Social Security used this information as well. The ID made out death certificates and called the Coroner when necessary. The ID also worked with the nursing staff when patients were absent without leave (also called AWOLs). This involved contacting relatives and the police, after a thorough search was made. The ID gave certain wards advanced warning when they were to receive visitors.

If patients failed to return, social workers notified family. The patients may have been placed on AWOL. If a patient was out on convalescence and was returned for some abnormal reason by the police, all leaves for that patient were revoked. By making these patients pickups and not AWOLS, there was a much shorter chain of command to go through to get the patient back to the hospital. In the case of AWOLS, the hospital had problems with the police. The different law enforcement offices seemed to give the hospital "the run around" when trying to find who was responsible for picking up patients.
It was the job of the Information Desk to know where the patient was at all times. It was the duty of the units and wards to provide that information to the Information Desk. Because of the breakdown in communication, many AWOLS occurred.

If a patient was taken off the grounds by someone other than a relative, a responsibility form was to be completed. If a relative took a patient off grounds, no form was needed.

Chaplain Department
Where: Old Main Building, Rear Center
Head: Chaplain David Richards

The hospital had three chaplains in the 1970s. Two were part time and the third was full time. Two were Protestant and one was Roman Catholic. Additional ordained lay volunteers and student ministers who were engaged in religious activities at the hospital. The student ministers were under the supervision of chaplains.

Until the 1970s, the chaplain was considered "peripheral" to the patient's care. The hospital was an asylum, a community apart from the regular population. In the 1970s, the view became that the religious needs of patients should be a part of their care. The chaplains were part of their care, but the focus was on restoring people to their homes and contact with their own ministers, rabbis and pastors. Religious services were a part of everyday life and visits to the critically ill were commonplace. Sometimes because of the training chaplains received, they were able to provide input on how treatment and religion together could help the patient. Chaplains also provided individual and

Persons under the age of twenty-one years will not be employed in any department of the Hospital.

AGE, HEIGHT and WEIGHT should be accurately given on date application is signed.

Misrepresentation in anything connected with this application, when discovered, will meet with prompt discharge from the service.

APPLICATION OF ....

FOR THE POSITION OF ....

IN THE

Central Indiana Hospital for the Insane.

Filed .... 190......

Employed .... 190...... .... 190......

WM. B. BURFORD PRINT, INDPLS.

READ THIS RULE BEFORE SENDING YOUR APPLICATION.

GENERAL RULE XIII.

As the Insane are confided to our care for PROTECTION as well as TREATMENT, no person will be employed here in any capacity who is not willing to do all in his or her power to aid us. Any ABUSE or NEGLECT of a patient coming under their notice, it will be their especial duty to report it AT ONCE to the Superintendent, who can always be seen for that purpose. Should it at any time appear that ABUSE or NEGLECT has been witnessed and not brought to the notice of the Superintendent or Medical Officer, it will result in the IMMEDIATE dismissal of all the parties concerned. Persons governed by the SO-CALLED "HONOR" that prevents reporting the abuse of a helpless insane patient are not wanted at this Hospital.

Left: Application for employment

Right: Contract signed by employees.

The signature of the applicant must be affixed to this Declaration, or the application will not be considered.

I hereby promise to obey the rules of the Institution; to faithfully execute the orders that may be given me by my superior officers, and to perform any duty assigned to me, although not of the kind for which I am chiefly engaged.

I consider myself bound to promote the objects of the Institution; to do my best to further the recovery of the patients; assist in all undertakings for their amusement, and to secure their comfort and safety.

I also pledge myself not to bring into the Institution, or the grounds thereof, any intoxicating liquors; to be careful of its property; to avoid all GOSSIP as to its inmates or affairs, and to endeavor by my own language and deportment to sustain its reputation.

I certify that I have read the rule printed on the back of this application and fully understand that it is my duty to report all cases of abuse or neglect of patients to the Superintendent, which I hereby agree to do.

I agree to give one week's notice should I wish to resign my position.

I acknowledge the right of the Superintendent to discharge me, without warning, for acts of harshness or cruelty to patients (either by language or act), intemperance, disobedience to orders, unsatisfactory services, violation of any portion of this agreement or other cause which may to him seem justifiable.

Name..

Signed this......................day of..............................190.....

group therapy.

Chaplains were involved in administrative duties through leadership and suggestion. They had to have additional work in a clinical setting. Protestant chaplains had to have the approval of the Indiana Council of Churches. The religious community wanted to ensure religious affairs were handled fairly and human rights promoted.

Richards stated, "The Chaplain department holds itself responsible to make representation against dehumanizing practices."

In 1970 the National Council of Jewish Women celebrated their tenth anniversary of service to the hospital by conducting the Arm Chair Travel Club.

In 1975 Reverend Earl Hoppert became the head of the Pastoral Department (12). Reverend Benjamin Friend was also on staff, and a rabbi was on call. Protestant and Catholic services were held weekly. On holidays such as Christmas and Easter, additional services were held.

Hoppert and Friend believed that they had an obligation to protect patients from religions which would do them harm. They heard of patients with a strict religious upbringing where who had been fed hot salt water to "purge them of the devil". They thought their work was good because there was still a stigma about the mentally ill and religion. Hoppert heard a sermon where the minister told the congregation that illness of any kind, including mental, was all because of sin.

The Chaplain Department also had students of divinity work with mentally ill. The "spiritual needs of the mentally ill are not that much different than the rest of the population."

THE UNFORTUNATE MISS RAEBURN

Miss Raeburn worked at Central State Hospital from 1909-1921. According to her, she worked 12 hour shifts and didn't take vacations many times because of staffing shortages. She worked her way up from attendant to a night usher (watchman). Her tenure ended in 1921 after she was discharged by Dr. Edenharter.

In a statement to the Board of Charities at the time of her discharge, Miss Raeburn said she'd come back from vacation early because staff was expected to be on duty on Thanksgiving Day. Dr. Edenharter called her into his office and presented her with a list of rules that were meant for her alone. She resented being singled out because she felt she was doing her job. Due to her position, Miss Raeburn was not someone who mixed with employees, although she believed she treated everyone equally. She was given privileges because of her service and position, and feared other people were jealous of her. She was to lock up at 9:45 p.m. and if anyone hadn't entered the building, they were locked out. Many times, Miss Raeburn said, she'd lock the doors when she saw people coming up the steps at 9:45 p.m. because they were late. She believed this gained her ill will.

Miss Raeburn also stated that Dr. Edenharter would employ Catholics and if you weren't Catholic, you were out of favor. She said Dr. Stockton was overbearing and had other physicians do her work, especially since she hurt her leg in 1919. In the same year, Dr. Stockton hurt her other leg and was bedridden, drawing a salary, but not working.

Nothing seems to have come of these charges. Miss Raeburn was not asking for reinstatement. She just wanted the Board of State Charities to understand what was going on in the hospital. Dr. Edenharter stated in Miss Raeburn's discharge papers that she had been in "violation of certain rules" and she had a "disregard for the instructions of the Superintendent." When she was called to his office, her "language was of such a character that I determined that the period of forbearance had been reached."

THE KIRKBRIDE WAY

Kirkbride advocated certain standards.. In his book, "On the Construction, Organization and General Arrangements of Hospitals for the Insane with Some Remarks on Insanity and Its Treatment", he advocated exacting plans and construction.

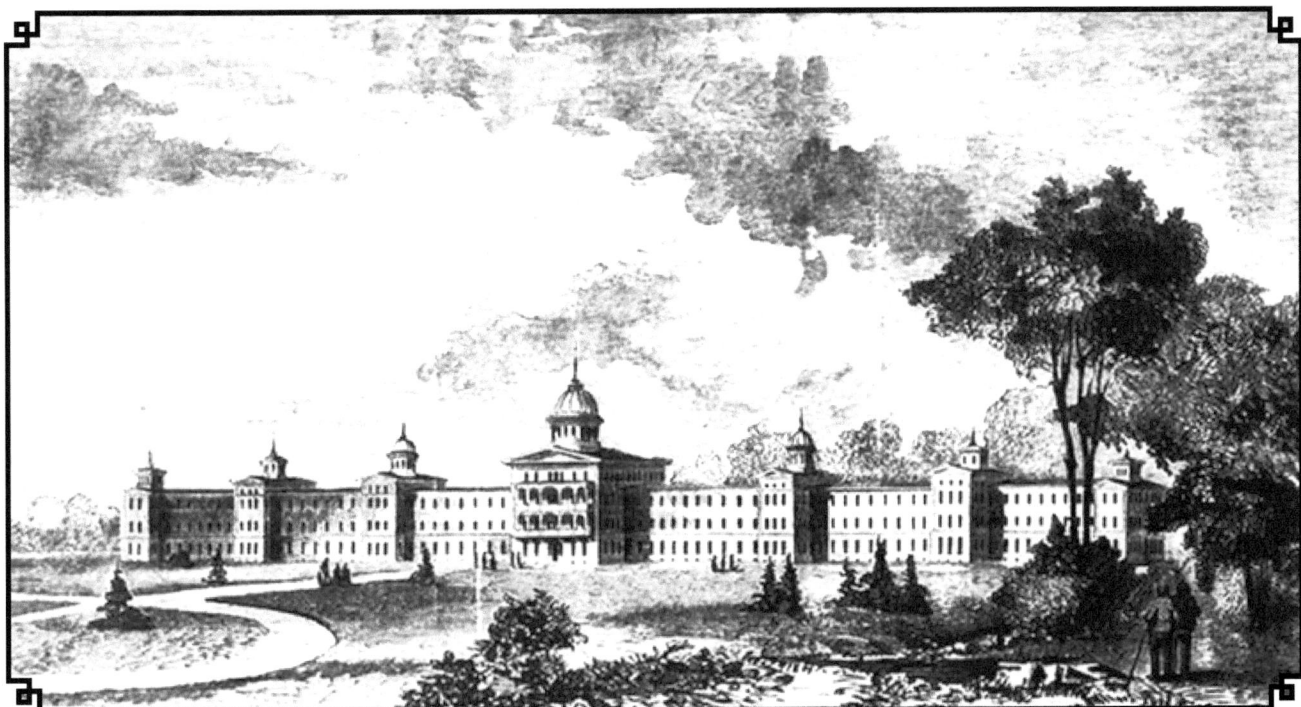

Top: A recommended plan for an infirmary ward.

Bottom: An etching for an insane hospital on the linear plan. Central State Hospital's first building for men was built on this plan.

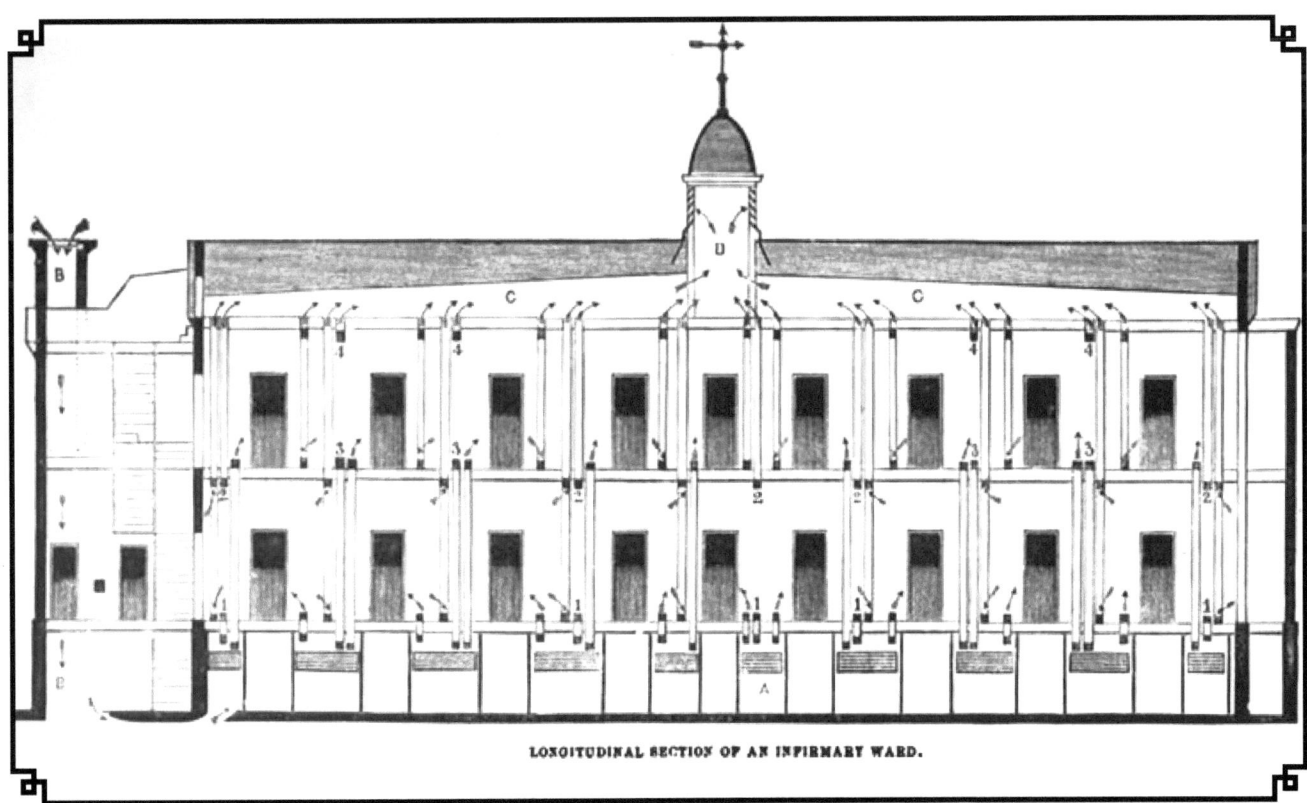

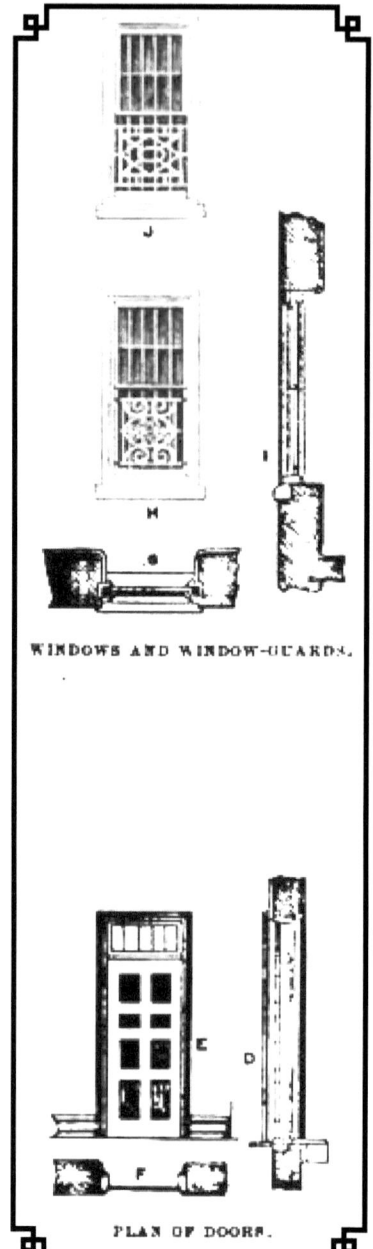

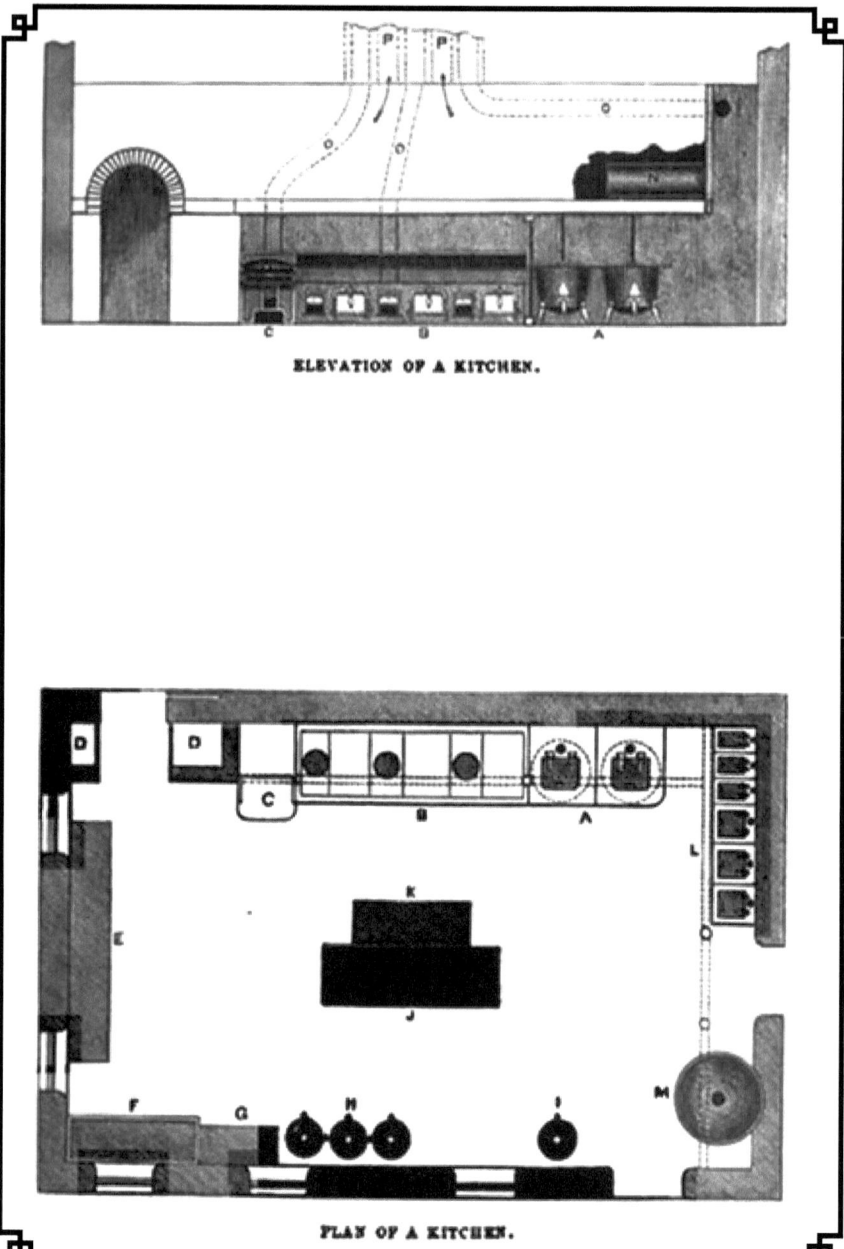

Top left: Plan for window and doors.

Top right: Plan for kitchens.

Six

TREATMENTS AND RESEARCH

Many people speculate on how horrible, cruel, and inhumane the treatments were at mental hospitals. They need to remember that in 1848 the mental health field was really in its infancy, especially from the aspect of useful, effective treatment. Just as we have experimental treatments today (think cancer), so they did for mental health patients. Not a lot was known about psychology or the brain, and throughout the history of mental health, the process of trial and error occurred.

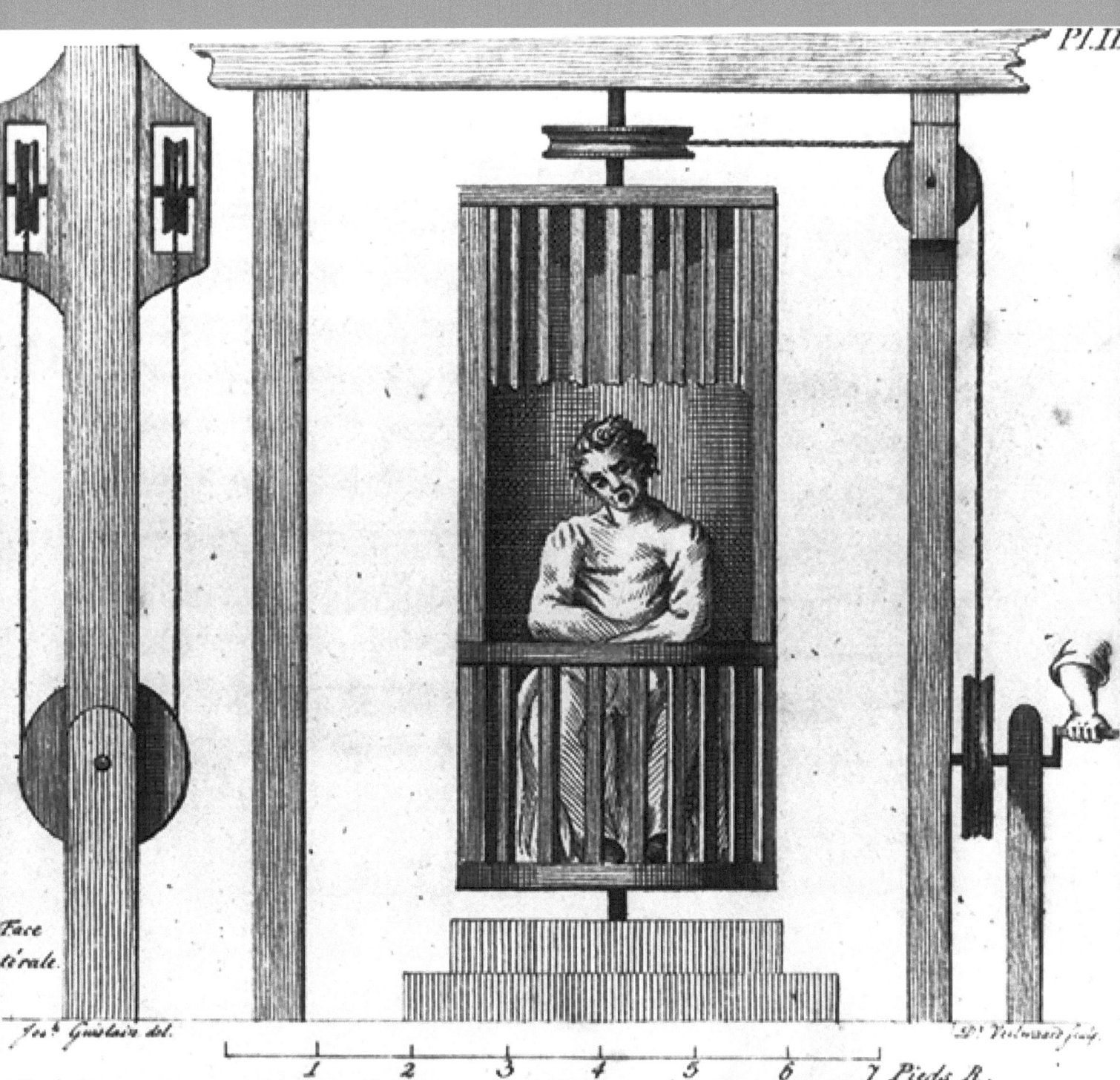

CURE RATES

When Central State was opened in 1848, the outlook for the insane had changed in the U.S. and abroad. Patients with the best chance of success (less than one year of insanity and an 85% cure rate) would be admitted first, then chronic cases (greater than one year of insanity and a 43% cure rate), then people who had applications on file the longest, and finally, the appropriate amount of people allotted each county would be taken into consideration.

By the end of the year, 104 patients had been admitted. Twenty left cured, four left improved, and 4 died (two from consumption, one from disease compounded by hypothermia at the jail before admittance to the hospital, and one from apoplexy.)

In the early days, doctors believed they had a 90% success rate in curing the patients. But by further looking at the statistics, this is impossible. By 1850 according to the Annual Report, 162 patients were admitted. 58 were discharged as cured, 4 as improved (but not cured), 4 improved and incurable, 1 eloped (AWOL) and 5 died.

Even removing every discharged, improved and deceased patients, 87 patients are still unaccounted for out of the 162. This means the "cure" rate is 54% at best. If the "improved but not cured" and the deceased are excluded, the "cure" rate is 36%.

However, these numbers for 1850 do not match a table in the 1850 Annual Report. The table in the report indicates 134 patients and 80 remaining at the hospital. If we use the same logic, the "cure" rate (minus all the discharged and deceased patients) would be 60%.

All of these figures are far below the 90% claimed by the 1850 annual report.

The next year they stated a 73% recovery on patients discharged and 80% on recent cases discharged.

In 1853 the amount of people cured was even calculated lower. Instead of calculating a yearly rate, the report stated 61% of total patients were cured or improved.

The hospital followed a formula set by the Worcester Insane Asylum and the State of Ohio Asylum. In this model, the percentage of recoveries was based on patients cured among the discharged instead of basing their numbers among the total patients and the number considered recovered. The hospital followed this model, because it was "customary" instead of following "our own convictions of what is the better mode of comparing results."

Seeing a decline in the "cure" rate, doctors now wanted to track readmitted patients. If patients were discharged and remained out for over three months, then returned, it was considered a second attack or subsequent attack. If patients were discharged and readmitted in less than 3 months, it was considered a relapse and they were considered "not cured" anymore.

The emphasis at this time was on "curing" the patient. Patients were also discharged as "improved". Later, as more became known about mental health, "cured" was no longer used and terminology changed to "discharged improved" and "discharged unimproved".)

Because doctors were finding that some patients were incurable, the hospital began to see a population of these patients growing in an already overcrowded hospital. To alleviate the problem, the hospital believed that any incurable patients could be sent to the poor farms. This reasoning was not because they were unfeeling, cruel, or uncaring. Doctors believed at the time they were achieving a 90% cure rate and that there were less than 500 insane people in Indiana. To the doctors, this meant that only about 50 people were incurable, leaving less than half of the county poor houses with an incurably insane person to look after. They believed that the 50 people would receive better care at a poor house than a busy institution.

After the doctors and administrators toured the poor farms and found them to be "anything but comfortable" and "abysmally run", they retracted their statement. To combat these issues, the hospital admitted that to make room for patients with a better cure rate, some cases were "prematurely" released and they were "under the disagreeable necessity of discharging few incurable cases who, too dangerous to be at large, or to be kept by their friends, have at least, we are pained to say, found a home with the criminals in the common jail…These things ought not to exist in a Christian community- they will not long exist in Indiana."

As a result of overcrowding, some chronic cases were sent home as "discharged unimproved" and some as "discharged improved. The hospital sometimes saw these patients back in the hospital and sometimes they didn't return.

Moral Therapy

When the hospital opened, moral therapy was widely used. This was based on treating the patient humanely and making their surroundings pleasant. Later, when more was learned about what causes mental illness, moral therapy changed into basic patient rights and other treatments were applied.

Industrial Therapy

From the early years of the hospital until 1968, industrial therapy through farm work was a booming treatment for Central State's patients. Many of the people who worked on the farm during this time were the chronically insane, whom doctors believed had little hope of recovery and whom would most likely be at the institution until death. It was thought the work would offer them enjoyment, fresh air and "as pleasant a life as was possible." Psychiatry had not reached a point of being able to show improvement yet due to its infancy. The Mental Hygiene Society wasn't making inroads in educating the public, or improving care of the patients, as most of the people involved were former patients. Further, the public still lacked the education (or seeming interest overall) to understand any improvements or have "improved" patients back in the population.

Early Drugs

Treatments at the hospital consisted of standard practices based on research from around the world including cathartics, narcotics and other sedatives, and moral therapy. In 1848 bloodletting ("bleeding") was not used. Mania, it was reasoned, could be controlled by warm baths, cold applications to the head, warm foot baths, mild cathartics and anodynes and nauseates. Doctors at the hospital believed bleeding calmed the mania, but brought it back ten-fold.

Cathartics (laxatives) were used. Doctors thought mild cathartics were better, because "drastic purging" had the opposite effect. One laxative was "Blue Pill" (also known as Blue Mass), a mercury based pill that was supposed to help improve mood, and cure tuberculosis, constipation, toothaches, parasitic infestation, pains of childbirth- and most importantly for Central State Hospital for the Insane- treat syphilis, which a large portion of the population had. Other laxatives included spiced syrup of rhubarb (widely used for children and infants), confection of Senna, aromatic tincture of guaiacum, and prescribed diet.

Narcotics such as opium were used. People with high manias may have had them prescribed under certain conditions. Tonics used included wine, whiskey, iron, and various barks and roots. In 1870, the hospital began using Chloral as a sedative and sleep agent.

During the 1800s bromides were used for sedative purposes. Chloral was used with ergot and potassium bromide in the violent sleepless stage of mania. Purging (inducing colon cleansing) was implementing "mechanical interference or hydraulic mining with a Davidson syringe". Also alkaline diuretic drinks including acetate of potash were thought to help get rid of waste matter and clean the kidneys. Warm baths were used to sooth and depurate the skin and body. Felseium, aconite, and veratrum viride slowed the heart and quieted delirium. Doctors advocated eggs and raw, hashed beef. Albumen and fibrin was also given to help purge waste, but if those drugs didn't work, doctors would put food in the patient's rectum. One man was fed this way for three months.

Stomach pumps were not used much as they were harder to administer than an enema. Salivation and stomatitis were treated with glycerite of borax and chlorate of potash. Exhaustion was treated with stimulants such as Quinia (quinine), an alkaloid of Cinchona. If a patient refused medicine, a suppository was given. Other treatments included carbon dioxide inhalation treatment to calm patients.

Hydrotherapy *(also known as Hydropathy)*

Hydrotherapy has been used since ancient times. Mineral baths such as those at French Lick and Paoli, Indiana claimed therapeutic properties. Therapy in the hospital however, didn't use mineral water. Therapies ranged from a simple bath in warm or cold water to specific baths for the head. Patients were also put into a warm or cold bath and a sheet was put over the top leaving their head and shoulders exposed.

Visitors

Early in the hospital's history, tours were given to educate the public. In the first five years of the hospital, 5,000 people visited during these tours. This did not always work as more chronic patients were admitted and housed at the hospital. At times, the more violent patients would abuse other patients or become unruly during visiting hours. This made the tours become more of a freak show than a way to view the hospital as a healing institution. The doctors in 1848 wanted to revise the rules so that the patients were never made to feel as though they were on exhibit. In 1860s, visitors were looked upon more favorably and visitors were welcomed into the hospital.

Malarial Treatment

Syphilis

Part of the problem at Central State is that many of the people who were admitted to the hospital had syphilis. Syphilis is a sexually transmitted disease that is spread through sexual contact or through mother to fetus during pregnancy or at birth, resulting in congenital syphilis.

Now, syphilis is diagnosed through blood tests, but back in the early days, doctors were unable to treat it. It was only with the discovery of the causative organism, Terponema pallidum, by Fritz Schaundinn and Erich Hoffman in 1905 that the disease could be cured. The first effective treatment was developed by Paul Ehrlich in 1910 (Salvarsan). This led to the malarial treatment which was used at Central State, and then penicillin in 1943.

Because syphilis causes dementia and nerve damage, many of the patients came to Central State with other problems coupled with the disease, or with a later stage of the disease which affected their mind and body. With no cure, these people were doomed to be part of the chronic population of the hospital until they died, most likely of complications due to the syphilis.

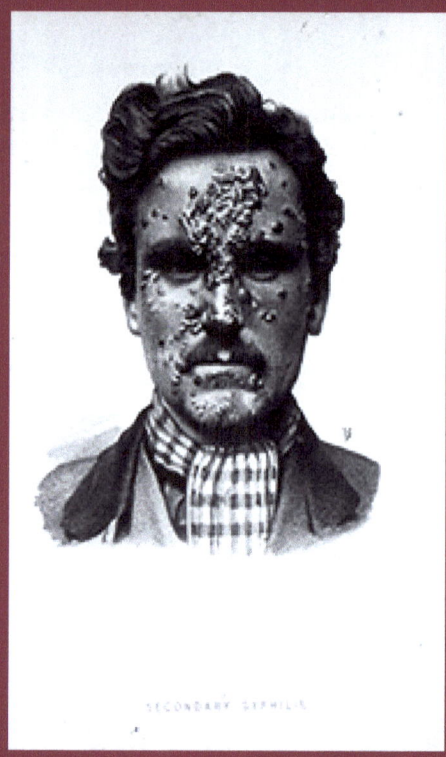

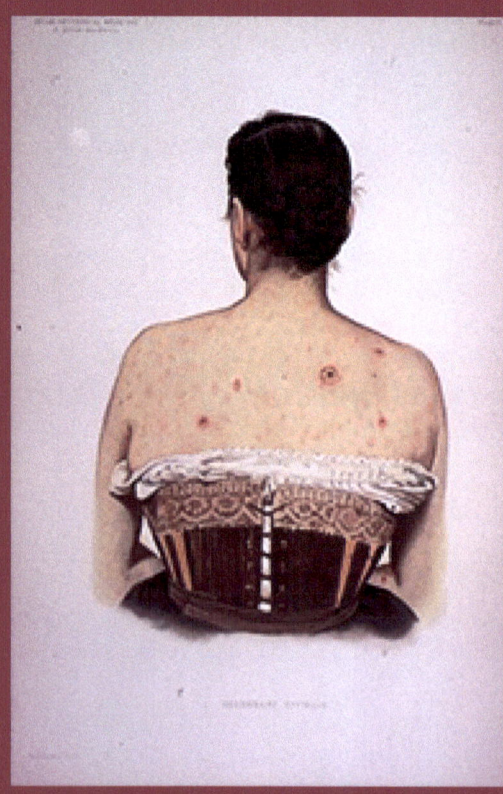

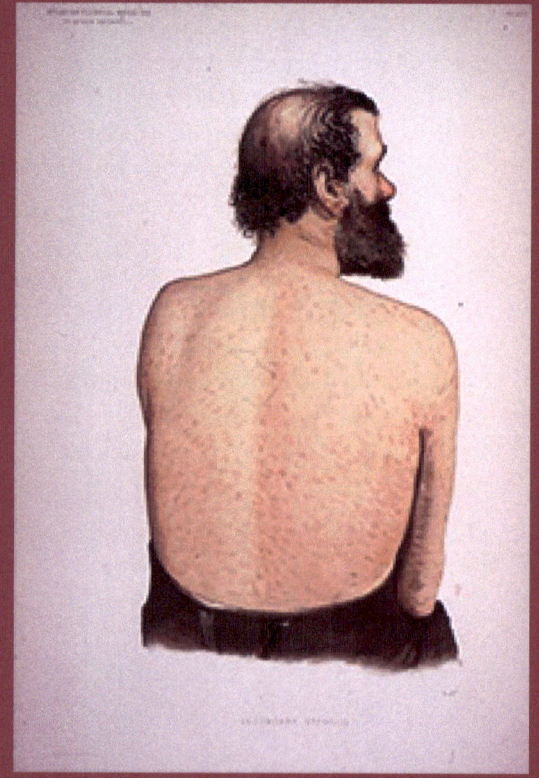

Top: Man with secondary syphilis.

Bottom left: Drawing of a woman with syphilis.

Bottom right: Drawing of a man with syphilis.

One of the major treatments to come out of the asylum system was the treating people with syphilis with malaria. The malaria would kill off the syphilis and then the patient could be treated for malaria. Although the cure rate was less than 50% due to the stage of syphilis and the efficacy of the treatment in general, it was better than letting patients languish when a cure might be possible. This treatment was used until the 1950s when penicillin was found to be a better cure.

Shock Therapy

Shock therapy (electric convulsive or insulin) were commonly used in hospitals around Indiana and the Midwest in the 1930s.

Electro convulsive Therapy

People misunderstand the use of electro convulsive therapy (ECT). Many of the issues with early ECT were due to staff being undertrained, misuse of the equipment, and improper administration of the therapy.

In the 1930s electro convulsive therapy was developed replacing Metrazol (cardiazol) shock therapy. ECT passed a current through the brain and induced an epileptic fit, which sometimes injured patients. It did, however, help some patients suffering depression. In 1930 160 were given electro shock with an average of 14 treatments per patient, mostly schizophrenic, and 57 were improved and furloughed from the hospital. No patients were lost due to death by any of these methods. Up to four nurses helped with "immobilization".

It is still used today in limited cases, mostly with severely depressed patients or in patients who pose a threat to themselves or others and doctors cannot wait for medications to take effect.

Insulin Shock (Insulin Coma)

Deep Insulin Therapy was used to treat schizophrenia at Central State Hospital, from 1938-1942 then it was revived briefly in 1951. It was once believed that schizophrenia was caused by high blood sugar in the brain. There was no set protocol for this treatment in the medical field and hospitals created their own. At Central State Hospital, insulin was administered until the body went into shock for one hour (2) . Then the patient was revived with sugar in tea or some other drink or intravenous glucose. Generally, patients went through many rounds of this procedure, many times 6 days a week. It was used with psychotherapy and sometimes ECT.

This was a risky procedure in which patients sometimes became overweight, brain damaged or even died. Overall, doctors from many institutions agreed that part of the improvement from the disease came from the treatment and part from the fact that with the other treatments given, the patients would achieve improvement anyway. With this

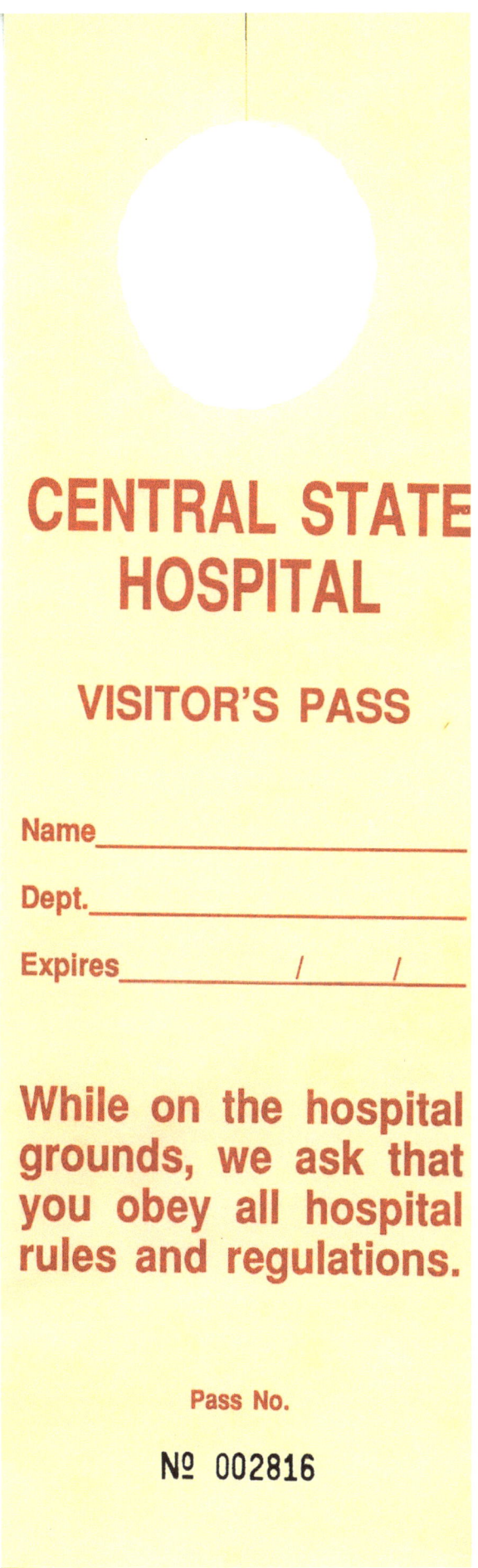

therapy there was about a 50% chance for success and a one to five percent chance of death.

Hypnotics, Stimulants and Other Drugs

The 1930s also saw an increase in sleeping pill usage for patients (hypnotics). These were used for sleep and to calm agitation. Stimulants were used to improve mood.

Therapies

Psychotherapy

Psychotherapy is interaction between a patient and a therapist, sometimes in a group setting. In psychoanalysis, one examines one's thoughts, feelings, and behavior. It is used to increase self-awareness and wellbeing. Cognitive therapy began in the 1950s and cognitive behavioral therapy (CBT) was developed in the 1970s. Acceptance and commitment therapy and dialectical behavior therapy developed from CBT.

Psychotherapy was integrated with medial and the social approach at the hospital. By 1939 however, the doctors didn't really believe in its helpfulness. "Psychotherapy has been employed treating the patients by individual psychotherapeutic interviews….. These efforts however, have not led to an appreciably greater discharge rate. For this reason we have no undue optimism with regard to the value of the intensive use of individual psychotherapy except in certain instances." By 1948 this thinking had changed and the doctors now believed psychotherapy "gave the patient the best possible care and gave the patient the belief that the hospital is interested in him." It also helped the relatives feel better about the institutions.

Occupational

Occupational therapy creates structure and has a focus on health and well-being. Many times patients would take classes focused on hygiene, coping skills, medication management, and social skills. As part of therapy, patients were taught dictation, transcription, and shorthand. They made hats and other items for the hospital. Additionally, they also learned farming, carpenter trades, animal husbandry and custodial skills.

Recreational

The treatment had been used in the east for three years, but Bahr felt that testing on efficacy had been inadequate so it was tested more fully at Central State Hospital.

Recreational therapy was started at the hospital in the 1950s and included a variety of recreational activities.

TYPES OF INSANITY: MASTURBATION

We know now that some of the types of insanity the hospital reported in the yearly reports are symptoms of mental illness or not considered a mental illness today. Each yearly report focused on one or two types of insanity and provided an overview and treatment for it. In 1851 and several other years, the subject was masturbation, which was believed a symptom of schizophrenia. The doctors felt they could not give the patients relief, citing Dr. N.D. Benedict, Superintendent of the New York Lunatic Asylum. Dr. Benedict believed that the first indication of masturbation was religious excitement because people afflicted with the impulse were worried about their immortal souls due to their actions. The doctor believed over years that the masturbator would become shy, timid, nervous, and unhappy. It was thought men were of small physiques; and the women became emaciated but had "gay and voluptuous manners".

Doctors believed one could tell if a man was a masturbator by the fact that he didn't want to do manly things (sports, walking, etc.) and would prefer to be "sedentary" and read "trashy" novels instead of running off "energy and excitability". All of this led to deterioration of the mind.

To prevent this insanity, boys were never to be in the same bed together or allowed to linger in bed. In 1858, the treatment for men was conium and iron, baths, and a flesh brush or a course towel to help "restore the body, but it is rarely permanent." Other treatments included mechanical restraints, aphrodisiacs (e.g. conium, camphor, and belladonna) for men and women. Additionally, there is some evidence that cauterizing the urethra was done elsewhere, but as no proof of efficacy was produced, it was not performed at Central State Hospital for the Insane. Cold baths and blistering were sometimes used.

Watching movies, walking, playing sports and cards were all part of the recreational therapy program.

Superintendent Dr. Max Bahr stated that the beauty treatments for women suffering from dementia praecox helped them to recover. By the ladies wanting to take an interest in their appearance, they overcame indifference and apathy. From 1952 the hospital had a barber shop and beauty parlor. In one year they completed:

- 6,416 trims
- 786 scalp treatments
- 3,461 Marcel waves
- 4,330 finger waves
- 6,063 shampoos
- 17 henna packs
- 785 facials
- 6,165 manicures
- 690 eyebrow arches

Musical

Music therapy started in 1953. Over the years, it included learning how to play instruments, music appreciation, choirs, and other music endeavors.

Art

Art therapy included creating art for personal pleasure and for the hospital. Large murals adorned many of the halls in the hospital.

Antibiotics

Penicillin for syphilis is the norm and older ant syphilitic drugs such as arsphenamine and bismuth are no longer used.

TYPES OF INSANITY: SPIRIT RAPPINGS

In 1851, a new cause of insanity, "spirit rappings" was entered into Central State's reports that year and for many years. People afflicted in this way were influenced by mediums and therefore they lost sleep, walked about in delirium, and approached dementia. Eighteen people (13 men and five women) were admitted for this affliction. They were treated with "very liberal use of tonics, as iron, wine and barks, combined in most cases with anodynes or narcotics of which the pure extract of the conium maculatum seemed to be the most beneficial." Eleven recovered entirely and seven remained in the hospital. From those seven, it was thought two would probably recover and five would not.

The doctors believed that the whole cause of belief in spirit rappings was "ignorance to scriptural truth….. Had the victims of this 'lying wonder' furnished themselves with a moderate degree of acquaintance with and adhered to a few of the plainest instructions of the Bible, the seductions of this error would have vanished before the influence of such truth, as the ghosts and fairies of fabled story fled before the light of day." Central State doctors likened this lack of attention to God and spiritual teachings to transcendentalists "who peep and mutter" to "spirits that have no more dignified mode of communication than a knock and scratch, to tip or move a table."

TYPES OF INSANITY: INTEMPERATE DRINKING

Another report indicated intemperate drinking was a cause of insanity. Doctors attributed the frequent occurrence of insanity from drinking to the strychnine, fishberries and other poisonous drugs used in alcohol preparation.

Leucotomy (Lobotomy)

The roots of lobotomies go past Central State Hospital. Dr. Egas Moniz, who conducted much of the research in the area of leucotomy, instructed Dr. Pedro Almeid Lima, who had worked with him on the procedure during the first procedure on a human in 1935. This consisted of drilling two holes in the patient's brain and injecting ethyl alcohol into the prefrontal cortex. Alcohol was used to destroy the neuronal tracts that were thought to give people thought. During the November 1935 and February 1936 they performed 20 lobotomies, revising the process as they went. In the published report, out of the 20 patients, 35% improved significantly, 35% improved slightly, and 30% were unchanged. No patients died, although many experienced a vastly different change in their conditions and mental state. By 1937 Moniz created the leukotome which was an instrument designed to do the job of the alcohol. It was inserted into the brain and moved around to severe the neuronal tracts. This practice was discontinued by 1950 by most institutions. By 1970 the practice was no longer performed. In all, it is believed in the U.S. that about 40,000 people had been lobotomized. Today, some forms of psychosurgery are still used in a small amount of cases.

Prefrontal Leucotomy (Prefrontal Lobotomy)

At Central State Hospital, the following was said regarding prefrontal lobotomy: The "curative program has been somewhat restrained. This is due to a shortage of registered nurses and surgical convalescent program." The doctors believed the procedure "produces results which are beneficial from the standpoint of total behavior" (versus attacking the mental illness). Additionally the hospital stated, "Until a regular program for the use of this method is established in the institution, the patients who are considered eligible for this form of treatment are usually released from the hospital to relatives. The family of the patient makes arrangements with a neurosurgeon in private practice for the performance of the operation. When the condition of the patient warrants it, a return to the institution is affected for the further management of the psychosis."

Additionally in 1901, Edenharter stated that the Sick Hospital was only for emergencies. He did not have faith in operations curing insanity. "I doubt whether an operation to cure insanity will ever be performed there. I believe in surgical operations for the relief of physical conditions in the insane just as in the sane."

Transorbital leucotomy (frontal lobotomy)

The first American (Freeman-Watts) transorbital leucotomy was in 1946 by Drs. Walter J. Freeman and James W. Watts with mixed results. An instrument resembling an ice pick was inserted through the eye socket piercing the bone between the eye sockets and the frontal lobe. The instrument went into the frontal lobe to sever connections with the brain between the prefrontal cortex and thalamus). Patients were usually under the effects of electroshock therapy or a sedative during the procedure. At Central State Hospital, the administration was "reluctance to recommend and go ahead with" this treatment. This was supposed to benefit long term patients who had already been treated by one or more of the numerous methods (psychotherapy, insulin and electric convulsive therapy). The long term results weren't known, especially with people with epilepsy. The doctors quoted Dr. Percival Bailey, Director of the Illinois Neuropsychiatric Institute, who discussed personality changes after the procedure and asked whether doctors had the moral right to alter a patient's brain. At Central State, 15 patients had the procedure done by 1951 after they were admitted. It is not completely clear, since access to patient records is limited, whether the patients who had the procedure once admitted to the hospital, had it at the hospital or through an outside source. Based on the information in the report, it is likely the majority, if not all, were done outside the hospital. Other patients who came to the hospital had the lobotomies before they came to the hospital. This topic was not part of any yearly report and no formal program was started.

WHO'S WHO OF LEUCOTOMY

Top left: Dr. Egas Moniz;
Top right: Dr. Pedro Almeid Lima
Bottom left: Dr. James W. Watts
Bottom right: Dr. Walter Freeman

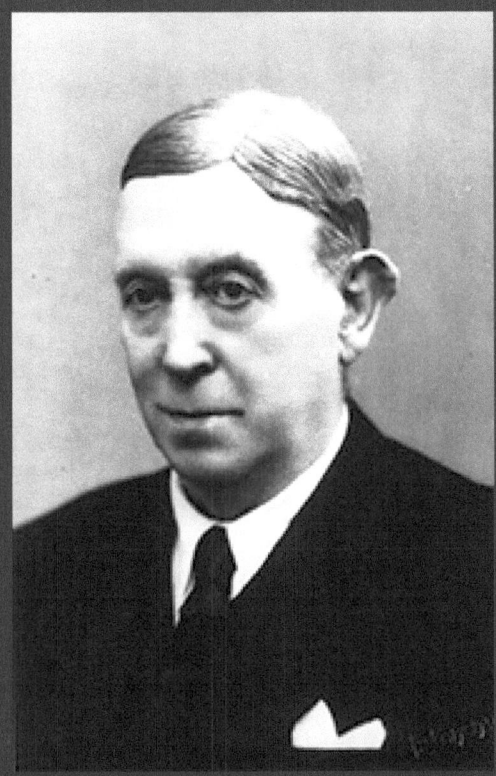
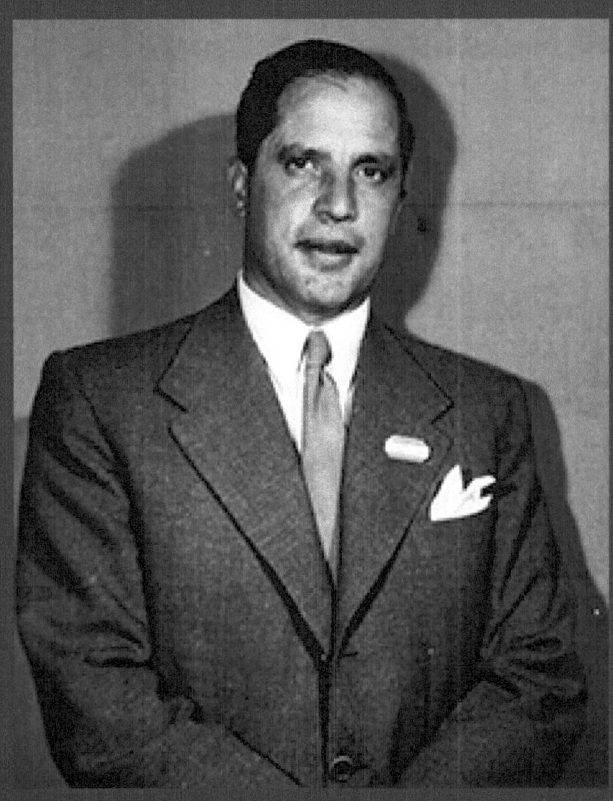
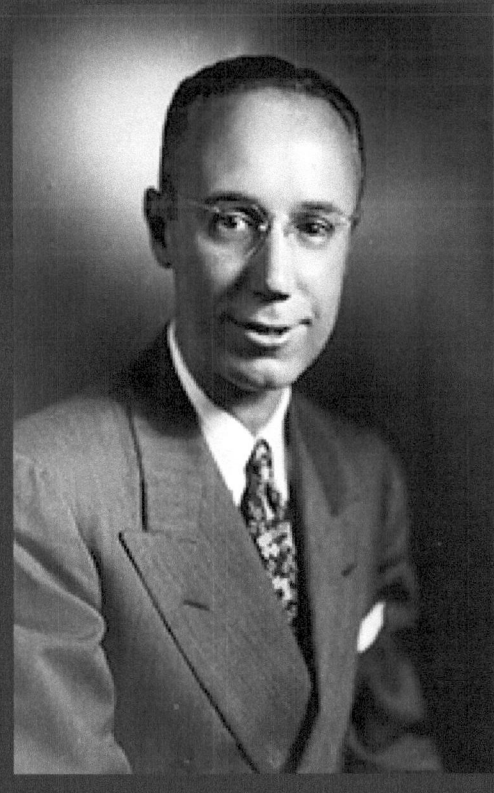
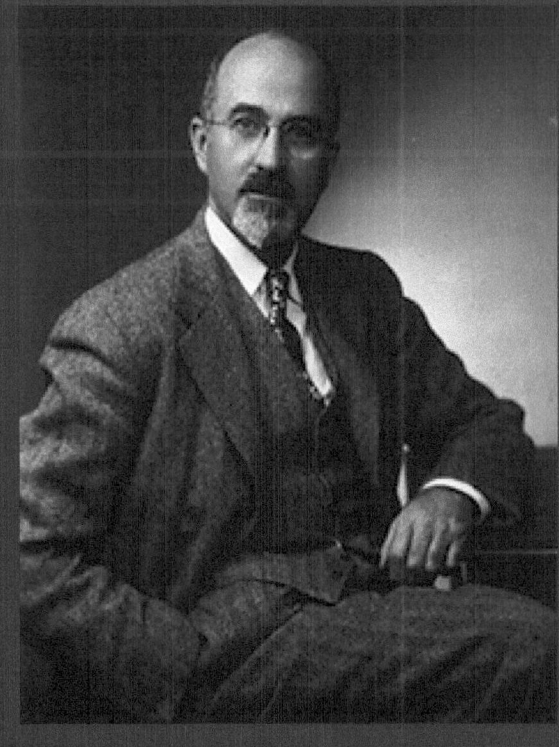

Restraints

Restraints used at Central State Hospital included the Utica crib (1), bed restraints, camisoles, fingerless gloves, hand mitts, and wrist, neck and ankle straps. In 1885, Dr. William B. Fletcher, Superintendent at the time, abolished the use of restraints, burning them in a bonfire at the hospital. Later Superintendent George F. Edenharter used restraints as sparingly as possible. Reports suggest camisoles and hand mitts were used occasionally.

Catalogue page from a 1920s hospital magazine.

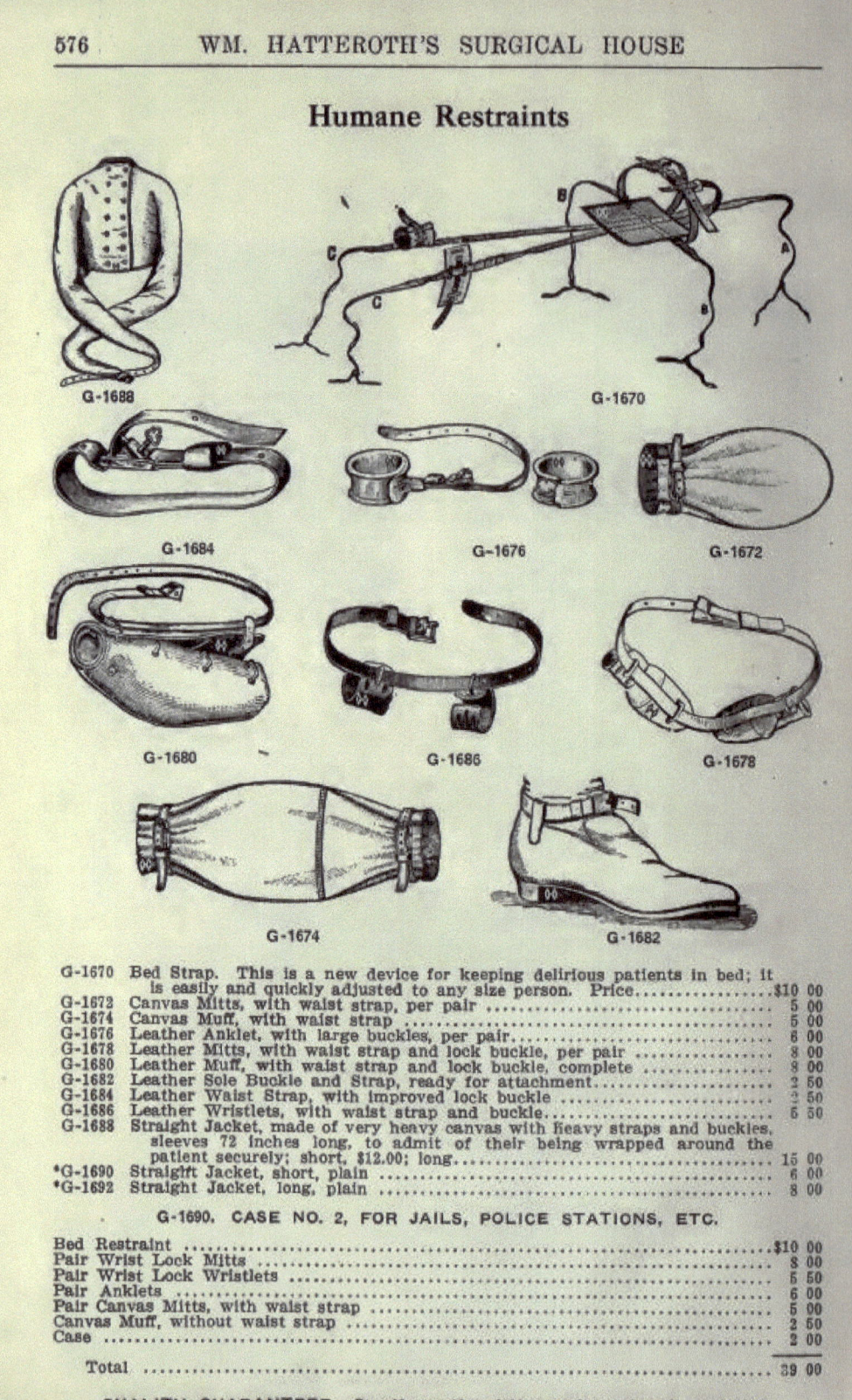

Psychotropic Drugs

Chlorpromazine, known in America as Thorazine, was available for schizophrenia and other mental illnesses. It was used to replace ECT, surgeries associated with mental illness and insulin shock therapy. Other drugs that were developed were Haldol, Trilafon, and Navane.

Other treatments

When the hospital first opened, all wards were closed. Patients ate and slept on the wards. When they went out, it was in a group. Later, cafeterias were built but largely, the wards were still closed and patients had no freedom to move about the grounds. Open wards were employed in the 1950s. Two patients were elected to ensure that the duties were done and the rules obeyed. It seemed to help patients. These patients were more likely to get furloughs and to be moved into the community faster.

Services for Children

One of the biggest changes at the hospital was services for children. It had been problematic whenever children were admitted because the hospital didn't have housing or programs for them.

In 1932 Dr. Bahr wanted to start a mental clinic for children. He felt if they could deal with mental issues in children, it might be easier to deal with them as adults or even curtail them. Emotionally disturbed children were housed at Central State Hospital in appropriate wards based on their behavior in 1961. Superintendent Clifford Williams asked for state treatment centers for the children but the state did not make appropriations for them. Representative John Mitchell opposed it because he didn't want "them to live in luxury out there."

In 1965 the Bahr Building was planned. It was to have a children's treatment center for the 86 children who were now in the hospital's wards and admission unit. The goal for this program was to rehabilitate them in a homey setting. The program was specifically designed for children who were "incorrigible," or "uncontrollable" and those with anti-social behavior. Initially funded by $100,000 in Federal money, the plan derailed into red tape.

Two years later, a Title 1 grant was obtained and a camp for 50 children ages seven to 18 was created at the Bahr treatment center. Kids could play sports, go to counseling, do crafts, nature study and go on field trips to places like Brown County State Park. But this didn't solve the problem.

In 1968, William Shuba, the Director of Education, reformed and improved the children's program. He claimed 10% of the kids were getting out of the hospital through reacclimation. Part of the program was giving children the opportunity to go into regular classes. Out of the 18 sent, 10 came back because they couldn't handle the stress. The other 8 were gaining ground on their issues.

Eugenics

Eugenics was a misguided attempt to create a better genetic quality of the human race. It advocated for more reproduction from people with better traits and a cessation of reproduction by people who were of lesser genetic material, including the "feeble minded."

People with intellectual disabilities included classifications for idiots, imbeciles, and morons. This led to classifications of moral insanity, moral idiocy, and moral imbecility.

In the U.S. these people were screened and sometimes forced into compulsory sterilization and abortion. Other countries advocated forced pregnancies, such as in slave breeding, and genocide, as advocated by Nazism.

In Indiana Dr. John Hurty, Secretary of the State Board of Health was a huge proponent of eugenics and Indiana was the first state to enact sterilization legislation in 1907.

Eugenics fell out of favor as more became known about genes, traits and heredity, and about the intellectual disabilities some of the target population had. For example, Thomas Hunt Morgan demonstrated genetic mutation outside of inheritance with fruit flies. He claimed this proved that not all traits were inherited. Additionally, some of the traits previously thought of as a case for eugenics came to be known as disease or a cause of a disease, such in the case of Down's Syndrome or haemochromatosis, which leads to an increased susceptibility to illness, and can cause physical deformities.

Ethics were also at stake. People believed that if one race was considered less intelligent or more intelligent, negative consequences could occur, as was seen in Nazism and the genocide played out with Jews in the WWII.

Later most of eugenics theology was dropped and people who were considered "feeble minded" were now called "mentally retarded", which fell out of favor as well. Federal statutes changed this terminology in federal circles to "intellectual disability" in 2010.

Not much is recorded about eugenics and its effect at Central State Hospital. Interestingly, there was no discussion of eugenics in the yearly report and it was most certainly a hot topic in Indiana. Indiana's eugenics law targeted, "confirmed criminals, idiots, imbeciles and rapists." In 1921 the law was declared unconstitutional but in 1927 the law was reinstated and amended to be "the insane, feeble-minded, or epileptic."

The total number of people sterilized in Indiana varies from 700 to over 2500, depending on the source. Also depending on the source is when the sterilizations stopped. The law was in force from 1907-1921 and from 1927-1974. However, some sources state that the sterilizations in Indiana ceased in 1909.

The 1927 law was targeted at people in state institutions, including mental hospitals. While it is very possible Central State did some involuntary sterilization, the number would most likely be small. Most patients who were considered "feeble minded", including "idiots" or "imbeciles", were sent to the Indiana Asylum for the Education of the Deaf and Dumb, which opened in 1846 and is now the Indiana School for the Deaf. The criminals and rapists were in prisons. Epileptics were eventually sent to the Indiana Village for Epileptics. Patients with tuberculosis were kept at the hospital, although Sunnyside Sanatorium was formed in 1917. It was not equipped to handle mental patients.

The idea that patients from these institutions would have been sent to Central State Hospital for surgery from the various institutions is unlikely as many of these institutions had their own surgery theaters and would also have worked with local doctors and hospitals.

However, anyone considered "feeble minded" was not sent to a facility outside of the hospital. The "the insane" mentioned in the 1927 and 1931 versions of the law, may well have been involuntarily sterilized, although the records for Central State Hospital do not mention these.

Clinics and Research

Medical care called clinics were offered for patients, from dental and eye to hydrotherapy and ECT. ECT was offered 3 times a week. Some patients were sent to other hospitals, including Methodist and IU Medicine to perform services for patients (most notably genito-urinary medicine, which may have included sterilization). Also, "The Lilly Project", which tested "new products in psychopharmacology" was conducted in Men's Cottage 3B under Dr. Ivan Bennett as a research psychiatrist.

Research

Central State Hospital was also "officially recognized " to do research by the National Committee for Mental Hygiene.

In the 1950s, the Psychology department did some testing in the Indiana School for the Blind and the Indiana Solider and Sailors Home. Additionally papers were planned and one was accepted for presentation to the American Psychological Association meeting in Chicago 1956. By 1958, several types of testing were done in Cottage 3B"

- 250 members of the staff were inoculated against Asian flu (50 of these volunteered and 93 state police also participated)
- At the Farm Colony Pitman Moore Co did a blood cholesterol test related to diet- personnel and patients participated.
- Another study was done on cholesterol in older women
- Drug therapy: a new tranquilizer was used on Ward 6 but other medications were more effective so it was stopped.
- Syringe breakage: study done on disposable syringes. Overall it was positive- less breakage and cost effective.

Seven

Patient and Attendant Experiences

Over the years, much has been written regarding experiences in the hospital. In this chapter are several patient and attendant experiences.

THIS PASS MUST BE SURRENDERED WHEN LEAVING THE GROUNDS

CENTRAL STATE HOSPITAL

VISITOR

WELCOME TO CENTRAL STATE HOSPITAL

WHILE YOU ARE ON THE GROUNDS WE ASK THAT YOU BEHAVE IN ACCORDANCE WITH HOSPITAL REGULATIONS. IF YOU NEED ANY ASSISTANCE CONTACT A SECURITY OFFICER ON DUTY WHO WILL BE GLAD TO HELP YOU.

1886 Albert Thayer

In the publication, "Rough Diamond" in 1886, Albert Thayer related experiences he witnessed while a patient in the hospital. Albert related a story about the early days of the hospital in which an unruly patient received a syringe of aqua ammonia in the eyes. One eye was destroyed and the other nearly so. Another story was about a married patient in pain who was forced to mop the floor. After a few hours, she gave birth. Although Albert admits these "unheard of cruelties" were not premeditated, they were the result of staff ignorance and carelessness. Unlike other deliberate acts of the attendants who would frequent a saloon in Mount Jackson and get in drunk to make the "cranks toe the mark."

These examples were intended to show that the mistreatment started in the early days and it continued up to 1886. Albert described the wards as keeping the worst patients in the back wards. Back wards were the back part of the hospital buildings and the parts the furthest away from the middle of the building where the public might come into contact with them.

Two attendants were expected to take care of the ward, to wash, scrub, set the table, give medication, bathe and take the patients out on the grounds, etc. Albert stated that no patients were given restraints. If some patients became unruly, a slap or two would suffice for them.

His experience in 1883 on Ward E (northernmost back section of the Department for Men) was in a back ward. During his time there, James Brady (who was later on the police force), Attendants Ballard and Pattison were his attendants. When Albert arrived at the hospital, he refused to sit in a chair, so they put him in a room by himself, without any physical abuse. Dr. Hubbard came in and told him he needed to obey the attendants and do as he was told. Albert sat in the chair, for hours, with no one to disturb him, take him outside, help him if needed, not even to use the restroom. All he heard was the ticking of the clock.

In the evening, as Albert sat there, listening to the tick tock of the clock, Pattison decided to conduct a lesson for himself on the violin, which Albert found "torturous." Albert stated, "If I could have been sure death would have been the result, I would have hurled myself headlong against the hard wall and ended all." Finally the lesson ended.
A patient, Hoffman, was beaten by his attendant. He had fits and as a result, he was put in a camisole, the precursor to the modern straightjacket, although he was never violent toward anyone. One attendant threw him on the floor, one "pounded and choked him", and Ballard held one of Hoffman's legs and "stomped on his abdomen." Hoffman tried to fight it, but eventually lay as if dead, with blood pouring from his mouth and nose. The terror became an occasional kick and finally, Hoffman was told to "get up and wash himself." Many times he witnessed a patient 'acting up' and receiving stinging slaps, or choking, accompanied by cursing. "A kind word in [Ward] E was a rare thing indeed."

Brady told Albert that Hoffman was a "very dangerous man." Albert didn't agree that a beating was necessary when Hoffman never appeared to be hurting anyone in his fits except himself. He believed Hoffman was beaten as a warning to other patients and that the attendants were fearful of the more needy patients. The beating of Hoffman to Albert was "an act of wanton, savage cruelty."

Additionally, Albert slept in a locked room with 12 other patients. No one came in during the night to calm disturbances but a watchman would look in every 30 to 60 minutes. Sometimes the patients talked together about what was happening at the hospital. Sometimes they would "rant" which was "fearful" for Albert.

"I am fully aware of the fact that the rules of the hospital require the attendants to bear in mind that those under their charges are demented and not responsible for their conduct, that they must be treated kindly; that any acts of cruelty on the part of the attendants will be punished. If found out, but dismissal and if possible by prosecution etc. I am aware of this and I am aware too that there is a Bible in every house in Indianapolis, but that does not prove that the people, generally, keep the ten commandments, not by any means. "

Albert gave the example of Dr. Thomas, who was in charge of the male department, did rounds twice a day spending about 30 minutes with 20 patients. Albert wondered, with this little time spent with patients, if Dr. Thomas found a patient "beaten into jelly" and if the attendants stuck up for each other, would there really be any consequences.

Eventually, Albert was moved to Ward C and treated more kindly.*

Dr. Fletcher responded to Albert's letter that was printed in the Indianapolis News. Albert asked him why he didn't admit the abuses existed instead of making a show of "denying the charges". In his letter, Albert suggested that all patients receive fresh milk, eggs and fruit as well as ice in hot weather. Additionally "a more intelligent class of personnel" should be hired and a doctor should supervise the attendants in their duties when they are on the grounds of the hospital. Dr. Fletcher, basically said the State didn't provide enough money to do as he suggested.

Albert went on to state that what Dr. Fletcher said was not necessarily the truth. He cited the yearly reports. In 1884 the State paid for 168 tons of ice ($384), and 4.000 gallons of milk in addition to what came from the 30 milk cows at the hospital ($340.72). Albert stated he was an inmate twice, once under Dr. Rogers and once under Dr. Fletcher. Neither time was he nor the other patients furnished with milk or ice. Dr. Hubbard asked for Albert to have milk twice, but he ever got any, except from a small quantity from Brady's own glass. When he was on Ward C (south center section of the north wing, Department for Men), a little ice was put in a pitcher for the ward, which wasn't enough to go once around. He also argued that Fletcher had seven rooms furnished at $1500 while Ward C in all was allotted only $500. His point was that there was a huge discrepancy between the doctors and the patient's furnishings, and it seemed that carried over to food. What was the point of the hospital if not to care body and soul for the patients?

The food was first served to the staff- doctors and their families, subordinates and officers, and attendants- then to patients. The food was good in Thayer's recollection. He did remember once, some bad prunes, and some "slightly tainted meat." There was never enough food, however. "the dining room itself was a small affair into which the patients crowded like hungry pigs around a swill trough to eat their meals."

Thayer stated that he believed that Dr. Hubbard and Dr. Thomas treated him with the "greatest kindness" and that Brady and J H Cressinger were good attendants. Other items he thought could use improvement included giving the patients treats (when some received goodies from home, others had none). Albert also thought the patients should also have "a good supply of pure, fresh, cold water". The physicians should eat with their patients to ensure their orders are being carried out.

"But little good results to the patients by turning out one superintendent to put in another. Nor should a superintendent be expected to perform the duties demanded of him with one hand tied behind him. He should have full power to appoint or dismiss subordinate physicians and officers as well as attendants and other help and then be himself alone be held to a strict account for the good management of the institution."

After the letter was written in 1885 to Albert by Fletcher, two patients were killed by other patients, several committed suicide (many by escaping to the "old woods" to hang themselves, believed to be the section of the land next to Cemetery Section 1) and many escaped to return home or disappeared with the masses. Two major fires broke out at the hospital.

However even Thayer was taken by the grounds. "The beautiful groves of forest and the shade green from which sound the sweet songs of happy forest birds, the shrubbery and flowers that boarder the smooth gravel walks. The countless beds of sweet smelling flowers among which the cunning ground squirrels burrow and play hide and seek; the dripping fountains where the young robins come to flutter and bath in the pools of cool, sparkling water….. make the place a delightful and cheerful retreat for them that are afflicted with disordered minds….."

Finally, Albert pointed out the Catholic Sisters of Charity were trained to do the work of attendants and they would not charge a lot of money to help. When he asked a priest why the nuns could not help as attendants or nurses at the hospital, he was told, 'Because the religious bigotry and intolerance of the times will not permit it." Apparently Catholics were not wanted at the hospital.

Albert also pointed to several other patient abuses, such as, dressing patients in ill-fitting clothing and then leaving them in a hall to be stared at by visitors.

Mrs. C., a patient, was someone everyone went to when they needed to talk. The attendants were jealous of this attention. Mrs. C. interfered when a patient was being abused. One attendant pressed Mrs. C.'s head to the wall and while another pulled her hair to the point that skin came off with her hair. Later, Mrs.C. was discharged as "cured".

Countless times, Albert saw attendants take a patient's hat and hide it, causing the helpless patient frustration and agitation.

An epileptic begged to not go with the others to breakfast, saying he was ill. The attendants made him go anyway. The patent requested a talk with Dr. A.J. Thomas but the doctor failed to appear. The patient became agitated. When he refused to put on his slippers, he was slapped, beaten and cursed. Then he was sent to another ward where the attendants said there would be a way found "to subdue him."

Captain James Buchanan who was a Civil War veteran for the Union was in the hospital because of brain damage sustained from a head wound suffered during the war. He was continually beaten, and had sores by his eyes and bed sores on his back. He limped and he was made to sit upright, although it caused him great pain. Finally, when an attendant "drew a stick" on him, but did not strike, the Captain said in a commanding voice, "Run me through and kill me. I want to die and end my sufferings."

Albert told his lodge about the incidents at Central State Hospital and recommended Captain Buchanan be removed. He also contacted Dr. A.J. Thomas and recommended that Captain Buchanan be treated kindly until his release. The doctor said Buchanan would be sent home soon. And he was -to die.

As a side note, many parents complained that Dr. Thomas was too brusque and that they were fearful of conversations with him because of his demeanor.

Clifford Beers

Clifford Beers, a former patient, also advocated for better conditions at the hospital. He made the comment that it was the patients needing the most care- the infirm, senile, violent and noisy- who were the most neglected and suffered the most. For example, between 1903 and 1906, 23% of patients were suicidal and 10% were homicidal. Almost all were considered delusional with psychosis and neurosis aggravated by a wide range of physical disturbances. Beers gave an example of one of the most difficult classes of patients. A twenty-eight year old man was admitted. Prior to this, he locked himself in his room for five months and preferred to be with just his family for fear of being drugged. He would only eat raw food he prepared himself and he carried all sorts of weapons. Even more difficult were aged, with senility and alcoholism related issues.

A Mother's Experience

In 1919 Louisa Mayer wrote a very long letter to the Board of Commissioners about her son Dave's treatment in Central State Hospital. She charged:

There was no heat in the entire ward.

She looked at patient named Thompson, who seemed ill. Louisa was told by the attendant that a doctor had been called. She was surprised the person hadn't been taken to the sick hospital. She went out the following Tuesday to see Thompson. The regular attendant was gone but an attendant from T ward was filling in. Thompson was still lying on a mattress on a cold wet floor.

She went to see Dave the same day and he was lying on the floor, also cold and wet. Louisa asked where the attendants where the bed was and was told, "He sleeps on the floor". Louisa became worried over the conditions at the hospital. The attendant quickly told her not to worry and that her son would have a bed.

Louisa went to the hospital again on Wednesday. Thompson could now sit up and her son had a bed- a rusty, filthy bed with springs so broken they were "worn and hanging on the floor". The attendant told her they 'did the best they could' and had tried to "tie them [the springs] up".

On Thursday Louisa went to the hospital again and looked in on her son. The bed was gone and he was back on the cold, wet floor. She asked if they were putting in another bed and was told no. Mr. Gibson, an assistant, asked other staff if her son, Dave, wet the bed and when told he did sometimes, Gibson took the bed away. "A good way to cure bed wetting," she wrote sarcastically. Louisa also noted that the heat was still off.

Dave was 25 years old and had been there three years. He had only been wetting the bed for four years. When Louisa asked him why he didn't go to the toilet, he said "I can't get there in time." He had had no medical attention since he arrived, with the exception of having teeth removed.

When Dave first arrived on S ward, he slept in a room with a "Negro". The man screamed and pounded all night. Dave became worse because of it and was removed to another ward. In the new ward, he began to wet the bed frequently and they put him in A ward, also in a basement and from there P ward.

Louisa stated Dr. Lyman (not listed in yearly reports) told her not to bother him when she tried to speak with him and instructed her to see the attendants. When she tried to make a complaint, she was told everyone was out. A few days later, she tried again and was told the same thing. She said she would remain until they returned. Mr. Gibson was in the next room. He came in and she told him of her issues with the doctor, with patients hitting other patients, and with attendants locking up patients "for doing nothing at all." Louisa also complained there was nowhere for them to sit in their rooms. It was sit on the floor or standing.

She also told of the following issues:

- When her son, Dave, was on S ward, the attendants made him shine their shoes. The attendant would spit on his head.

-

- An old patient, Dave Taylor, would talk to himself and Attendant Flint would kick him until the patient fell to the floor and the attendant would slap the patient in the face.

-

- In T ward, a "feeble minded" boy, Gentry, was brought in. Although he was sitting quietly, an attendant would pester him. When the boy became noisy or excited, he was thrown on the floor and the man stood on him. When the boy would scream, the attendant would pick him up and choke him.

Louisa concluded by saying, "Now gentlemen, I am stating these facts not on my son's account but for the sake of humanity. You or your son or your father or brother might be the next one to go there. Can you imagine them lying on a cold wet floor with rats, mice, bed bugs, flies and mosquitoes for companions?... These unfortunates couldn't be treated worse if they were surrounded by Huns. We call Indianapolis no mean city, Indianapolis to the front, while at the very gates of the city we have an institution that is a disgrace to the city and the state."

It is unclear if any of her complaints or observations were investigated or corrected.

DEFINE CRUEL TREATMENT

2/8/1901: William Schwartz, a lawyer sought to divorce his wife, Mary, on the grounds of cruel treatment. He alleged that she would "fly into a passion", broke furniture and threw her teacup at him. Mary Schwartz' brother helped fight this case by stating that the cruel treatment information had been used to place Mary into Central State Hospital. He stated that the reason William wanted a divorce was to marry his stenographer and housekeeper, Tillie Gisler., who was the wife of Frank Robinson. He shot her in Schwartz' office in 1900.
The judge dismissed the case.

ASTRAL PROJECTION

One particularly strange occurrence of astral projection with a patient was documented in the book, "Doubles: The Enigma of the Second Self" by Rodney Davies . On June 14, 1854 Alexander Ferguson was readmitted to the hospital because he'd once again become unpredictable and violent in New Harmony (Posey County, Indiana), which is 181 miles south west of Indianapolis. He was 46, unmarried and he'd been a farmer. He was also a big man which made it easy for him to intimidate people. He was described by Dr. E.V. Spencer, one of three doctors who examined him, as "not wild but is a shrewd cunning fellow by looks."

Ferguson had actually been in the Lunatic Asylum at Lexington, Kentucky from 1838-39 where he escaped. He was later deemed "much improved both mentally and morally." This was probably from not drinking so much, rather than from being put in a large barrel and pouring cold water on his head.

Ferguson was the sixty eighth patient in Central State Hospital in 1849, and he was released as "recovered" in 1850. Ferguson went back to his old ways. He was readmitted in 1854 at the request of his guardian, H.C. Cooper after trying to hurt his brother, Ashberry Ferguson, and other members of his family.

Ferguson refused medication again and became homesick. In March 1855 according to Dr. S.B. Brittan, the hospital administration had a surprising visit from Posey County authorities. Posey County officials received complaint letters from people in New Harmony that stated on February 27, 1855 Ferguson was seen "wandering at large in the neighborhood near his old home." The people of New Harmony were afraid of him. They wanted Ferguson returned to the hospital and an accounting as to how he had escaped.

Dr. John Athon, the Superintendent of Central State Hospital for the Insane, said either the Posey County folks were mistaken, or this was a practical joke. Ferguson had not been released nor was he missing. This was confirmed by the hospital staff.

The next day, Dr. Athon received a letter from H.C. Cooper stating that Ferguson had been seen in the area of New Harmony and Cooper wanted to know when, and why, Ferguson had been. Dr. Athon told him that Ferguson was at the hospital and had not been allowed out since his arrival.
In reply, Cooper gave a detailed account of where Ferguson had been and what he'd done, stating, "his movements were closely observed by several persons who had been familiar with him for years. The witnesses concurred in saying that he did not look well, that he was pale and that he was indisposed to converse; but not one entertained the slightest doubt of his identity."

Dr. Athon was perplexed and interviewed Ferguson. When asked when he'd been in New Harmony, Ferguson smiled mischievously and replied that he'd made a "flying visit" to the area three weeks before. When the doctor gently pointed out that this was impossible, Ferguson stated, "I tell you that I did go. My spirit flew down their [sic] quick and left this pair of clothes and the rest of me that you see here in the ward to take care of the Antichrist and keep the Devil out of the bathroom."

Ferguson went on to describe where he'd been, what he'd done and whom he'd seen. This included a visit to a distillery where he drank quite a bit. Dr. Athon was amazed and incredulous. Many of Ferguson's actions were ones reported to him by Cooper and the authorities.

Ferguson continued, "I didn't see anybody on the road- I was so high up; came with the pigeons' they was a'cheering me- ha! Ha! Ha! And didn't make no time at all; I got home first; I'm going back tomorrow. The whisky…

made my head swim-run against the lightning, which singed my whiskers, coloured 'em red. The truth is, Doc, they are all crazy." It was suggested by the author, Davies, that Ferguson's "insanity somehow made it easier for his double to vacate his body along with his consciousness."

Anna Agnew

Anna Keyt Agnew was a patient at Central State for six years. She was born in Moscow, Ohio, in 1836 as the daughter of middle class parents. Her father, Nathan, married her mother, Martha Keyt, after his first wife died. Apparently, there was animosity between Anna and her mother. Martha's mother was a great deal younger than Nathan and only 19 when Anna was born. She believed Anna had a very bad temper (probably an early manifestation of her disease).

In 1870, two years after her father's death, Anna married David Agnew. After the birth of their first son, Nathan, in 1872, they moved to Seymour, Indiana. Here, Anna had William and David, her other children.

Anna seemed to have a happy marriage until she started having more noticeable bouts of depression. Anna also experienced some psychotic delusions. For example, when she would sit at a table to eat, she believed her food became alive. "I could not put those vile things in my mouth." Her manic episodes included laughing, screaming, using profanities and feeling as if she was out of control.

What led to Anna becoming a patient at the hospital was swallowing chloral (used for sleep and sedation) and sugar until her tongue, throat and stomach were "in ulcers." She went to two local doctors and told them of her wish to kill herself and that she was afraid she would hurt someone else. They told her "You might put a quart of poison on that mantelpiece with perfect safety. Persons who are contemplating suicide don't advertise the fact."

Months later, these same doctors attended to Anna after she swallowed strychnine. Anna said one of the doctors stated, of her condition that, "it was perfectly wonderful what had gotten me into such a nervous state." The doctor believed the problem to be hysteria and prescribed several large doses of bromide of potassium. (Strychnine causes convulsions. Bromide was used to counteract them and as a sedative.)

Anna's husband didn't believe she was suicidal either. He never understood, according to Anna, what she was going through. She said her children were "her idols". She never blamed her husband for her plight.

Part of David's harshness may have come from his time in service during the Civil War. Any man who couldn't deal with the war and complained of mental illness was a considered "malingerer". Therefore, Corporal David Agnew dealt with his problems and kept on with his service in the 98th Ohio Infantry. He was described as "a young man of delicate frame" and may have looked to Anna as an older, strong wife to help him in his life. When she "failed", he became sour and punitive towards her.

According to her autobiography Anna endured all sorts of indignities at Central State Hospital: poor healthcare from doctors and attendants, pain from restraints, and the curious citizens of Indianapolis who flocked and sometimes jeered the patients. During her time, the wards were open from 10a.m. to 5p.m. and anyone could come in and look around. It was as if the patients were "entertainment." If the visitors didn't see a display of the crazy people doing something abnormal, they left disappointed.

While at the hospital, Anna's husband's actions became quite clear to her. Anna had been extremely low until one day, her husband came to see her. At first, she said, "I think I was never so happy…. It was his first visit to me…. But now my husband had come and he did care something for me…."

Anna's joy was short lived. As David stood there, speechless, she asked him to say something. Looking into her eyes, he asked, "Were you insane when you were married?" She replied that she was not, but then stated, "I have changed my opinion since then, materially and willingly, I admit I was insane. And my most profound symptom was that I married him."

Anna asked for news of her children. David said "inhumanely" and "tortuously", "Your children? Why I hadn't presumed to think you cared to hear from them. You don't certainly presume to profess to love them?"
Anna replied, "I did not dare to see them"
David sneered, "Very well, I will never bring those children to see you until you ask me to."
Anna stated she thought he'd lost all his regard and affection for her. Her husband replied, 'Oh, no, Anna you are quite mistaken. I love you as well as I ever did." Then he demanded more answers to questions that left Anna little doubt as to his "purity". Later, he sent her a letter stating, "But after all, I must remember she is the mother of my children."
Anna charged one doctor mistreated her. She wrote to her sister that she was "fast becoming an imbecile" and was put in with epileptics. She wore the same calico dress for years until it was in tatters and still the doctor said, "Don't give her a dress till she asks for it." She stayed on the epileptic ward for a year, then returned to her old ward, where one of

the attendants said, "Look, the devil is back!"

Having a phobia of white things, Anna did not like touching her blanket. An attendant acclimating two attendants who used to work on other wards said, "You two girls are used to devils on your ward so I want you to make "Old Anna" fold her spread tonight. I don't care you half kill her so you don't leave any marks where Mrs. Rogers [ward matron] can see."

That night, the attendants stuffed blankets in Anna's mouth and said, "So you are the high-toned lady, who won't mind her attendants, are you? Do you know we are going to choke the life out of you if you don't get up this minute and fold your spread?" They dragged her out of bed and onto the floor. Anna screamed for Mrs. Rogers. They beat Anna with a shoe until one attendant said to stop in case Anna would tell Mrs. Rogers. The attendant believed, "…no telling what these damned crazy things will do."

Many times, Anna was forced to eat even though looking at the plate, it became "live, creeping, squirming vermin".

As part of Anna experience, she recollected speaking with a woman on a regular basis about suicide and what happened after death. She wondered if the person allowed to come back and where did they go. At this time, suicide was considered an unpardonable sin. Anna believed she had a perfect right to choose whether or not she stayed on earth. Her friend said, "Well, my friend, you and I have had pleasant, enjoyable times together here, but I must believe that suicide is the unpardonable sin! Since for this there is no repentance. So, if I should kill myself tonight. I believe I should go right to hell! I don't presume in that case I would be permitted to return neither do I suppose you would care to receive a visit from a lost soul! But just as surely as spirits are allowed to return, I will return to you."

In the morning, the woman Anna spoke with was found "stiff and stark". Anna said the woman appeared to her many times afterwards, not as the "stooping fragile body" or with a "care-stamped face" but rather with "the springing, buoyant step and bright laughing face of her early married life, so often talked about…."

Not everything about Anna's stay in the hospital was bad. She thought Superintendent William B. Fletcher, and his wife were marvelous people. She was also allowed a wage and worked in the sewing room during her last year in the hospital. This helped her keep her out of the county poor house where her husband wanted her sent.

Anna worked tirelessly after her release to improve conditions in the hospital. She asked the General Assembly to close the hospital to the public. The visits from the public angered her so that she wished the world had one neck so she could "strangle the life out of it." She posed the question, "what if their families were the ones in the hospital?" She believed people should have kinder hearts and compassion for the patients instead of mocking them.

Anna's husband refused to let her send items to the children, or to contact them. "Let them forget your last days spent with them! Let them forget if they can!" However, Anna was a fighter. After Anna left the hospital she went to Aurora, Indiana, where David was living to see her children. Her sons rushed into her arms "with tears and smiles, struggling for the ascendance, repeating over and again, as though glad of the opportunity to use the dear name of Mother, 'Mama, mama, don't cry so, we are so glad to see you." Anna had been denied the opportunity to see them for seven years.

Again, Anna's joy was short lived. Her remission ended and her illness returned with a vengeance. She was sent to Western Pennsylvania Hospital for the Insane (also known as Dixmont State Hospital) on January 5, 1894. Her brother-in-law George Irwin took her there and provided for her care, ensuring it continued even after his death. Anna died there on March 25, 1917. By that time, some of the reforms she had begged for in Indiana had been established in Central State Hospital, most notably women physicians and a nurse training program.

Civil War Veterans

Eric T. Dean, Jr. wrote a book called "Shook Over Hell: Post-Traumatic Stress, Vietnam, and the Civil War". Many documented cases came from Indiana and many of these veterans were in Central State Hospital.

Owen Flaherty (Company C, 125th IL Volunteers): Described as a "well adjusted, normal person" as he entered the Civil War. After the Battle of Stones River in Murfreesboro, Tennessee, he requested a furlough that was denied. He began to change, becoming "far away" and "homesick." He began to have nightmares, mumble in his sleep and be paranoid. When he returned from war, he became a blast furnace operator, but couldn't concentrate and seemingly needed to "be on the go." He would become furious whenever anyone would speak about war or politics with him. Eventually, he was put into CSH, diagnosed with "mania", and after a short stay, deemed incurable. He suffered from delusions, was "highly suspicious of strangers" and had bursts of anger and violence. He was later given over to a guardian and placed in the Vigo County poorhouse. His guardian advocated for him and Owen was awarded $72 per month compensation as a disabled veteran.

James P. Green (69th Indiana Infantry): Not much is known about this soldier except that he participated in many battles, including the Battle of Richmond, Sherman's assault on Chickasaw Bayou (near Vicksburg), and Grant's siege of Vicksburg. He was also captured by Confederates after the Battle of Richmond, but later released. It is not known what he experienced personally in any of these instances, but his unit suffered casualties in battle and through numerous diseases. When James returned to Indiana, he could not work and tried to kill himself. He would not talk except to say "'terbacker out" (meaning he was out of tobacco). In 1878 he was sent to CSH and diagnosed with "mania". Sixteen years later, his family applied for a veteran's pension.

Erastus Holmes (quartermaster sergeant, 5th Indiana Calvary): He was taken prisoner by confederates and held in Florence, South Carolina and later Andersonville, where he was ravaged by disease and forced to sleep in a hole partially filled with water. He went in at 160 pounds. When he escaped, he weighed 85 pounds. He no longer slept at night and would be very emotional in his retelling of his escape from prison. He even had a replica of the prison dugout area in his yard and would show it to people. He went to Central State Hospital in 1885 and stayed there until his death in 1910. His behavior was quiet, except when he would talk about the army and his experiences.

Lt. Co. John A Keith (21st Indiana Infantry): He suffered as a result of many gunshot wounds when bone particles surfaced and was alcoholic. He was sent to Central State Hospital twice for alcoholism.

ATTENDANT EXPERIENCE: CARRIE WHITE LIVELY

Carrie E. (White) Lively (1871-1957) taught school and worked as a maid before becoming an attendant in Central State Hospital. When she walked into the Women's building, she had high hopes. "It seemed I had been born anew to do and be competent."

Her orientation included Dr. George . Edenharter, Superintendent, speaking to her about rules and duties of attendants. She was given a book to read. "It seemed to me that if one [rule] was broken, that was the end of it… some of those rules seemed trivial, but I was sure I would do nothing wrong."

Carrie was in for a surprise. In the next few days and weeks, the staff rules were broken and no consequences were to be had "so long as Dr. Edenharter did not hear of it or the supervisor did not learn of it." When staff would come in late once the doors had been locked, Carrie reported "the most deceiving attendants" talked to doctors "with the sweetest smile." Their primary concern was not getting "eaten up."

One of the worst wards Carrie worked on was Ward 21. Patients afflicted with everything from anxiety to 'raving behavior" were kept in the same area. Carrie learned that the more excited patients had to be carefully monitored to protect other patients. She also wrote that staff newcomers were put on the bad wards because they had to pass an unwritten test. If they could survive the worst, they would be promoted to better wards. For Carrie, it was much more than she ever expected. When she asked Dr. Sarah Stockton if something could be done for a woman who moaned day and night, the doctor laughed and replied, "You let Miss Hart attend to that patient and don't let your sympathies spoil your work here." Dr. Stockton followed up by saying the woman's pain was "imaginary." Carrie watched the old woman and began to suspect the patient's problem was something females sometimes experience, "The uterus would not stay in place." She felt her job would be in danger if she spoke up again, so she "relieved" what she could and whatever couldn't be helped, she "let alone."

In her autobiography, Carrie charged that once people were put into Central State that very little was done for pain. However, she learned that most conditions were considered "mental ailments" although they manifested as physical ailments, and that cures were made and people were sent home.

Throughout her time at the hospital, Carrie tried to become "hardened" to the suffering around her. She felt once she got a paycheck, it would be bearable. She remembered a Negro patient, Clarissa, singing and an attendant throwing water on her to make her stop. When the patient, was asked about what the attendant, Marie, had done to her, Clarissa smiled and said, "She cooled me off!"

When Carrie went to an attendant, Marie Hart, about the transgressions of another attendant, she was advised not to report the cruel attendant because she was told they stuck together. However, "Miss B.", the most horrible of all attendants, made Carrie's life unhappy. Normally four attendants were on the ward. One patient, Mary, was "crazy as crazy could be" but was largely a help with the cleaning. One day, when the ward patients went to the dining room, Carrie noticed Mary was not in attendance. Miss B. said they "couldn't get the stubborn thing to move. Go on and we will attend her."

Carrie was afraid that Miss B. would pull one of her tricks such as wetting a towel and slapping it on Mary's face or worse, drawing it tightly from behind.

After they attended to Mary, Carrie went to clean items in the bathroom. Mary had always "willingly helped," but she wasn't there, and Carrie worked alone.

Suddenly Miss B came in and said, "Mrs. White, will you come and look at Mary?"

Mary was found gasping for air. Carrie yelled at Miss B., asking her to call a doctor, but Mary died before one arrived. Carrie could not prove Miss B. killed Mary. The doctor called it heart failure.

Attendant Agnes Stritt used to be left on the ward to care for patients who weren't well enough to go to the dining room. When Carrie looked at Agnes, her suspicions that Mary still roamed the halls were confirmed. Agnes said later, "I can't work in that bathroom. It always seems I can hear Mary say in her old way, 'Say fellows, come on bring your vessels.'" Mary always addressed everyone as "fellows."

Later, Miss B. noticed Carrie avoiding her and tried to find out why. Carrie replied, "I know a few things about Mary, I guess, and when I get it cleared up, I'm reporting it."

Miss B's face "turned a grayish color." Then the pair had words. Carrie recalled, "She reminded me of a cornered tiger."

That evening, Miss B developed "nervous chills" and the doctor advised her to go home for a rest. After Miss B. left, Carrie was sent to Ward 9 with Attendant Marie Hart. It was still a difficult ward and she needed to learn her patients' "ways and hobbies." One example was when she heard a commotion and found an old woman whimpering in her room. The old woman's roommate said, "That'll teach her whose bed she can get into." From then on, Carrie remembered to help the old woman into her bed, as the woman was almost completely blind.

When free time was allowed, Carried did enjoy some of her experiences. When she had time off, she would walk the grounds. "The grounds were beautiful and we could go anywhere on the hospital grounds and we could sit on a swing with a friend and just rest and talk." She even found a bit of companionship with a former childhood chum, Jack R, who also worked at the hospital.

Carrie's tenure ended one time when Carrie's friend, Zella and her beau got a day off with her but Jack R. did not. Jack asked Carrie to call the hospital and say a friend was at the station once she'd gotten off campus. She was to see if he could get off to pick him up. Carried did, was caught out, and Carrie and Jack lost their jobs.

Carrie went back home to be with her mother, who was watching her children. Later she got a job at several other state hospitals, East Haven (Richmond) and Logansport. She described her experiences at East Haven as much better than at Central State. Carrie felt everyone was nicer and the patients were better treated there.

Although she kept in contact with Jack, they never reconnected. After corresponding with an old sweetheart, Tolbert Lively, they got married in 1902 and she resigned from her job.

September 13, 1959

The new Central State Hospital kitchen won best in nation. It replaced the 1870s kitchen and dining halls. In the old areas, the floors were eroded and pitted and couldn't be properly cleaned. The equipment was old, some dating to the beginning of the hospital and was hard to clean. The new dining area was a one story brick building with a loading dock at the rear. Vegetables, precut meat portions and dry goods were stored in the storage area and in walk in refrigerators. The kitchen had five areas: Receiving, storage prep serving and cleaning. Floors were quarry tile and walls had glazed facing tile making them easy to clean. Stainless kettles and steamers were hung on the wall to clean under them. Employees had lockers and washrooms. A hose at the end of the cabinets made washing easy. Garbage disposals were installed at strategic locations. A large "china clipper" dishwasher was installed. An electric oven and refrigeration for salads with a double opening to allow people get premade salads for themselves was installed.

A typical evening at the kitchen included preparing vegetable dishes and meat. The menu would be posted and delivered to the wards or various dining rooms. Food carts and sterile dish carts were taken to the loading dock and wheeled to the ward/dining room and plugged in to maintain heat. There was a special cooled unit for cold items such as salad. Each food cart had beverage urns. Trays and plates scrapped of leftover food and put back onto the carts. The employees received the same food as the patients. Their dishes were carried by conveyor to the kitchen where they were washed. Four large carts held food for 1,540 people. Eight smaller carts, served 400 more people.

Gladys Roberts

Gladys Roberts worked many places in her life, but preferred the infirmaries. Miss Rogers, part of the Central State nursing staff, described her as an "expert in psychiatric nursing care and unusual in her devotion to the inform patient whether young or old". She worked the day shift in North (part of Seven Steeples) for $325 a month. Her hours were from 7a.m. to 3:30p.m. five days a week. She worked with a couple other attendants. Their goals were to take care of the patients and keep the ward clean. Only 12 of the patients could dress themselves. They were given two baths and a shampoo every week. Many required medicine or treatments according to the doctors, who visit the infirmary every day. Thirty four of the patients could go down stairs for breakfast, although one had to be restrained with soft strips of material and fed. Wheelchair bound patients ate on the ward. After lunch some patients took a nap and others went outside.

Every day 54 beds had to be made and the entire floor area of the ward cleaned and disinfected. Beds and chairs were washed each week "Somebody has to take care of these people," Roberts said "I'd rather work here than any place in the hospital because I feel I might be able to help."

On her days off Gladys thought about the patients and when she went on vacation she looked forward to seeing how they were when she returned. "There was one little old lady in her 80s that no one came to see. The doctor gave me permission to take her home with me on my day off. She sits there so pretty while I put my dinner on the table. What's rough about the job was not having enough help. We could have done more with the patients if there were more of us attendants. Theoretically, we had five on the day shift but because of days off there were often only two of us. [We could have done more] if we had help with window washing and floor and all the other cleaning we do. You need a strong back to work here. I think the hardest thing was lifting some of these old ladies out of their wheelchairs and into a bathtub with high sides."

ART AND PATIENTS

Jon Mangold , Psychologist, began an art program for the patients. "I found some real talented guys," he said. One patient, Mark Foust, was "especially talented." Mark had been at Central State Hospital for seven years and was transferred to another facility. For Mark, he just started the program in an extra room and didn't talk much about how therapeutic it was. "because it seemed so obvious." Patient Hugh Hoskins agreed, "You didn't have to think about being sick all the time." One of the last projects the group did was with Carol Tharp-Perrin, a muralist. It was a six foot by twelve foot landscape. It was in a locked ward for violent patients. Mark said that the closure of the hospital was "an amazingly sad experience."

A.E. CORY AND JACOB SCHMITT

Ward O (minimum security; best patients)

Mrs. A.E. Cory lodged a complaint about her husband. He was admitted March, 29,1913. Three weeks before the complaint, Mrs. Cory said she found her husband's throat swollen. Her husband said Attendant Johnson choked him and shoved him against the wall. A week after this, she found her husband's hand hurt. He said the same attendant kicked him. The attendant was present when Mr. Cory made this statement but did not respond. Mr. Gullett, the supervisor, tried to find out how Cory's hand was hurt and reported to Mrs. Cory that he was unable to find out if her husband had been kicked.

Additionally, Mrs. Cory furnished all her husband's clothing except underwear. but was asked not to do so and later found him in ill-fitting clothing. She found her husband chronically in soiled shirts. She inquired and was told his clothing was in the laundry. When she visited again, she saw him in a new shirt and it had never been laundered.

Mrs. Cory was initially afraid to complain, especially when the attendants were known to retaliate against the patients. She charged that her husband's mental and physical condition had worsened since his stay and she said he wasn't receiving proper treatment. He had also been in the Sick Hospital with head and body lice. This made him think he's contracted a "loathsome disease". When Mrs. Cory spoke with Dr. Wiles, she received "gruff, unsympathetic" treatment.

What is even more interesting is that Mrs. Cory's friend, Mrs. Jacob Schmitt lodged a complaint about her own husband on August 7,1912, before Mrs. Cory complained. Mrs. Schmitt's husband was admitted on July 27, 1912 and was also in ill-fitting clothes. Mrs. Schmitt was told his clothes were burned. Mrs. Schmitt offered to send new clothes but the attendants said that was not necessary. A few days later, Jacob Schmitt was still in the same clothes. Mrs. Schmitt was told the new clothing had come, but not been marked with his name yet. A few days later, she visited and found Jacob still in the same clothes. She was told again that the clothing hadn't been marked. Finally, on the day she filed the complaint, Jacob got his new clothes.

Jacob was diabetic and in need of special diet and medical attention. He told his wife the food was not good and there was never enough. Breakfast was hash or potatoes, bread, and coffee. Sometimes not everyone got coffee or other parts of the meal. When asked about this, Dr. Everman said "that there was just so much coffee for the ward and they had to do the best they could with their allowance." Dinner was boiled vegetables, meat, bread and water.

The Unruly Catherine Taylor

In a letter from Dr. WB Fletcher's Sanatorium, Catherine Taylor was committed to Dr. WB Fletcher's Sanatorium by her father and her Attorney, Judge LC Walker. Later she was removed to Richmond by the same. Taylor tried to shoot her aunt and believed she was being pursued by enemies.

Fletcher's Sanatorium believed Taylor was permanently insane but that she was harmless, mainly talking "profanely and threateningly" at times. While at Dr. Fletcher's, Taylor kept to her room most of the day. The next day, she disappeared. That evening, she was removed from the Monon train at Westfield and returned to family.

Taylor fought Sergeant Hagerdorn, who brought her back to the Sanatorium, "rigorously" and attacked Dr. Fletcher. In his letter to the Board of State Charities, S. Edward Smith, Medical Superintendent of the sanatorium, wrote to Central State Hospital. He stated he could hold her for two to three days as a "charity case," but that he couldn't hold her longer. (The bill to date was $150 and he'd been paid $50 so far). Smith was "certainly very anxious that the transfer be made."

The vegetable was usually beans or cabbage. The bread was served with preserves. Jacob said the attendants were not around during meal time and patients would steal food from others.

Mrs. Schmitt said
- it was two weeks before her husband was shaved and five days before he was given medication. His insanity, she said, stemmed from alcohol. He had improved in mind since he'd been at the hospital because she didn't think he could get drink there. However, he was weak because of the lack of and type of food and medical attention.
- one Sunday when many family members came to visit there was no one to issue passes. Many disappointed and frustrated people went home without seeing their family and friends.
- she was afraid to make complaints for the same reasons as Mrs. Cory. She felt he was already being punished for her speaking up at the ward level. She said Dr. Edenharter stated that if she wanted her husband furloughed, "she need not come to him about it because he would do nothing for her." Mrs. Schmitt felt this comment was unnecessary because she had not asked to see Dr. Edenharter and just wanted to talk to Dr. Everman about her husband being able to go outside on the lawn.

As of the time the letter was written, Mrs. Schmitt's husband had not been out nor allowed to go to Sunday school, although he asked to go. Dr. Everman was reported to have read Mrs. Schmitt's letter and stated that it was all "a lie." He stated to her husband, "You made trouble for us, now we are going to make trouble for you." A barber told Jacob, once he found out what had happened, "You won't get out of here for six months."

On September 14, 1912 Mrs. Schmitt's attorney said things had improved and unless "some gross abuse occurs," Mrs. Schmitt would take no further steps.

The Strange Case of Abraham Cook (1907)
Cook was very violent and had been camisoled a few times. He died of pneumonia, but at the time of death, many bruises and broken ribs were reported during the autopsy. An inquest was done and an investigation was undertaken to see if the attendants had been rough with him. A man named Dempsey Disney (Demsey Disney in some records) was in the habit of beating Cook.

The Sad Case of M. Elizabeth Miller
A letter dated June 13, 1890 regarding Mrs. M.Elizabeth Miller: Two attendants, Miss Christie and Miss Cain, were negligent in their duties and provided insufficient care by inflicting, and not reporting bruises on Mrs. Miller's body.

Additionally Dr. Adams, the assistant physician, failed in adequate care of the patients under her charge and in her duty to the hospital in that she did not mention the bruises in her daily report, nor rigorously investigate the causes of the bruises. The letter was signed by the Board of State Charities and its secretary and the attorney for Mrs. Miller.

Despite Science-George Brumemer
On January 31, 1902 instead of fancy treatments, George Brumemer was cured of insanity by a blow to his head. He'd been in Central State and released. A few days later it appeared he would need to return to the hospital. While the officers were on their way to pick him up, George got into a fight and was hit on the head with the butt end of a whip, which caused a deep gash. He was patched up and from this point on, George did not have any signs of insanity.

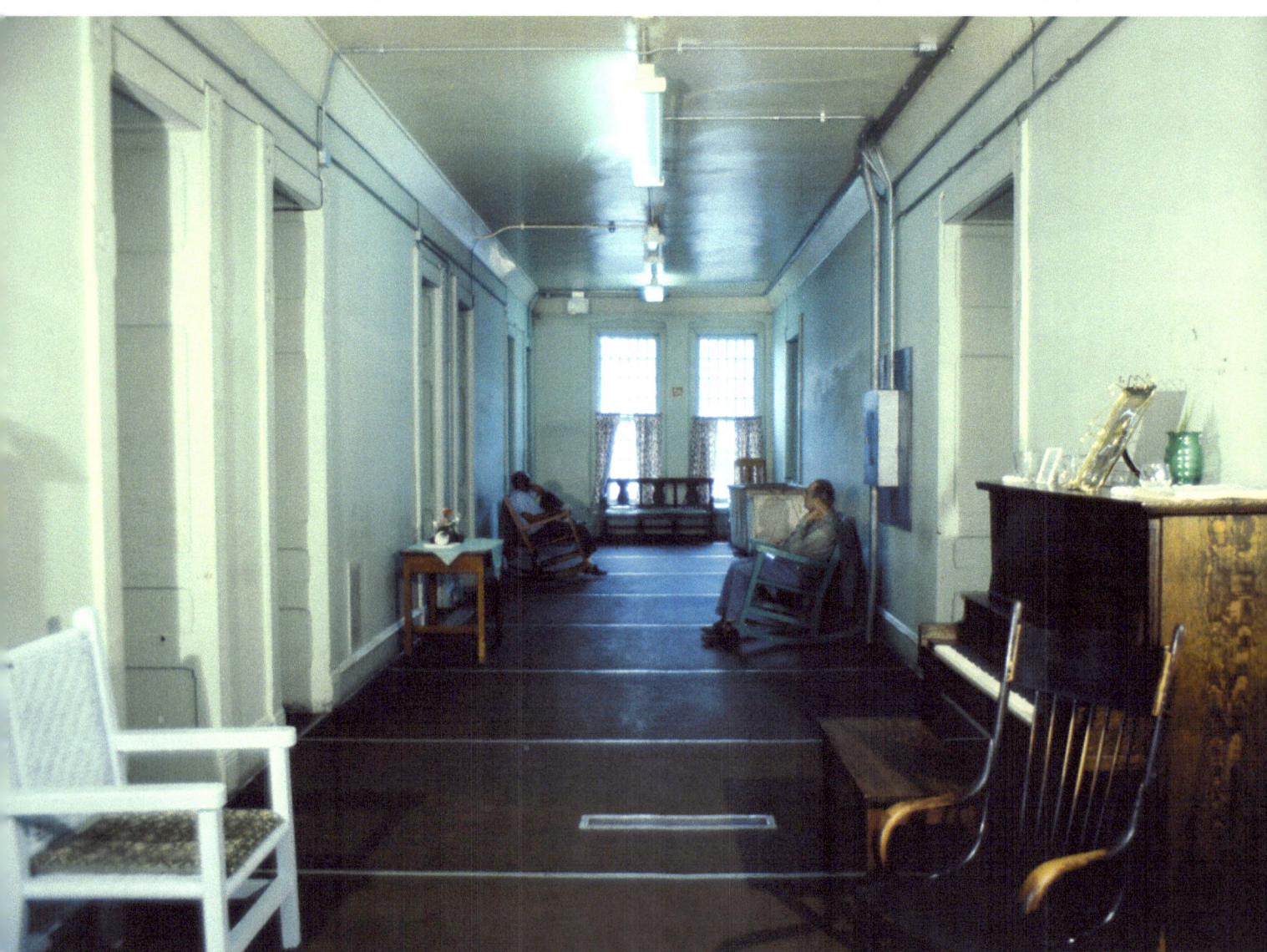

Department for Women, also known as Seven Steeples. Although intendend for women, while the Department of Men was razed and cottages built, men were housed in this building.

EIGHT

INVESTIGATIONS INTO THE HOSPITAL

By the 1880s, the hospital had grown to include the Department for Men, the Department for Women and several outbuildings used to run the two massive buildings. These included kitchens, dormitories, and maintenance buildings.

With the additional buildings came more staff. The various departments were responsible for providing a report of their activities to the Superintendent. Any money paid out required a receipt to be submitted to the steward.

Between 1879 and 1880, many people and the newspaper had vilified the hospital alleging abuses and mismanagement of money and power. According to yearly reports, the claims were unfounded and the hospital administration felt vindicated. However, the truth is that indifference and abuse were prevalent. There were only a small number of physicians responsible for a great number of patients, and a poorly trained and educated staff, who didn't know how much they didn't know, so treatment could not be very good.

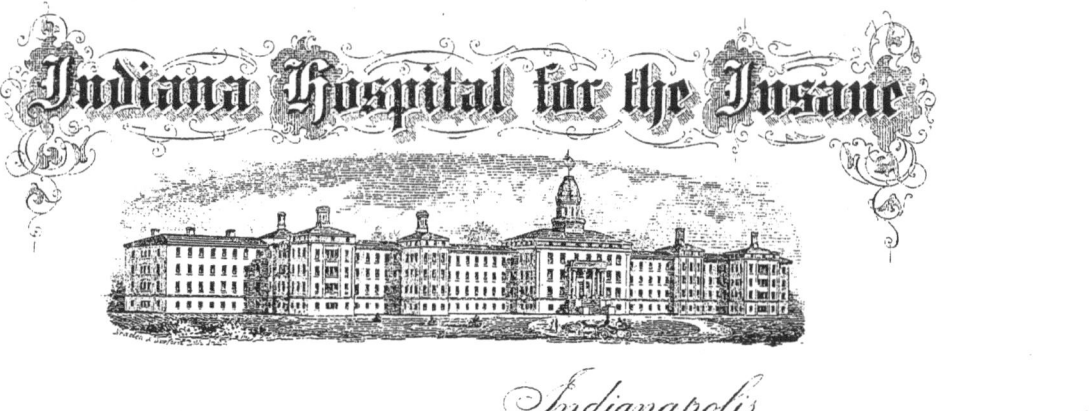

Sometimes asylums were likened to their early counterpart, the prison. "It is too common a belief that hospitals are prisons, and the superintendents only keepers; and the friends of the insane will look for every other help before they will trust an insane asylum. (1)"

Additionally, the superintendents didn't help matters. Many admitted to "a gradual yet inevitable accumulation of the chronic and incurable class in hospital populations…" They believed this "affected their reputations unfavorably as agencies of cure." Central State Hospital superintendent believed, "…recoveries are much less likely to occur than I once believed…. I do not believe more than 24 of every hundred get well." This goes against very early claims that boasted of 80 to 90% "cures" (2)

In later years, Central State answered such charges. As with any large organization (and some small), corruption became a part of everyday life (3). Three times in 1887, 1889, and 1899, the hospital was investigated. Three times the hospital was found negligent in some of its internal processes, with patients, with vendors and with the State and its citizens.

Some reasons for this were that custodial patients were generally made comfortable, as it was highly unlikely that they would ever be discharged as improved. These patients led to a population which required more care than other patient populations.

Additionally, violence between patients or even between patient and attendants was sometimes untraceable. Records were scantily kept despite rules to the contrary, and many daily logs were not filled out. Examples from other hospitals include information such as, "Fourth Ward, April 6, 1882. CS received blow on the nose from Mr. C; Mr. C. was sitting on a bench in the yard when S kicked him. Mr. CC then struck him on the nose. Witnessed by attendant EA Williams." Central State Hospital records are incomplete, but the records that do exist do not contain many detailed daily accounts. When situations like the one described happened at Central State Hospitals, superintendents and physicians had no time and were not very keen to correct these situations. The cases that were investigated were generally put aside. The attendants stuck up for each other and evidence was not easy to obtain. Patients were not believed or feared retribution (4).

To cut down on care and brutality, many asylums employed restraints. A waist belt was wound around the patient and a chair. The patient's hands were bound by leather straps which were attached to a metal ring on the belt. They could feed themselves, but not do much more. Leather mittens (4) were used on patients who abused themselves, such as with a scratching affliction. These were fastened around the wrist by a lock. The camisole was an early straight jacket. Made of canvas, it restrained the hands and arms, which prevented patients from "getting into mischief." The muff was another restraint where the patient's hands were placed into it. The covered bed, (the most famous one called the Utica crib) was originally used for children but later adjusted to adults. It was basically a wooden box, with bars resembling a crib. The top of the box contained hinges and a lock.

Part of the problem with these restraints was although they kept patients from harm, they were also used in a punitive way. Sometimes patients were kept in these devices almost all the time.

In addition, too few and untrained staff on all sides of the hospital did not help the situation. Staff didn't know what to do in some situations, and even if they did, they didn't have enough people to do the job properly. Those who should have been on top of the hospital and all situations were so stretched for time, they simply couldn't keep up.

"Adventures in Social Welfare" by Alexander Johnson in 1923 states:

> "Things certainly had been pretty bad. The condition of the Central Hospital for the Insane was one of the causes of Cleveland's defeat for president in 1888. The hospital had been investigated in 1887 and the 790 pages of testimony had disclosed an incredible amount of fraud, corruption, abuse of patients, a conspiracy of officers, trustees and contractors to rob the state- and the party that was in control was so discredited that it lost the next election. If the 15 votes of Indiana, instead of going to Harrison had gone to Cleveland, he would have been elected. That investigation had been one of the causes leading to the creation of the Board of State Charities.
> That year saw a Republican victory and William Fletcher, the Democratic superintendent of the hospital, was ineffectual at best, despite his prominence."

When the Board of Charities was formed, its goal was to ferret out abuses and help bring reform to asylums and other institutions. Unfortunately, boards like these were not necessarily equipped or motivated to be equal to the task of providing decent, let alone quality care. Many members were political appointees who were given their positions by a grateful governor for their endorsements. Some positions were held by the "well-to-do" of the community who expressed a want to be philanthropic. These positions were considered full time or part time, salaried or unpaid. Unfortunately, many of the people on the Board of State Charities had other interests of jobs, so the time needed to oversee, advocate for, and complete the work was inadequate. The board seemed to have very little effect in confronting these issues, because they were essentially addressing their peers and they could not get many of the staff to turn on their own.

1887 Investigation

The Board of Trustees was appointed under the "Brown" bill. Dr. Thomas H. Harrison (5) and Mr. Hall, the bookkeeper for the hospital at the time lobbied heavily for its passage. Dr. Thomas H. Harrison admitted that it was only for his "selfish" purpose of obtaining the presidency of the Board of Trustees that he worked so hard. He admittedly cared little for the running of the hospital. The Board of Trustees was to help investigate the allegations about the hospital and generally oversee the administration in the future.

The findings from the 1887 investigation into the operation and management of the hospital included the following conclusions:

Board of Trustees
- Dr. Harrison drew a salary of $1,600 instead of his $900 as dictated by law.
- No rules for governing the hospital were made until two years after the trustees had been appointed.
- Between November 1885 and October 1886 Phillip M Gapen, Treasurer, engaged in a private enterprise (a sawmill in Arkansas) and was not available to work, yet he still drew $50 a month for his Board of Charities duties.
- Dr. Harrison, President, and Mr. Burrell, the Secretary, should not have allowed Gapen's money to be drawn and should have reported his actions to the Superintendent.
- Only Democrats and people of certain religions applied for work because two thirds of the people were recommended by members of the Legislature.
- Gapen cashed a $64.77 check from Mellen & Co (New York) and used it for personal purposes instead of giving it to the Superintendent as per procedure.
- The Board of Trustees allowed unwholesome goods to be provided to the hospital.
- The 1886 Board of Trustees report was falsified in the amount of money actually on hand. It was much smaller than reported.
- The current Board of Charities should be removed.
- Any new Board of Trustees member would go through a rigorous appointment process.

Hospital
- Adopted bylaws were not followed which impaired the institution.
- Dr. Harrison tried to suppress testimony against him by securing witnesses from Lebanon
- Dr. Harrison had a conflict of interest, being a personal friend of John Sullivan, who was to supply produce to the hospital.
- D.P. Erwin & Co had been given a great many contracts for dry goods and Mr. Gapen had a son-in-law who worked there.
- Due to cruelty to patients, Dr. Fletcher wanted stricter behavior of attendants enforced, but it was never uniformly enforced.
- Elopement was rampant, with no records kept of who escaped or who was returned. Patients had gone missing and died because of this. Additionally when Jonathan Allen escaped and went home, his family sent a letter asking about his condition. They received a postcard back that he was doing well, even though he had long since escaped.

Staff
- Mr. J.S. Hall was allowed to be chief accountant although he had no training for this and the books were in a deplorable state. He was an apprentice clerk at a pharmacy and a teacher before coming to the hospital.
- Mr. Roth, Assistant Steward, had his salary reduced because he wanted to bring the inferior goods to the attention of the hospital. It was restored after the investigation started.
- Mr. Stacey, Mechanical Engineer, was fired after he refused to pay for inferior iron for the buildings.

- The matron was paid $1000 per year. The committee believed it should be $600 per year.
- Unqualified doctors and unqualified and abusive attendants were hired.
- Abusive attendants abused patients by not stopping patient on patient violence, one attendant stating, "Some of these wards are run by patients and not by the attendants."
- Abusive attendants kicked, knocked down, and struck patients with a club, or pitched them over a fence.
- Attendants were chosen because of their ability to do political work, or because they'd done political work in the past.
- The position of housekeeper needed to be abolished.
- Employees should have more modest quarters and, with the exception of attendants, should fix them up at their expense.

Products
- Bidding was rigged towards favoritism. Lower bids and better products overlooked for other contractors and special consideration. Inferior products included bad or maggoty butter, spoilt meat and milk, and bad produce.
- Pigs with cholera were served to patients. Employees routinely did not eat the meat because of that. Pigs without cholera were housed in the same area as the pigs with cholera that died from cholera.
- Many times when the Superintendent asked for inferior goods to be returned they were sold back to the hospital. This included bad butter and fish. The offending provider continued to be awarded contracts.
- The boiler iron was inferior and Mr. Stacey was removed for talking about it.
- Butter from July to September 1886 was inferior, and sometimes spoilt. It sometimes had skippers in it and was stored in the sewers. This same butter passed inspection in the storeroom and was put on the table for patients and staff. Mr. Hall ignored Mr. Roth and Dr. Fletcher's orders for its return. John Sullivan furnished this butter.
- Inferior groceries returned by Dr. Fletcher were often sold back to the hospital after Dr. Fletcher had gone about his business.

Record Keeping
- The storeroom books had a lot of errors, erasures, and pages removed
- The supplies for the hospital should be requested under the blind and deaf institutions.
- The books must be kept up to date

Ethics
- Spirits were being used for patients without a doctor's order and by staff although it was prohibited.
- Mr. Hall asked the employees to give money for political purposes.

Recommendations
- Remove the Board of Trustees (6).
- Install a woman on the new Board of Trustees to "increase its efficiency."
- Institute a policy that staff cannot participate in politics except to vote.
- Hire only women doctors for the Department of Women.
- For the Department of Men, have a man and a woman as attendants
- Enforce a new set of rules.
- Enforce rules against liquor.
- Reduce farm hands' salaries.
- Mr. Hall should be fired and a "thoroughly honest man" replace him.
- All supplies should be ordered with those of the Asylum for the Deaf and Dumb and the Asylum for the Blind.
- The books of the hospital should to be kept up-to-date.
- Examine the boilers and fix them.

The Minority Report (7) refuted almost all of these charges. It stated that basically no charges had been brought against anyone and for all the charges brought against the people named in the investigative committee's report, there was something to negate them.

1889 Investigation
Committee on Investigation of the Affairs of the Indiana Hospital for Insane, February 25, 1889, Room 52

- Daniel Leslie of Winchester, Indiana and Captain R.A. Fuller of New Albany, Indiana were accountants who made the examination of the hospital's bookkeeping.
- The committee consisted of Senator Frank B. Burke (Chairman) and Representative M.W. FieldsFields (Secretary), under the direction of the General Assembly.
- Representatives George S. Plesants and Theodore Shockney were on a subcommittee to review books and accounts.
- Representatives C. G. Conn, Fields and William A. Brown and Senator Timothy E. Howard had a subcommittee to examine the management of the institution.
- Meetings about the investigation were at 1:30pm Monday through Friday. Examination of witnesses by the Chairman and by a subcommittee of Senator Silas A Hays, Rep E.G. Henry.
- Any member of the committee could ask questions.

Food, Care and Cleanliness

The subcommittees visited the hospital twice. They found that the offices, halls and wards of the hospital to be clean and well-kept and in good working order and "discipline prevails." They visited once during mealtime (8) at the Department of Women and found nothing amiss. The tables were clean, food was "plain but well-cooked and of sufficient variety consisting of boiled beef, vegetables, bread and milk. The food was cooked in large kettles and pans and was clean and well prepared."

Ethics

- The general store was kept by Storekeeper Mr. Hyde. The subcommittee found that Treasurer P.M. Gapen (9), for part of his employment with the hospital, was in the employ of John E. Sullivan, a contractor at the hospital. Gapen became an employee to Sullivan at $25 per week in December 1887.
- Superintendent Galbraith was reported to have been handpicked for his position. He was told that as long as he didn't interfere with supplies or the Board of Trustees, and as long as he hired Dr. Howard (without knowing his qualifications), that he'd have a job. Galbraith neglected his duties by turning his eyes to abuse and not making improvements to the way the hospital was run and to patient conditions when necessary.

Illegal Loans

- During the time Gapen was employed, each month between $1,000 and $8,500 was withdrawn each month and given to Sullivan, or others as loans, which was in violation of the law. When the loans were not repaid, this left Treasurer Gapen in debt to the tune of $17,694.98, $3,000 of it to him personally, and people who had legitimate checks couldn't cash them because the treasury had no money.
- Superintendent Galbraith was found to have loaned $1,000 on two occasions to John E Sullivan at the behest of the Board of Charities. Treasurer Gapen did the same four times under the direction of State Treasurer Lemcke. The committee "condemns this practice as unlawful and recommends its discontinuance."

Bid Rigging

- Some of the bids were not done properly. When bids were received that the board didn't like, they wouldn't award anything to any of the bidders, but would authorize someone internally to find the materials "without any restrictions or limitations as to price, quantity, or quality."
- When bids were accepted, they were mostly to John E. Sullivan and certain other vendors, even when lower bids were submitted.
- The subcommittee believed the Indiana Board of State Charities was in collusion with the suppliers to supply inferior goods.

Money and Goods

- When goods at the hospital were sold or disposed of, instead of collecting money, they were given as pay-

ment on account (instead of money being put into the State Treasury, as was the law).
- A large discrepancy was found in the prices paid for butter, eggs, poultry, sugar, coffee and tea. The subcommittee believed some of this was due to substandard product being substituted in months when funds were short. Additionally, the amount needed to pay for produce from Sullivan kept increasing until it was $1,000 over what was needed to actually supply the hospital.
- Larger quantities were paid for than what the contracts called for. Examples included March to December 1887. The following items and quantity were bought during this time at smaller quantities than the next year, although lesser amounts were really needed: tea (2,200 pounds), sugar (13,822 pounds). In 1888 3,047 pounds of tea and 39,825 pounds of sugar were bought.
- An extensive system of waste was found. When requisitions were requested, there was no record that the goods got to the location that asked for them. Additionally, there was no systematic means to requisition supplies or account for them.

Insanity Trust 1901

Due to more worries from the public that people were being declared insane illegally and erroneously put into the hospital, in 1901 the Board of State Charities conducted an "Insanity Trust." Its purpose was to determine if anyone inside the Indiana mental hospitals was really sane and if any such cases were found, make suggestions for changing the laws to improve the process for commitment.

The Board looked at 27 cases plus two that were submitted by private individuals. Of these, no one was found to be sane and all patients were found to have been in the hospital out of medical necessity. The Board made this determination by reviewing reports from staff at all levels of the hospital. This was done in conjunction with the Attorney General of Marion County.

The Board suggested that judges hear commitment cases in chambers versus a public hearing. It also suggested that no insane person be held in jail before they could be transferred to a hospital as it exacerbated their condition.

Additionally, the Board tried to right wrongs. On August 3, 1901, Dr. Edenharter sent a letter to the Board regarding Sarah Younkin. He'd received a letter from A.J. Rousch on behalf of R.L. Cook, Younkin's daughter. According to the letter, Younkin was admitted January 27, 1880 and taken out of the facility on October 24, 1889 by David D. Long, her supposed guardian. Long put her into a home run by the Little Sisters of the Poor in Indianapolis, which was tied to the County Poor House of Marion County. The Board said it had no way of knowing how it happened, or if she was still there, but that her guardian had to file an accounting of her money every year. If he had not done so, he could be brought up in front of the Circuit Judge of Marion County. Younkin's daughter was concerned about her mother's welfare and location.

On January 11, 1902 James E. Richards, a patient, died and it was suspected that he hadn't had proper care. He had a bruised throat, a cut on his right temple and a cut under his lip. He had acute mania and his cause of death was "exhaustion of acute mania." The death report was written on a Department for Woman form, and signed by Drs. F.M. Wiles and O.J. Watters (10).

Another patient, N.O. Weakly, Z Ward died under mysterious circumstances in 1891. Attendant John M. Bates

> "This is an asylum and not a hospital. They need environment, the conversation, the encouragement."
> ~ Dr. Edward J. Kempf, 1912

and Attendant Albert Bridenstine testified that there was nothing amiss and that they did not hit him, administer a cold bath without permission or use towels to subdue patients. They said Mr. Kogler, was not abusive. They said that another patient gave Weakly his black eye. They and patients agreed that Weakly was "nasty." He would become violent and "approach men."

Samuel Stork, a former attendant, remembered Weakly. He stated Mr. Kogler struggled with Weakly and Weakly fell in the day room.

Leo E. Hudson, another former attendant, remembered Weakly having a black eye after he came to the ward. He said Mr. Kogler struck Weakly on the back of the neck with his fist and he fell face first to the floor. Hudson also stated Mr. Kogler stamped J. Greene on the neck until he was unconscious and Greene remained that way until he was taken to the bathroom and cold water thrown on his face.

Walter Housten, a patient, stated Bridenstine struck Weakly several times, as did Kogler and Bates would hit Weakly with a bathing brush.

Charles Young, a patient, stated Kogler hit Weakly several times with his fist and kick him on his hips and sides. Bradenstine hit Weakly in the ribs with his fist. Afterwards, Weakly was kept in the dorm so the doctor couldn't see him. Kogler and Bridenstine would wrap a towel around Weakly's neck to strangle (11) him.

In 1900, the State Board of Charities reiterated Dr. Joseph G. Rogers' view of the institutions stating that "our insane hospitals should not be allowed to become too large. The herding of human beings is not right. It is not beneficial. The best results cannot be obtained and it is to the discredit of any state when such conditions come to be. There should be no more in any one institution than can receive proper individual treatment and care. It would be wise to make provision to colonize the chronically insane a short distance from the existing hospital but not too far removed to be without the control of the management. To these colonies take the able bodied, harmless, chronic cases. They could be quartered in inexpensive buildings and employed so as to be in a large measure self-supporting. They could be readily transferred to the hospital in case treatment was needed. And others could be brought from the hospital to take their places."

1912 Investigation

In 1912 Dr. Edward J. Kempf was fired after "instituting a revolutionary movement against the management. This consisted in talking with some friends who were physicians in Indianapolis and obtaining their support in an effort to bring about better conditions at the hospital". Kempf made the following accusations:

- Charged that one third of the women employed died of consumption In the autopsies done in the 18 months Kempf was there, 47% had tuberculosis. Seven women came to work during that time. With nothing to teach them how to protect themselves against TB, five left with it (Gilmour, Frank, DeGulyer, Robbins, Morsey). At the time of Kempf's charges, two women had already died.
- Charged that the staff was overworked and that no one could possibly adhere to all the rules and see to all the patients' needs because of the patient/doctor ratio. When he brought it up, Dr. Edenharter, the Superintendent, would just bluff and bluster, and bring out letters from other institutions showing what a good job the hospital was doing.
- Stated that autopsies were incomplete and unscientific.
- Was shocked that the tuberculosis patients were not separated and that there were no voluntary commitment patients.
- Said the lab and the surgery weren't used and one quarter of the hospital was not used. Said the hospital had no graduate nurses and no system of training.
- Witnessed a cuspidor of sputum flung down the hall by an attendant.
- Accused hospital administration of putting "boisterous" patients in the sick hospital for weeks, despite the patients being seemingly to be in good physical health.
- Said that patients weren't really examined thoroughly. Because they were not examined an accurate diagnoses not made, doctors took chances in sending patients to a ward. If the ward wasn't the right one (e.g. sending a calm patient to a violent ward) , you simply moved the patient. No paperwork was done before or after. Kempf said that many patients had nothing in their files despite being there for years.
- Charged there was too much paperwork and no time to do it.

- Charged there were no staff meetings. Kempf spoke with Doctors Link, Eastman and Barnhill about it. One immediately called the superintendent. Kempf also talked also to Doctors Emerson and Bryan.

Kempf was discharged a week later for disloyalty. Drs. Bahr and Evermann stated, "The whole place was a big joke." They stated that Edenharter didn't know what to do, and that he had "millstones" such as Doctor Waters, Niles and Stockton.

Kempf's argument was "it [the hospital] does not have an active, living, progressive system. It throws the whole system on one man, and if he fails, the hospital fails. It does not have a system of nurses. It does not have a system of voluntary commitment and those coming of their own free will. There is no inducement in the State to get such patients in their incipient stages. No encouragement. The only provision the State has made is to take care of them [the patients] after they are hopeless. … we have to have some system which will catch the patient early."

Kempf and Dr. Bahr sent for temperature charts from New York and changed them to suit their work. Fifteen hundred were printed, but never used because the hospital didn't have chart boards. After Kempf was dismissed, these boards were given to the nurses, per Superintendent Edenharter's instructions. Kempf said he had over 400 cases and could do very little for any of the patients.

Some sources suggest that Kempf was whistle-blowing because he was fired not for disloyalty, but for spending more time trying to test his theories on patients than doing the day to day work. Others suggest he brought to Indiana's attention the same issues that were apparent in other institutions. In either case, he went on to a distinguished career, writing several books focusing on mental illnesses (12).

1921 Investigation

Otis E. Browning was a former supervisor at the hospital, who in his opinion, was discharged without reason. He sent letters to Governor Warren T. McCray and the State Board of Indiana Charities asking for Governor McCray to conduct an investigation into the hospital "so that at no future day the Republican party can be blamed with any responsibility…" Browning believed Dr. Edenharter should not be the Superintendent because:

- Edenharter's ideas were those of an "old fogy" and the institution was not using modern methods.

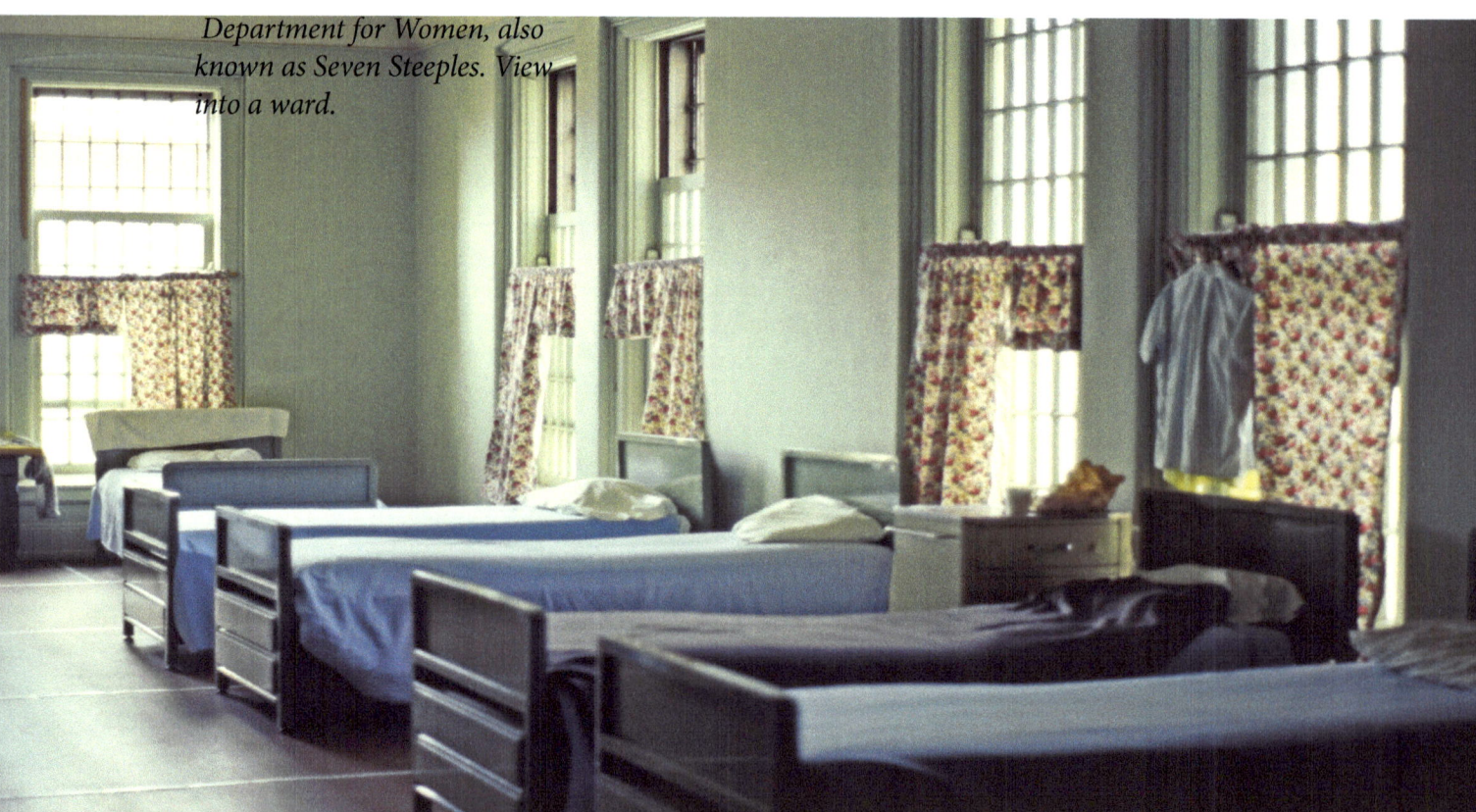

Department for Women, also known as Seven Steeples. View into a ward.

- Edenharter did not walk the wards and hadn't for the last five years.
- Edenharter didn't concern himself with the patients or staff.

Browning also hinted at some sort of scandal between Dr. Buehl writing about a patient, Frank Deglo. The State paid hospital florist, Walter Lewis. Browning asked the governor to find out what Lewis was doing with Deglo, where the florist was most of the time, and who was paying for the work Deglo did. He intimated that the florist was doing side work and using Deglo to help him with work outside of the hospital.

It was also suggested that the Governor speak with Lee Ragsdale, Dr. Edenharter's former secretary, to see what he could tell about bad management of the institution.

Effects of the Investigations

After the 1889 investigation, the Board of State Charities was comprised of six men split down political party lines. However, it never really achieved true bipartisanship. The Board of Indiana Charities advocated for the hospital, but seemed, as time went on, to relegate itself to infrequent visits and pleading in yearly reports. The public didn't seem too concerned about the hospital, or its dealings. The media didn't report much about the hospital.

In 1932 the duty of supervising Indiana State charities was taken from the Board of Indiana Charities and given to the newly formed Department of Public Welfare. As part of this change, the Division of Mental Health was also created. They began to supervise the mental hospitals.

What this really meant, as the mental hospitals were supervised by the Department of Public Welfare, that the Division of Mental Health served in a consolatory capacity. Because there was a dual control of the hospitals, there was a definite problem in having its recommendation implemented which led to ineffectual supervision of the hospital. This lack of efficiency and efficacy helped Central State continue toward its own demise.

Insanity Trust Patient Cases

Below are a sampling of the cases reviewed during the insanity trust hearings.

Case #30: Mrs. Sarah V. Rawley; Admitted: 1899;
Doctor: Dr. Stockton.

The patient was brought into the hospital because she was in bad physical condition and irresponsible. According to her husband, Sarah was unable to think properly and had bad judgment. Some days she was in a stupor. As an example of this, Sarah said that she and her husband were married after they knew each other two weeks. Her husband, Charles Rawley, said they were acquainted for 16 years. They have a child named Bell Marie.

The doctors say her husband is in bad condition as well. He came to visit and fell asleep on the ward. He is often drunk. The attendants couldn't allow him to be alone with his wife because he hugged her excessively and fondled her thigh. Bell Marie told Sarah that she had a new mama.
Charles petitioned to have his wife released. The doctors, including Dr. Edenharter, agreed that discharging Sarah to her husband would have to have a nurse for her day and night. The Board of State Charities was not satisfied with that. It stated if Dr. Edenharter let Sarah go home, the Board would have him removed as superintendent.

In her condition, the entire Board believed Mr. Rawley did not have her best interests at heart, rather that he wanted her "for the pleasures" he could get from her. Mr. Ellison from the Board of State Charities said, "I think her condition not a little due to his conduct. "(13)

Case #31: Martin Zimmerman;Diagnosis: Unknown
Doctor: Dr. Wiles

The doctors believed Martin did well at the hospital but when he left the hospital, he would get drunk and wild. His wife, Mrs. Rebecca Zimmerman believed Zimmerman's problems started when he was hit on the back of his neck by a tree branch that was torn off by a cannon ball during the Civil War. He also liked morphine and alcohol. Zimmerman had been in and out of the Northern State Hospital prior to his arrival at Central State Hospital.

When Zimmerman had furlough, he was violent towards the children and almost killed one. He also threatened his wife's life. His wife felt obligated to take him back because rumors in the area stated that her husband was not insane and she was keeping him in the hospital because she didn't want him anymore. The oldest sons, 18 and 21, refused to stay at home once Zimmerman was sent home. According to Mr. G.C. Forsinger, a neighbor agreed "if there ever was a lunatic outside of an Insane Hospital, that man is one. I do not regard him as a safe man to be at large."

Martin Zimmerman was born in Zimmerman, Ohio on November 21,1843, one of eight children. The family moved to Indiana when he was 15 years old. He served in the Civil War from July 8, 1862 to June 10, 1865. He ended his military career in Washington D.C. He married Rebecca Ann Carmichael on March 19, 1868. They had 13 children. He died on April 19, 1911 and is buried in Crown Hill Cemetery in Indianapolis, Indiana.

Case #32: Dr. U.L Blue; Diagnosis: Unknown
Doctor: Dr. Watters

Dr. Watters said when Dr. Blue was received, he was depressed, irritated, and excited. His clothing was in bad condition and he was physically and mentally in bad condition. At the hospital, Dr. Blue improved considerably.

A business acquaintance, W.E.Popen said he didn't believe that Dr. Blue was insane. Dr. Blue came to his business every day for the past six years and he never acted insane. He thought the issue with the doctor was his "fits of temper." He believed the doctor should be released and would give him $15 to get him started. He said the doctor had been fighting his wife as she wanted a divorce and the doctor mentioned if she would get him out, she could have the divorce.

The Board of State Charities talked to Lillie Bootes (daughter) and Elizabeth Blue (wife). Dr. Blue's daughter believes him insane but his daughter based her opinion on opinions of others. She said she could not take care of her father and her infant if her father was released.

Dr. Blue's wife said she did not believe her husband to be insane. She believed Dr. Blue was shafted by Dr. Boynton, whose anger was "aroused" against him because he cured a patient of Dr. Boynton. She believed it was "a piece of spite work." Dr. R. Boynton denied this and said that Dr. Blue was a "tolerably capable" physician. Dr. Boyton also said he was unable to care for himself. He said a friend of Dr. Blue's called him because he "recognized the need for immediate steps being taken" and Dr. Boynton called Dr. Fletcher, who made the recommendation Dr. Blue be recommitted.

M.C. Willis, an undertaker, knew Dr. Blue for over twenty five years and said he believed Dr. Blue to be insane. He said Dr. Blue was rational at times, but had frequent "spells of mild insanity." His information matched Dr. Boynton's.

Mr. Edward Gilbert from the Plymouth Building and Loan Association knew Dr. Blue for many years and believed him insane. He felt in Dr. Blue's insane periods he was violent and a spot in Central State Hospital was be the best place as it would be inhumane to let him out considering the pain Dr. Blue was in mentally. Mr. Gilbert offered to help persuade Dr. Blue to stay in.

On July 21,1901 Dr. Blue wrote a letter from Central State Hospital, asking to be released. He was sure he could find a place to stay for a month and had about $60 to live on. He also had patients that were willing to employ him as a doctor. He wanted to get out and provide for his family, although his wife owned a boarding house on New York Street. That contradicted what he told his friend about getting a divorce. He stated "I am getting no treatment here and the confinement with some of the horrible cases of insanity in here would soon derange the soundest mind so confined." He asked to be at least taken to the poor farm for a time.

Nine

PATHOLOGY DEPARTMENT

With scientific advances in the late 1890s, laboratories were built to learn more about the causes of mental illness. Before the Pathology Department at Central State Hospital opened, only Bellevue Hospital in New York City had separate facilities for labs (1).

Over the course of its life, the Pathology Department at Central State Hospital provided training and education and conducted groundbreaking research, some of which is still useful today.

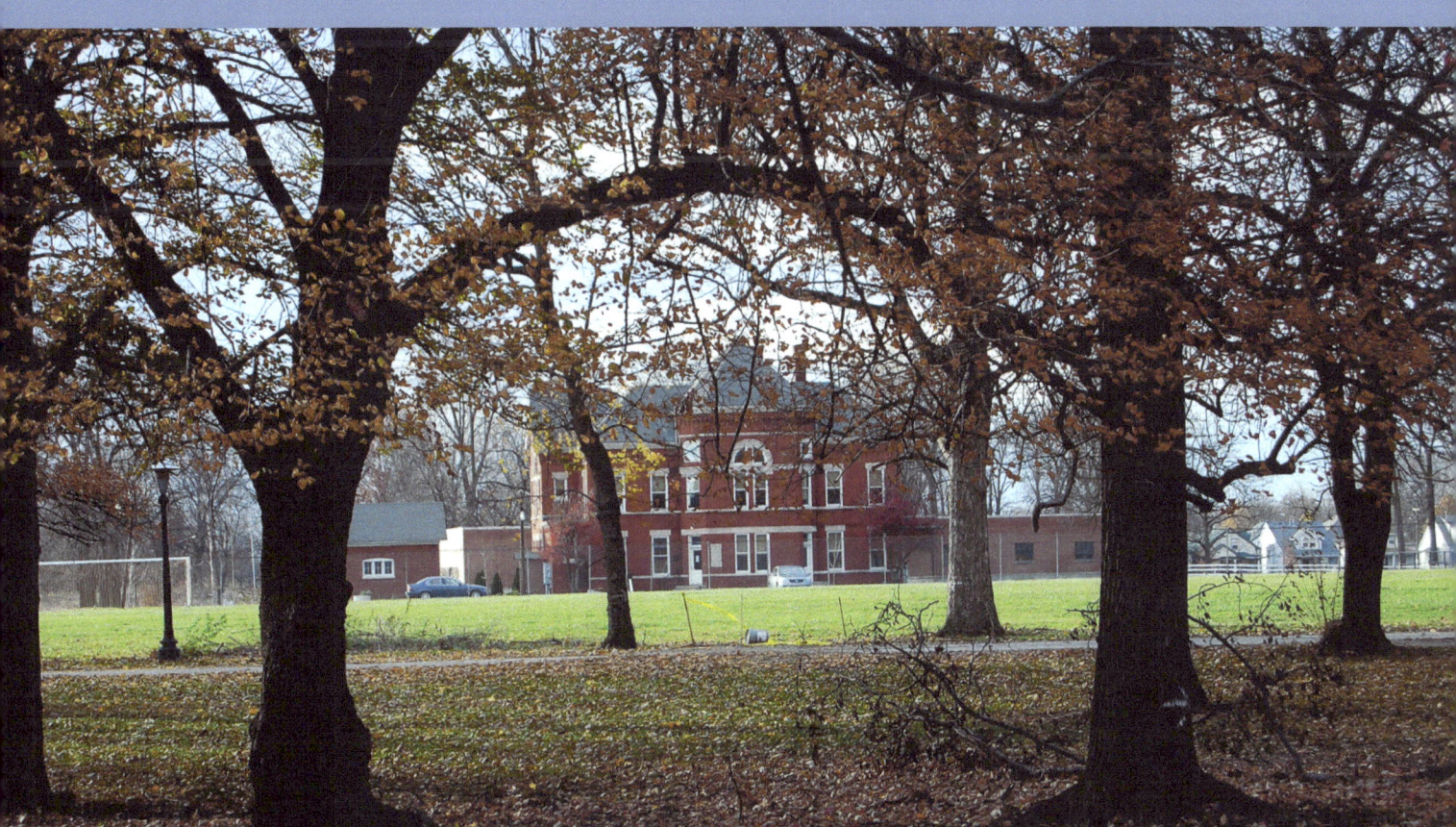

Neurologists

In the 1870s and 1880s, neurology was a new practice in medicine. Neurologists disagreed with psychiatric doctors on studying the pathology of mental health, in addition to ongoing care provided. They wanted to make the laboratory part of the emerging mental health system of care.

To neurologists, psychiatry was a subset of neurology. They believed that doctors had not found anything significant to further the field through clinical observation and rudimentary pathology. Neurologists also sought to improve record keeping to help patients and document patterns of care.

Additionally, neurologists at Central State Hospital also believed enlarging and overhauling the State Board of Charities, by replacing the majority of business men with doctors and attorneys. They also wanted to expand the Board of Commissioners power and systematically research the physiology of insanity through autopsies, which the doctors believed should have been a legal requirement.

Some of these requests were implemented and others not. For example, the State Board of Charities was overhauled and many replacements made. The Board of Commissioners had expanded powers as well and was overhauled. In the short term, these changes seemed to be good, but long term, they were unimpressive. The State Board of Charities was out of power by 1935 and the Board of Commissioners did little to make the changes needed (or convince the State of Indiana why the changes were needed) to keep the abuses from happening again. Autopsies were conducted with the permission of family members (or without if the patient had no family).

Pathology Department Need

Some doctors, including Superintendent George F. Edenharter wanted to emphasize the biological aspects of mental illness. He wanted to have a facility in which pathological research, teaching, and learning could occur. He believed a lecture hall, research and presentations, a medical library and labs, as well as facilities for autopsies would all play key roles in accomplishing his objective.

Unfortunately, the State of Indiana did not understand the need for or the impact the facility could have. It is believed that Superintendent Edenharter used money from the regular operating budget to fund the building.

Superintendent Edenharter was determined to improve conditions at the hospital. Originally, he envisioned a four room single story structure, but the building's final form was two stories, with 19 rooms. These rooms included

The Architect

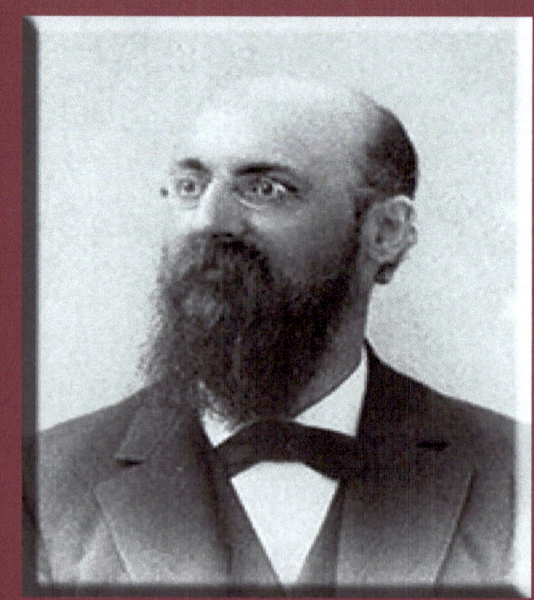

Adolph Scherrer designed the Department for Women (also known as Seven Steeples) and the Indiana State House. He was chosen for this project, too. In 1895 the John A Schumacher Company began construction and two years later after completion, the total cost was reported as $15,000 (9).

Scherrer also was responsible for designing the Tipton County courthouse (Tipton, Indiana) and the Maennerchor Hall and the gate at Crown Hill Cemetery, both in Indianapolis, Indiana).

a morgue, viewing room, records room, numerous lab rooms, an amphitheater, anatomical and pathological museum, photography room, library and offices.

THE PATHOLOGY DEPARTMENT

On December 18, 1896 a state of the art Pathology Department opened at Central State hospital to study the causes of mental and nervous disorders. It was the newest, most modern facility in the United States and out shined all others. The Indianapolis Sentinel stated, "Physicians who have studied in the pathological laboratories of the Old World say they have seen nothing to surpass it." The lab contained facilities for pathologic anatomy, bacteriology, clinical chemistry and histology. This research helped physicians to understand the natural causes of mental illness. The lab also contained a gravity drinking fountain (10), a 500 volume library, electric lights and a telephone connected to the city (versus an internal switchboard connected only to the hospital).

The formal dedication attracted over 150 members of the Marion County Medical Society and guests. Speeches were given by a variety of people, including Dr. Ludwig Hektoen, a professor of pathology at Rush Medical College in Chicago. A Bausch and Lomb microscope was given to Superintendent Edenharter for use at the facility. After the last speech, the group retired to the hospital's chapel, for coffee and cigars.

All was not rosy, though. Until 1924 the lab had a hard time retaining pathologists. Money was slow in coming from the state. From 1913 to 1917, Mrs. Frederick C. Potter, the wife of the head pathologist, wrote autopsy reports, compiled statistics and did secretarial work for the department. Early on, the pathologists carried out tests for the assistant physicians. These included blood, urine, spinal fluid and tissue. Food was also examined. Sometimes the assistant physicians did their own tests if the workload was high for the pathologist. Dr. William B. Fletcher and Dr. Sarah Stockton worked in the lab (7).

THE SUPERINTENDENT

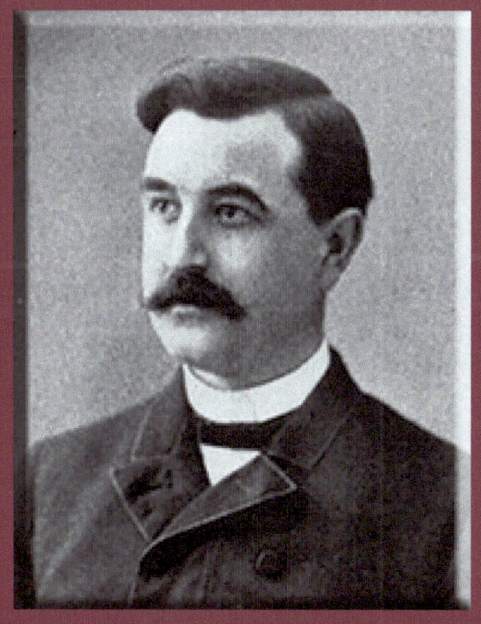

George F. Edenharter was born June 13, 1857. He grew up in Ohio and came to Indianapolis when he was 21 to work in the John Rauch cigar factory. He graduated six years later from the Physio-Medical College of Indianapolis in 1884 and received his M.D. in 1886 from the Medical College of Indiana.

His medical carerr began as chief of staff of the Marion County Infirmary and as a doctor for the city workhouse. Later he became the superintendent of the City Hospital and then he was appointed superintendent of the Central Indiana Hospital for the Insane until his death in 1923.

He was also responsible for the opening of Madison State Hospital (Madison, Indiana) and the Indiana Village for Epileptics (New Castle, Indiana).

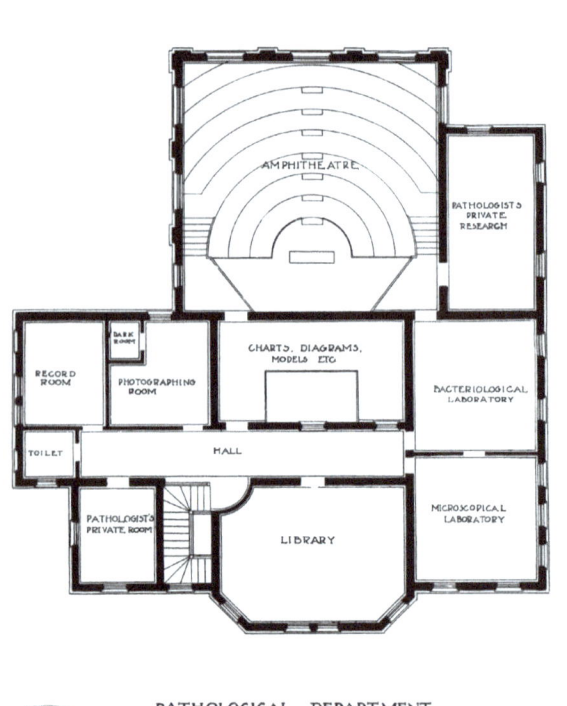

Left: Floor plans for the Pathology Department

TEACHING AND LEARNING

The Pathology Department solidified Central State Hospital's reputation as a teaching hospital for neurology, psychiatry and even early forensics. Professors from the Medical College of Indiana, and the College of Physicians and Surgeons taught courses there (8). The classes included lectures, autopsies, and patient observation. From 1907 to 1956 the Indiana University School of Medicine taught neurology and psychology classes at the building.

In 1898 mandatory staff training required a review of histology, bacteriology, chemistry, pathology and microscopy. Resident medical staff spent two hours every other day studying these topics. The pathologist offered one-on-one support. Sometimes evening classes, such as "Clinical Anatomy", "The Finer Anatomy of the Nervous System," and "Infection" were held. In 1899 "Outlines of Practical Histology: A manual for students" by William Stirling, MD, was required reading. The Marion County medical Society also used the building for meetings.

The work done with students prepared them to recognize and treat mental illness, and increase their understanding and ability to assess patients as sane or not. Training also helped them become interested in the field.

By the 1960s students no longer came to study and autopsies were viewed at Methodists Hospital. The lab closed in 1968 after Dr. Bruetsch retired.

CLINICAL EVALUATION AND EDUCATION

In 1898 Dr. Max Bahr developed a plan for clinical evaluation of patients. He used medical science from the day to back up his findings. This information was disseminated to colleges and universities across Indiana and the United States. He was also the first doctor at the hospital to have formal training as a psychologist, obtaining a doctoral degree in 1909 from the University of Berlin.

From the 1880s to 1930s doctors were trained in this way to take care of patients. The Pathology Department stated in an annual report that a "vast number of letters from institutions and universities received copies of the pathology report and commented on how valuable the information was."

In 1923 Dr. Bahr became superintendent of the hospital. He recruited Dr. Walter Ludwig Bruetsch to be the pathologist. Under their leadership, students continued to come to classes at the lab, even during WWII.

In addition to changes from inside the lab, the Flexner Report (5) ensured changes to the medical teaching profes-

Opposite:
Top: The beautiful wood staircase to the second floor.
Bottom: one of the many steam radiators.

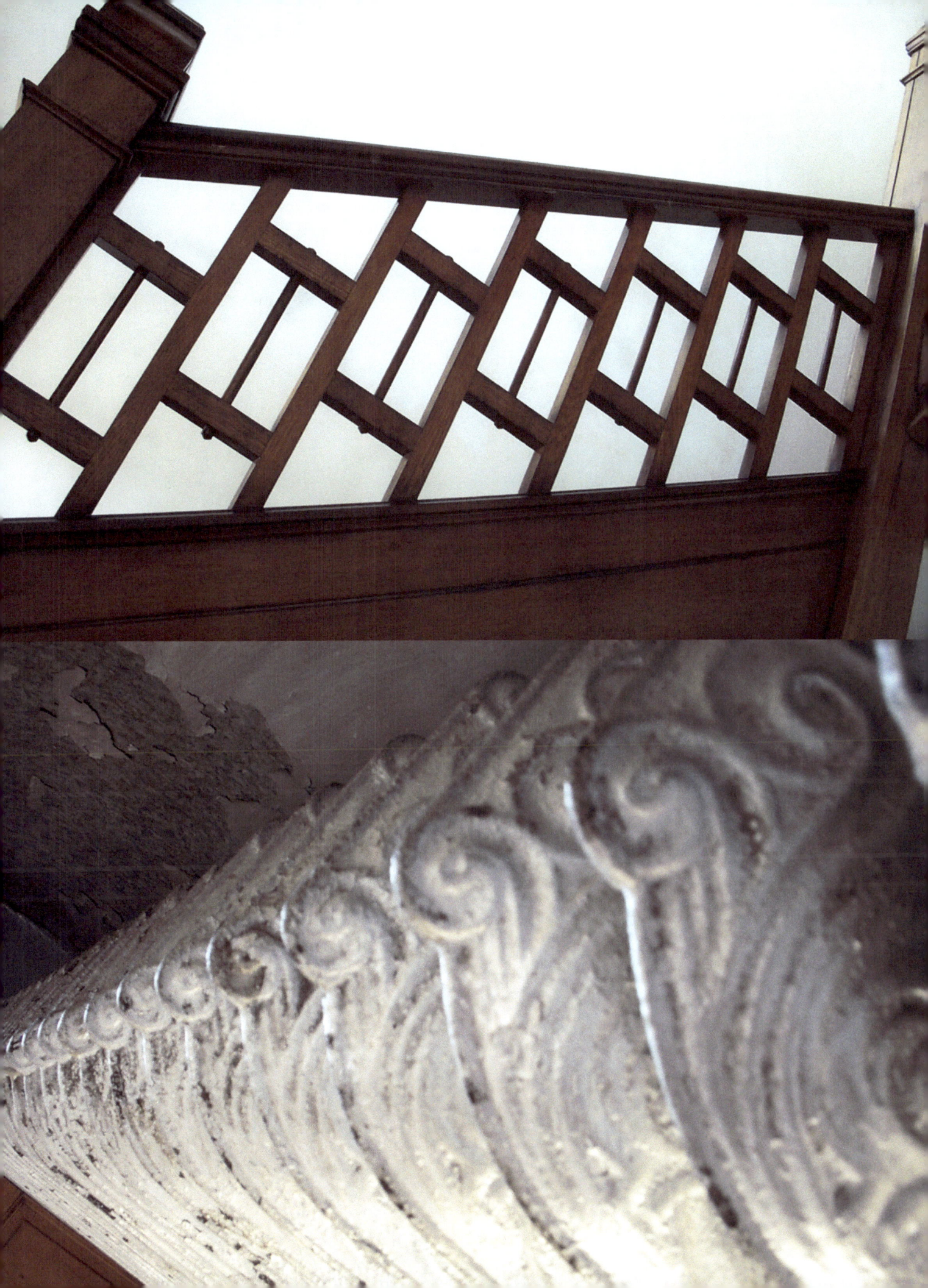

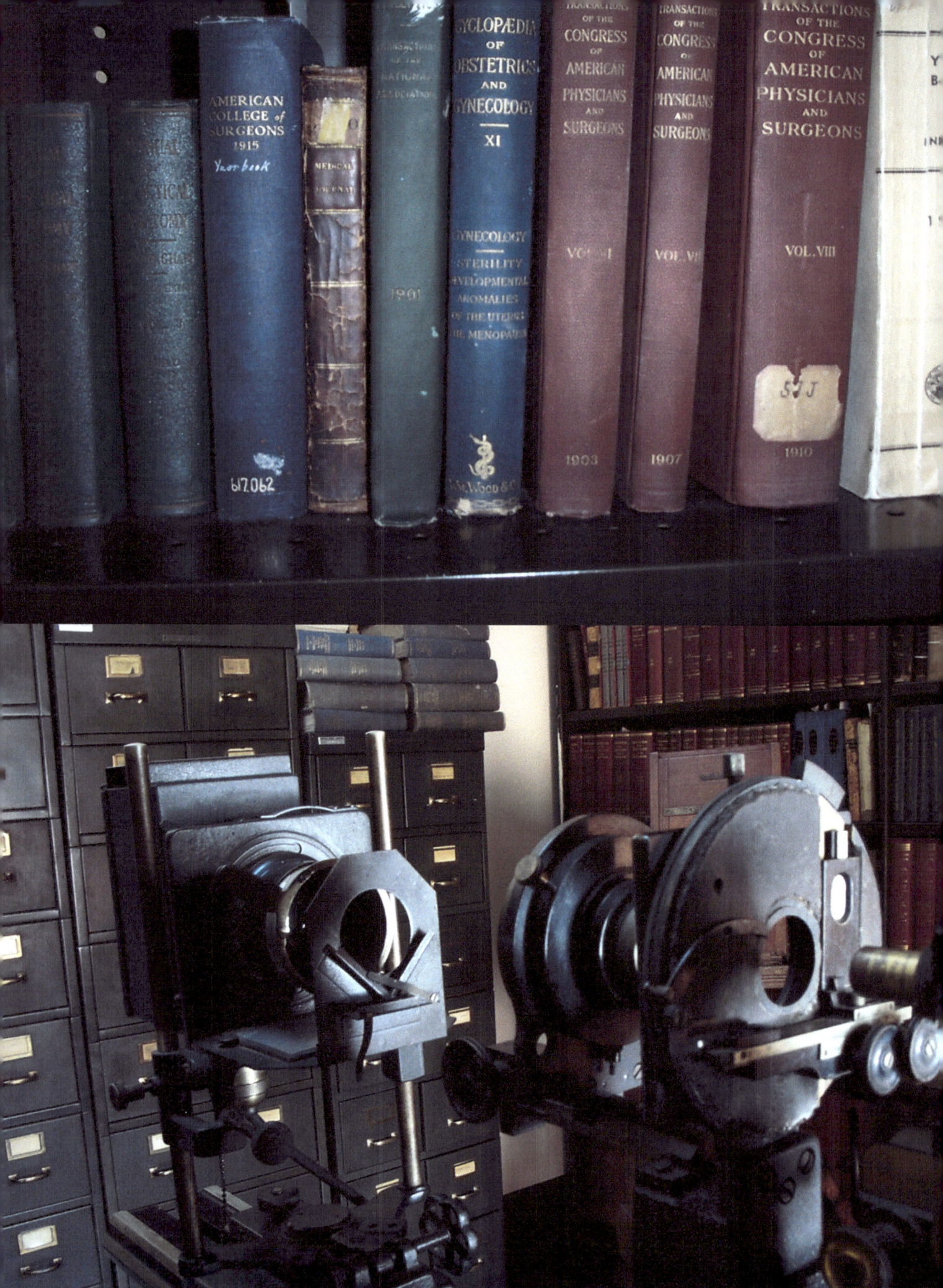

sion. Standardization, clinical procedures, and research were introduced into the education program. State licensing laws and higher standards for medical students were enacted. During WWII, accelerated programs were offered due to the need of doctors. The curriculum was covered in three years instead of four (6).

Until the 1950s students continued to come to classes at the lab. Every Saturday, a two to three hour class on neurology and psychiatry was conducted by Bahr and Bruetsch, with Dr. Larue Carter and Dr. Albert Sterne lecturing occasionally.

Bruetsch was remembered for his thick German accent. It was so thick that the students could barely keep up with understanding the concepts, let alone creating notes. The enterprising wife of one student would attend the lecture, transcribe her notes and sell them to other students for a quarter apiece. The first half of this class was lecture, followed by examination of patients. Slides and specimens were used, but students did not actually conduct tests or have hands-on practice.

Other organizations and students also used the lab's resources. From 1940 to 1960, medical residents studying for examinations given by the American Board of Psychiatry and Neurology used the lab's slides and specimens for study. Social workers and ministers used to attend lectures in the building. Lawyers came to classes on mental jurisprudence. Psychology students from Indiana University, DePauw University, Purdue University, and Butler College (now University) came until 1940.

Autopsies

During a typical year, the Pathology Department would report on how many people died and how many autopsies were performed. Information recorded included the gender, cause of death and any disease or anomalies with the body. The pathologist and assistant physicians attended these procedures. The organs and tissues were studied and sometimes put on display in the anatomical museum for teaching purposes.

Generally, this work was slow in the beginning because not many families wanted autopsies done on their family members and because staffing the lab was a problem. Research on the causes and prevention of mental illness was minimal. Case studies were often used instead of research being done at the facility.

During one year, 180 people died at Central State Hospital. Only 18 of them were autopsied. Each one had their brains removed. Five thousand, one hundred sixty –seven microscopial preparations were made from autopsy material for use by other medical facilities for research. Slide sets were prepared for candidates taking the examination for the American Board of Psychiatry and Neurology, as well as for other schools around the county. The lab did a study on late cerebral sequalae of rheumatic fever. Dr. Bahr and Dr. Bruetsch also made several presentations, and the staff consulted at hospitals and schools.

Malarial Treatment of Syphilis

The most significant research done at the Pathology Department was the malarial treatment of syphilis. Syphilis is a brutal disease. It starts as sores, which seem to improve, then it comes back and it can attack the heart and central nervous system, causing dementia or paresis. This results in the loss of power and mental abilities, which leads to death. In 1930 30% of admissions were due to syphilis, which was the most common form of insanity at the time (3).

Early treatments included arsenic or mercury- neither was effective.
- 1905: The bacterium that caused syphilis was isolated but it didn't lead to a cure.
- 1909: German doctor, Dr. Paul Ehrlich created "606" (Salvarsen), which was a huge hope, but still arsenic-based and required multiple injections before eradicating the disease.
- 1917: Austrian psychiatrist Julius Wagner- Juaregg found that if he injected patients with malaria, the syphilis was killed. Then, after an incubation period, quinine cured the malaria. He received a Nobel Prize in 1927 for this work (4).

Bahr and Bruetsch worked on the malarial treatment by researching it at Central State Hospital. Bruetsch also studied syphilitic optic atrophy in which the eye degenerates because of syphilis. Dr. C.P. Clark, head of the hospital's eye department, determined that the malarial treatment was as effective as, or better than surgery.

Opposite top: Some of the many books contained in the medical library.

Opposite bottom: Camera equipment to make specimen slides.

In the first 100 people treated with the malarial treatment at Central State Hospital, 25 were discharged as improved, 21 returned to their former lives, and 12 were expected to be discharged. Fifty cases had no improvement and 32 of these showed a decline. However the researchers said "untidy" patients now kept themselves neat and attacks of excitement either disappeared or lessened in severity, which was overall an improvement. Five patients died- two because of the malaria, two from complications of late stage paresis (2) and one from pneumonia. Of the 100 patients, 18 died within two weeks to 18 months of treatment. Those who died had late stage paresis.

Bruetsch believed in cases of success, immune cells in the brain attacked the malarial parasites, versus destroying the organism that caused syphilis which was the common believe. He demonstrated this and won recognition for it. In 1931, the hospital won international recognition for improvements in malarial therapy technique in syphilitic patients. For this type of work in 1938, the Pathological Department at Central State Hospital was considered one of the Top 20 research facilities nationwide.

In 1940 a new quartan strain, which caused seizures and fever every four days rather than every third like the standard tertian strain was introduced to Central State Hospital. It was used for treating African American syphilitics, as well as Caucasian patients who were unresponsive to the tertian strain. The Pathology Department became a world leader in this type of treatment. From 1930 to 1945, 1846 samples were sent for study to different doctors around the country. Bruetsch and Bahr created an exhibit called "Neurosyphilis and the Malaria Treatment of General Paresis" and traveled with it. Dr. Wagner- Juaregg was in attendance at one of the presentations.

The beginning of the end of this treatment began during WWII. Java, who was the supplier of 90% of the world's anti-malaria drugs, was under the control of Japan. Therefore, the Pathology Department and Eli Lilly & Company began testing other anti-malarial drugs. This effort was hampered by home front constraints.

The Malarial Treatment became obsolete when penicillin became available after WWII. Bruetsch agreed it was a superior treatment.

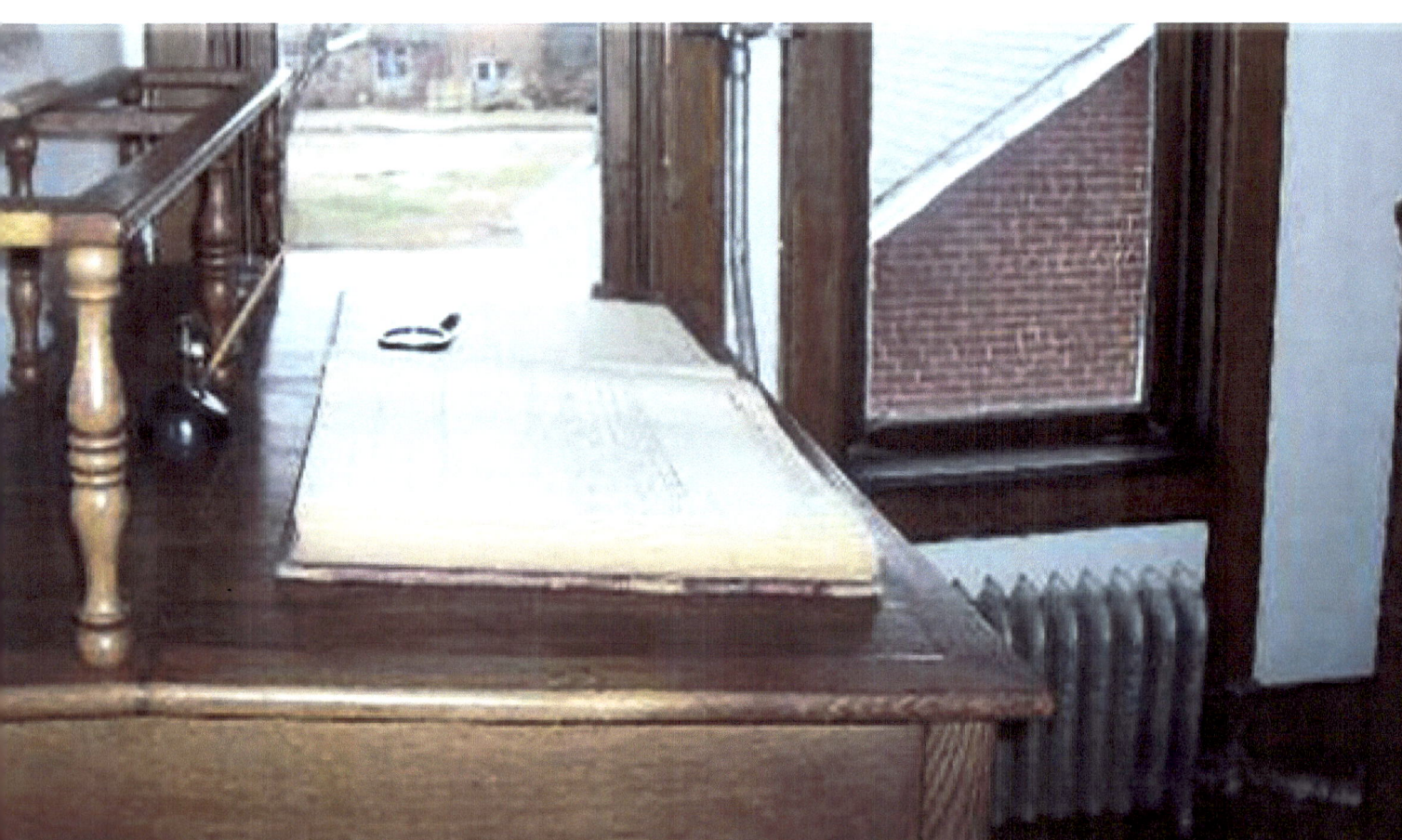

Bottom: A transcriber would stand in the Records Room and listen to the information being send through the speaking tube. The transcriber would record the information in the book on the desk. The autopsy results were sometimes included in yearly reports to the State of Indiana.

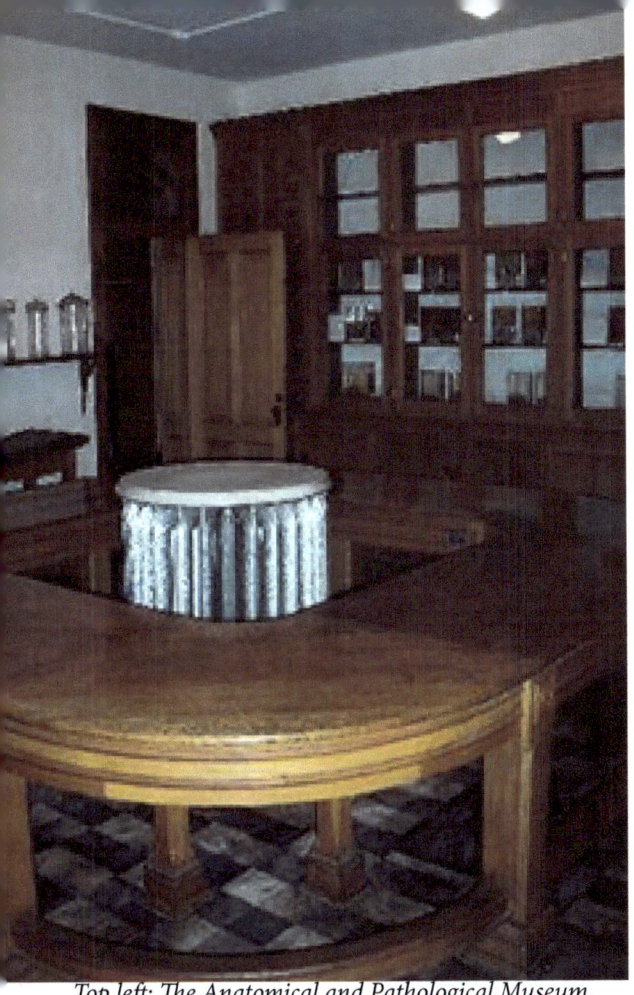
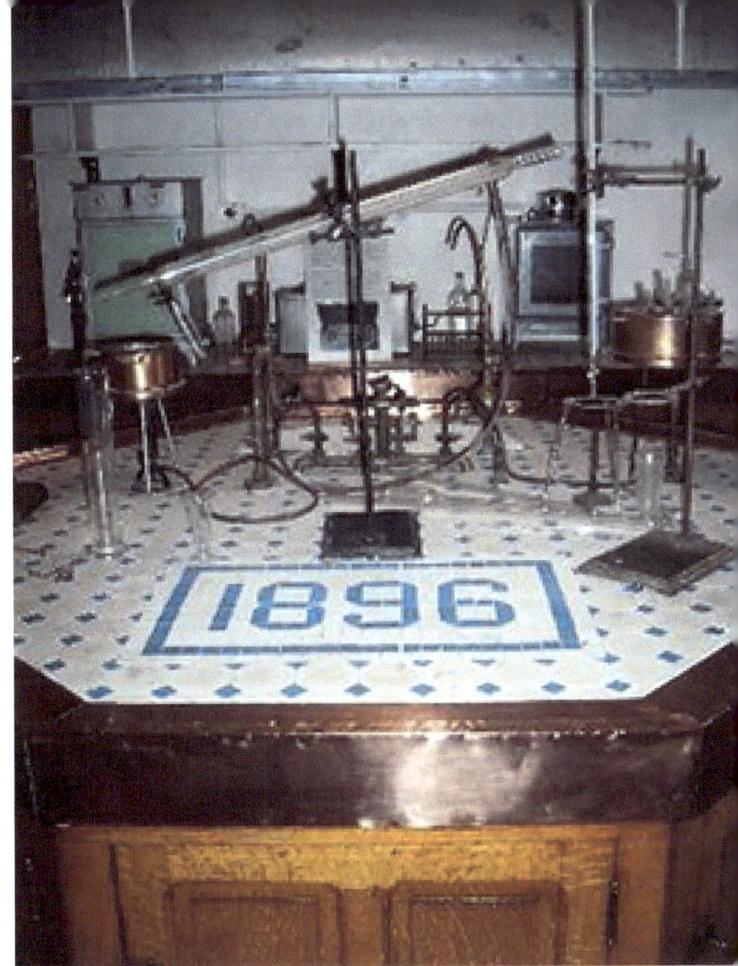

Top left: The Anatomical and Pathological Museum.
Top right: The Chemical Laboratory.
Bottom left: Amphitheatre where student and other lectures were held.. Much of the equipment and chairs are original.
Bottom right: Gravity drinking fountain.

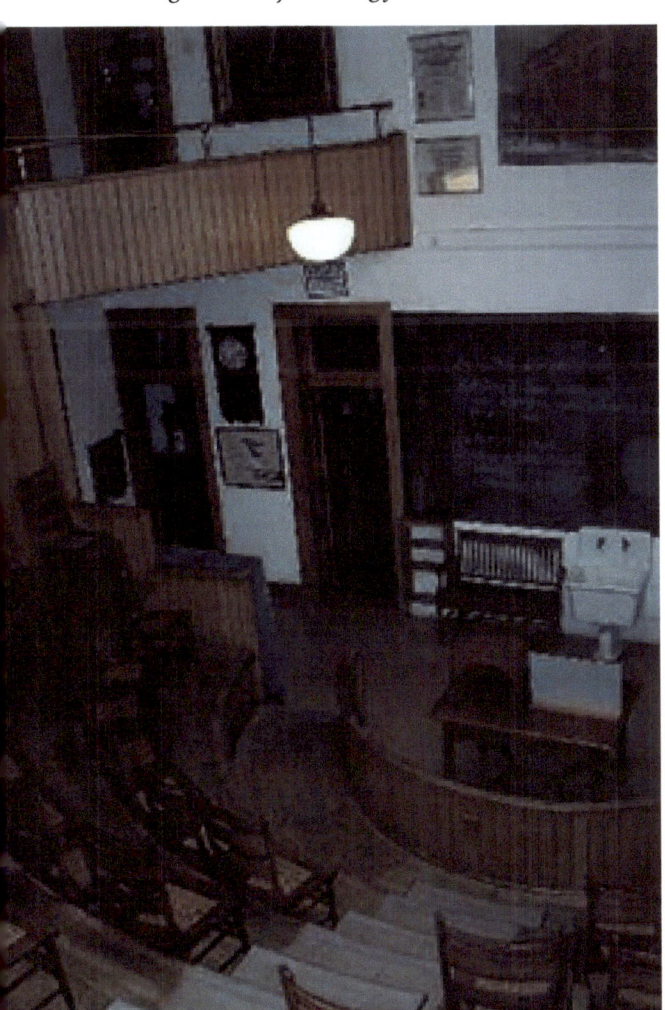
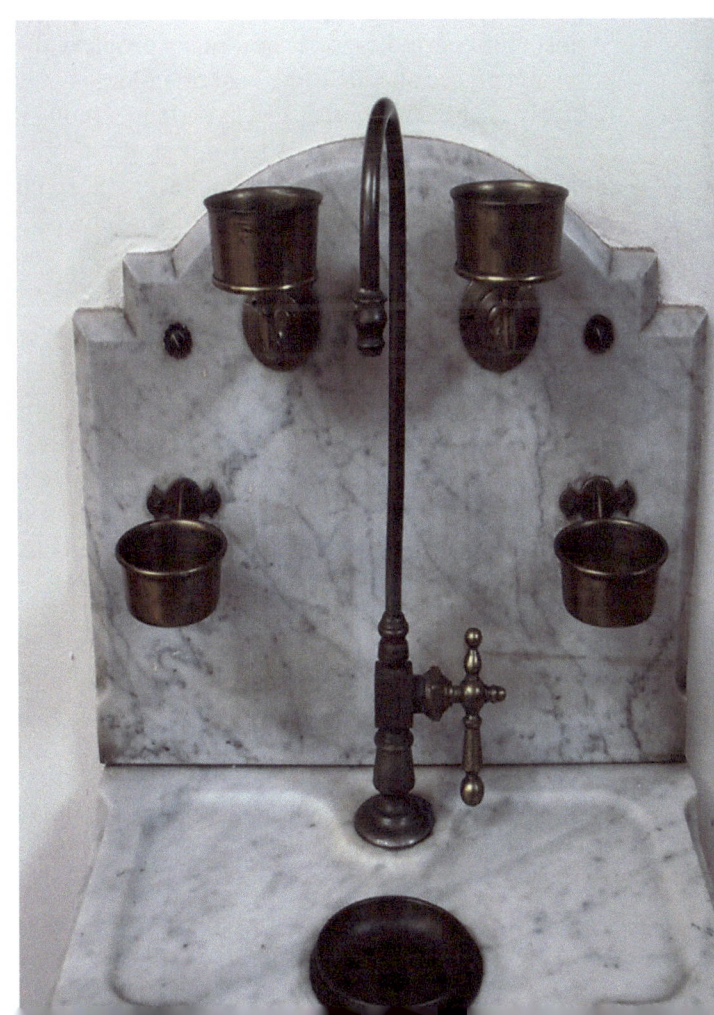

Spinal Fluid

In addition to syphilis testing, spinal fluid research was conducted. The most used test was the colloidal gold test. Sodium chloride solution and spinal fluid were combined in 11 test tubs and colloidal gold reagent was added. Within 23 hours the samples changed color. The sequence of colors in the eleven tubes indicated whether a patient was suffering from one of the stages of syphilis, or from another disease, such as meningitis.

Rheumatic Brain Disease

Bruetsch also studied rheumatic disease in the brain. After a streptococcal infection, the antibodies produced to fight the infection can attack the body's tissues, producing rheumatic fever. The result is severe damage to the heart and kidney, and lesions and inflammation of the arteries. Bruetsch believed it could damage the brain as well.

He believed in "rheumatic epilepsy." When people had rheumatic brain disease, sometime they suffered seizures. Dr. Bruetsch believed the seizures came from the lesions. In 1941 he received an award from the Layman's League against Epilepsy for his research.

Additionally in November 1936 the National Committee for Mental Hygiene asked the hospital to participate in a study of dementia praecox (schizophrenia in today's terms). Doctors at the hospital did post mortem studies to see how many people with dementia praecox had rheumatic brain lesions.
Today, rheumatic brain disease is no longer thought to be a cause of mental illness but this study still shows the dedicated research doctors did at the hospital to finding new insights and cures for mental illness.

The Ralston Needle

Dr. John D. Ralston, a psychiatric physician, created the Ralston Needle. It differed from the earlier 1868 Duchenne Needle that only sampled the muscle tissue. The Ralston Needle provided an electrical recording of the muscle. Dr. Charles Bonsett, a retired Indianapolis neurologist, said the needle was first used on steak, which they found was not the same as human tissue. Now, donated tissue from multiple sclerosis patients is used.

Decline and Rebirth

By the 1950s the lab was becoming antiquated. When Dr. Bahr retired, Dr. Clifford Williams became the next superintendent and was reportedly not

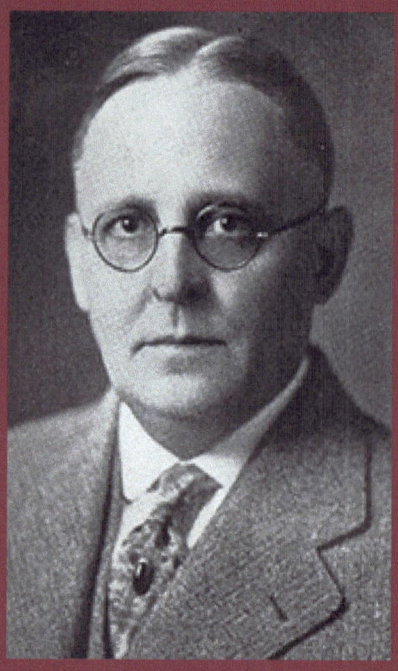

Dr. Max Bahr
(Mar. 21, 1872 – Jan. 24, 1953)
Bahr received his high school education from Shortridge High School and later his medical degree from the Central College of Physicians and surgeons in 1896. Bahr began working at Central State Hospital in 1898 and in 1923 he was appointed superintendent. During his early days, he realized that American psychiatry was not as advanced as Germany and he educated himself to bring new knowledge to the hospital. Additionally, he earned a degree of Doctor of Psychological Medicine from the University of Berlin in 1908 and began practicing as a clinical psychiatrist at Central State Hospital.

Bahr also had a fascination with the tie between crime and mental illness. As a result, Bahr conducted the first courses in America for lawyers in forensic psychiatry. He was very dedicated to his work and became the president of the Indianapolis Medical Society. He was instrumental in changing the name of the hospital so it on longer contained the word "insane". He retired March 1952.

as involved in the Pathology Department as Bahr had been. In 1956 Indiana University stopped sending students to the lab for classes because the school wanted the hospital to add full time doctors to the lab for classes and other tasks, which the hospital could not afford. Instead, students went to Larue Carter Memorial Hospital, which was opened for the treatment of acute psychiatric illnesses, clinical research and teaching.

By the 1960s, Dr. Bruetsch and Dr. Charles Bonsett were the last doctors working at the lab. Dr. Charles Bonsett maintained an EEG laboratory and the Indiana Neuromuscular Research Lab.

The labs weren't enough to keep the doors open. By 1969 the Pathology Department was no longer functioning and the building was in danger of the wrecking ball. Dr. Bonsett and other physicians and citizens established a not-for-profit to preserve the building and put it on the National Register of Historic Places (NRHP). Some of those people were:

- Dr. Charles Bonsett
- Dr. John U. Keating
- Dr. Dwight W. Schuster
- Dr. William M. Sholty
- Mrs. Donald J. White
- Dr. E. Vernon Hahan (and a bequest that allowed the amphitheater to be restored, and allowed the building to be added to the NRHP)

The Indiana Medical History Museum (IMHM)

The IMHM began in 1969 and the Pathology Department building was put on the National Register of Historic Places in 1971. In 1986 the State of Indiana gave the organization a 99 year lease of the building and the surrounding five acres. The museum building is one of the few pathology lab buildings in North America and is the oldest surviving example in the United States. It contains most of the original equipment used during its time as a lab. Medical specimens such as brains and skeletons reside in the anatomical and pathological museum. The morgue and lecture rooms, with original and period chairs and equipment, show visitors what the functions of the building were. Outside is a medicinal garden that is used to demonstrate the type of natural medications used in the 1800-1900s, some of which are known to be lethal today. According to the museum's website, its mission is to interpret and preserve the building and educate the public on health care, health careers, and life sciences in Indiana during the nineteenth and part of the twentieth centuries. The museum offers tours of the lab facility, exhibits, and provides the public, medical professional and researchers, schools and businesses with educational opportunities.

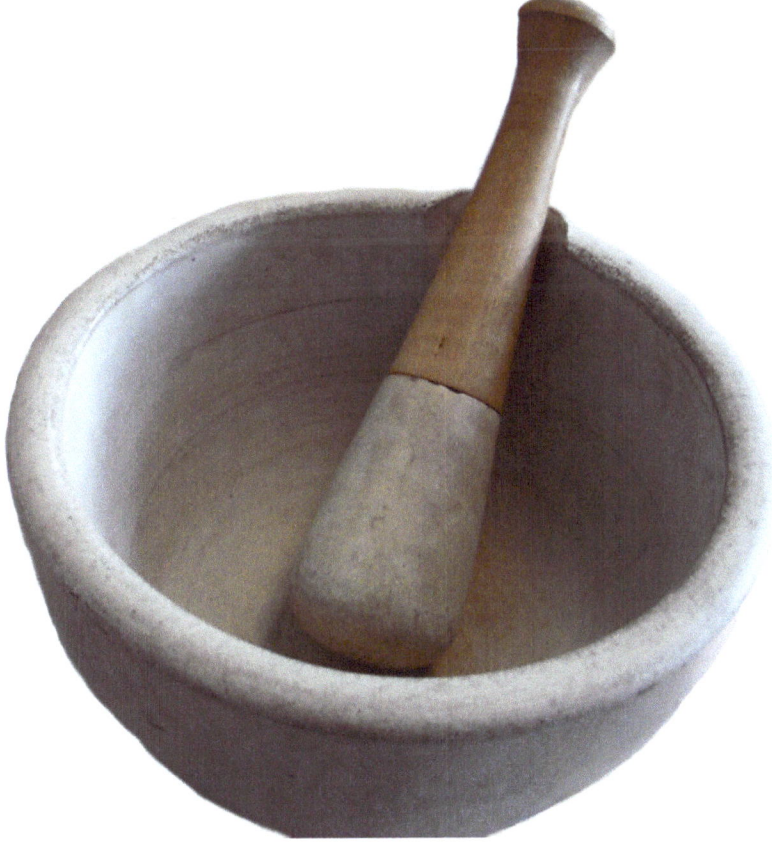

Left: A mortar and pestle for mixing from the Chemical Laboratory.

DR. WALTER BRUETSCH
(Nov. 25, 1896-Jan. 31, 1977)

Dr. Bruetsch was born in Heidelberg, Germany. During WWI he received a debilitating spinal injury during the Battle of the Somme. He was treated by Dr. Babinski, a noted neurologist. After the war, he started his studies to become a physician and received his degree in Freiberg, Germany in 1922.

Two years later, he immigrated to Indianapolis and began his research on the malarial treatment of syphilis in 1925.

From 1955-1957, Dr. Bruetsch was out of the lab because he contracted tuberculosis. When he returned, he continued his research in the hardening of the brain's arteries, rheumatic endarteritis (inflammation of arteries due to rheumatic disease). He was internationally renowned for his neurosyphilis research.

Interestingly, in the 1990s, technology made it more possible to study Bruetsch's theories on immunological methods, and fever treatment of paresis and its effects on the brain. His study on the effects of streptococcal infection in the brain is still being explored. Most recently Indiana University's Pathological Department has been using Dr. Bruetsch's research to look for schizophrenia markers in patients with mental illnesses.

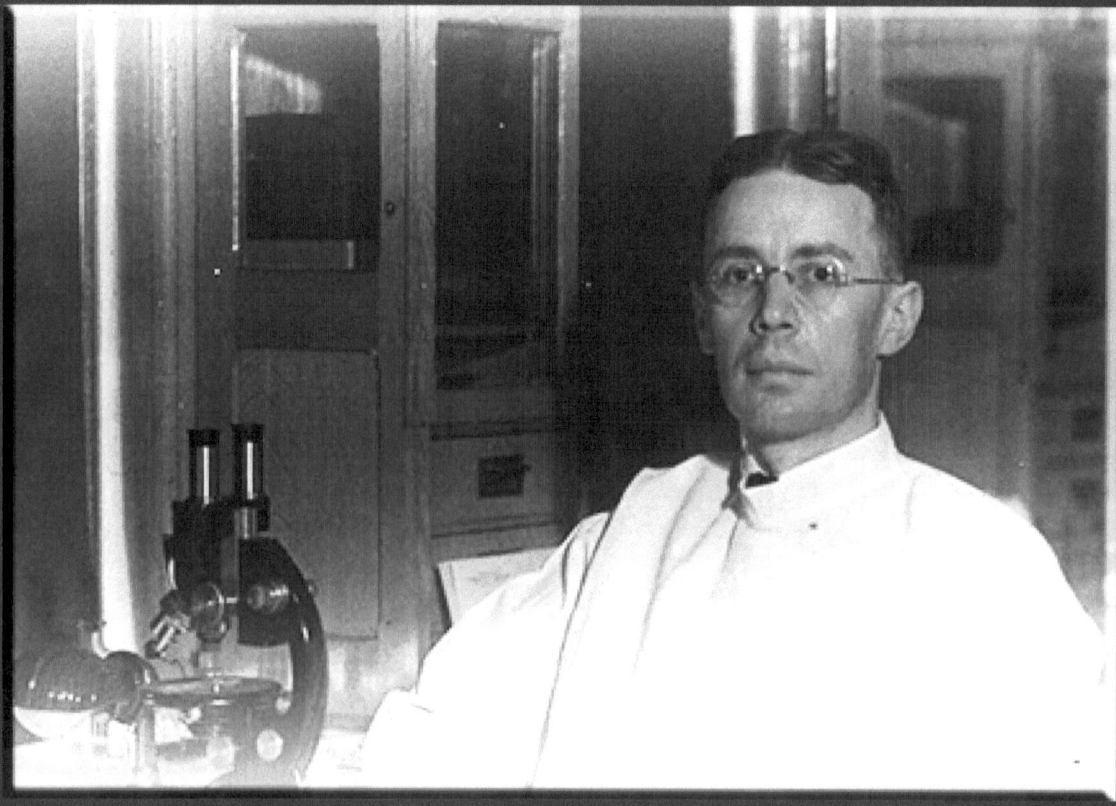

Above: Dr. Walter Bruetsch

Opposite top: The Bacteriological Laboratory.

Opposite bottom: The Anatomical and Pathological Museum.

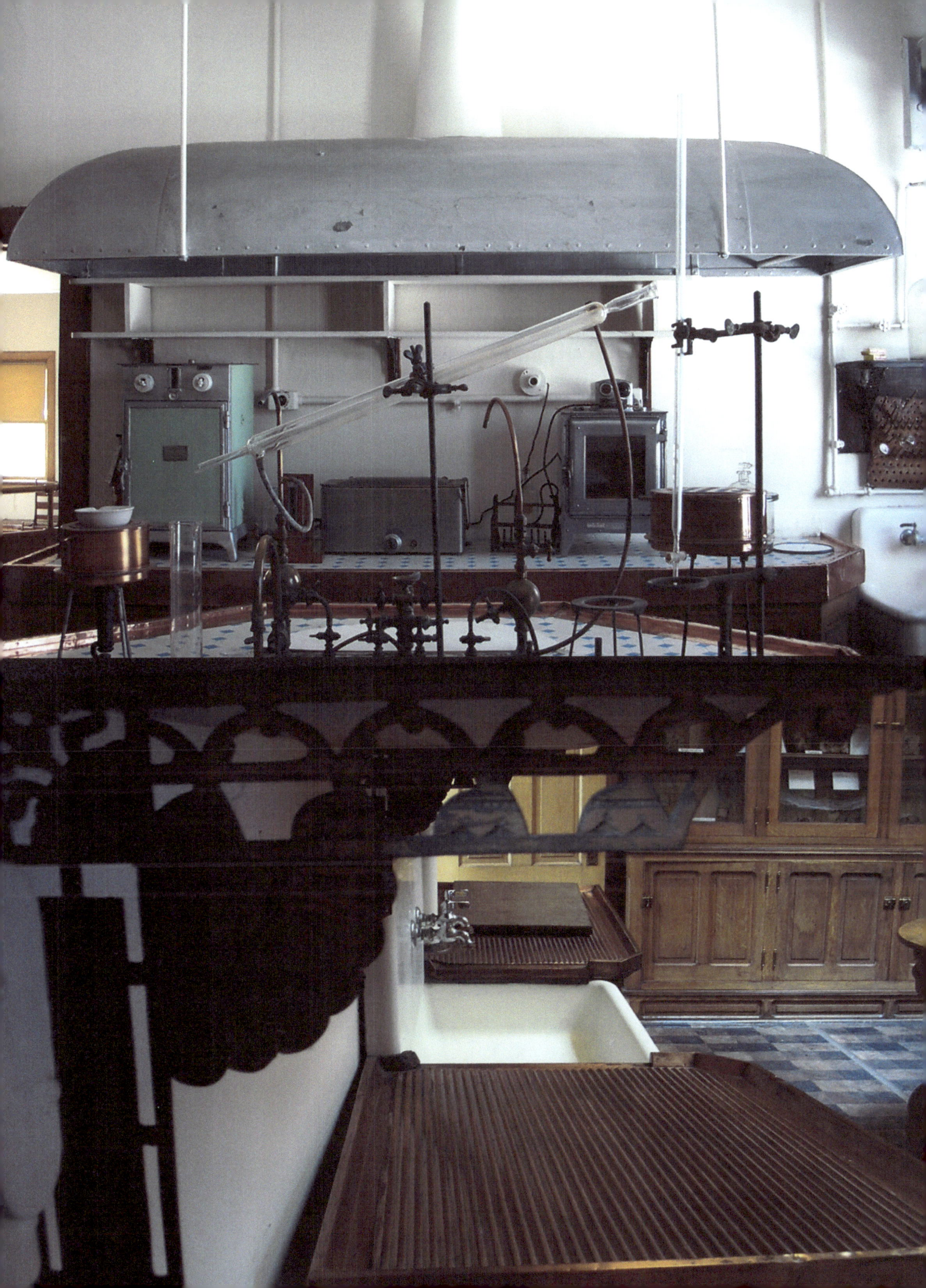

"SADIE" AND "MAXIE"

In 1989 a box of mementos and letters from a female patient named Sadie was found in the Indiana Medical History Museum. The contents of the box provided a view into a patient's life that is normally unavailable. Sadie was believed to have worked as an assistant or custodian as part of her occupational therapy. She was admitted to the hospital in the late 1890s and lived on Ward 11 in the Women's Department, which was medium security. Her letters were found in a crawlspace in the Pathology Department in 1941. Her unread, unmailed letters were filled with religious imagery, elation and darker messages: "October is a great love month. For me the same as March. So much more beautiful." And "Beware of mad dogs." Another letter states that the dentist at the hospital stole her gold fillings.

Sadie wrote of passes to see her father and of dances at the hospital at "The Grove", where the attendants would dance with the patients. She also wrote letters to Dr. Bahr, who was often referred to as "pet" or "Maxie".

Sadie's thoughts and diagnosis seem to point to schizophrenia. During her time at the hospital, schizophrenia was treated with insulin therapy. On October 14, 1940 Sadie wrote a letter to Dr. Bruetsch asking to go home, and she asked him to put the matter to the Board of Trustees. She died shortly after the letter was written.

Letters, along with tiny tubes of crimson lipstick, were also found wrapped in a handkerchief in the box. They were given to Sadie's daughter, who was only ten years old when her mother went to the hospital. To have a piece of her mother back was priceless.

Below: The morgue, also known as the "Dead House". This is where the patient bodies were stored until family claimed them or a burial took place. Opposite: A corridor in the Department for Women.

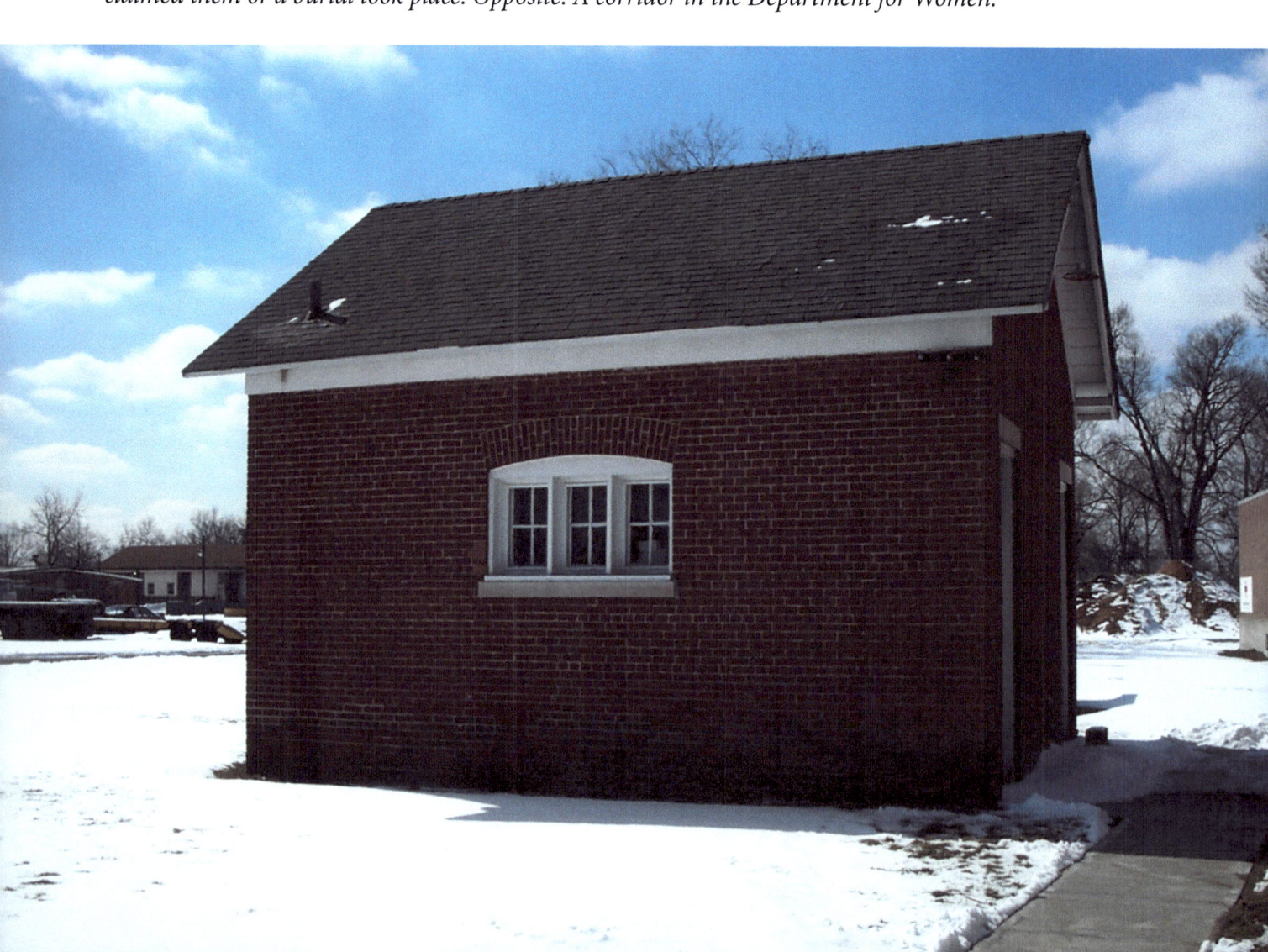

Ten

BUILDINGS

After Central State Hospital closed, treasure hunters used metal detectors on the area to find artifacts from the hospital. Additionally, soccer teams played on the east side and in the area of the Department for Women. Many people would jog or walk pets through the haunting wooded area. The police also housed horses and the overflow vehicle pool at the hospital. SWAT practiced in the Evans and Bolton buildings.

Unfortunately, due to heavy trespassing at night by thrill seekers, who stole items from the hospital and further damaged structures, the grounds became off limits except for people visiting the Indiana Medical History Museum.

This book contains a listing of all buildings according to the time period in which they were built. Because of appropriations, delays and some misinformation in certain non-source materials, the exact date they were opened may differ from other sources. This information was taken from 1897, 1898, 1914, 1915, 1936, and 1956 Sanborn maps, historic Indianapolis GIS maps, visual verification and annual reports. Not all minor buildings (such as old pump houses and cisterns) are accounted for.

Also, not all the information was available for every building. Sometimes wall thickness, material or equipment for one building is given but not another building.

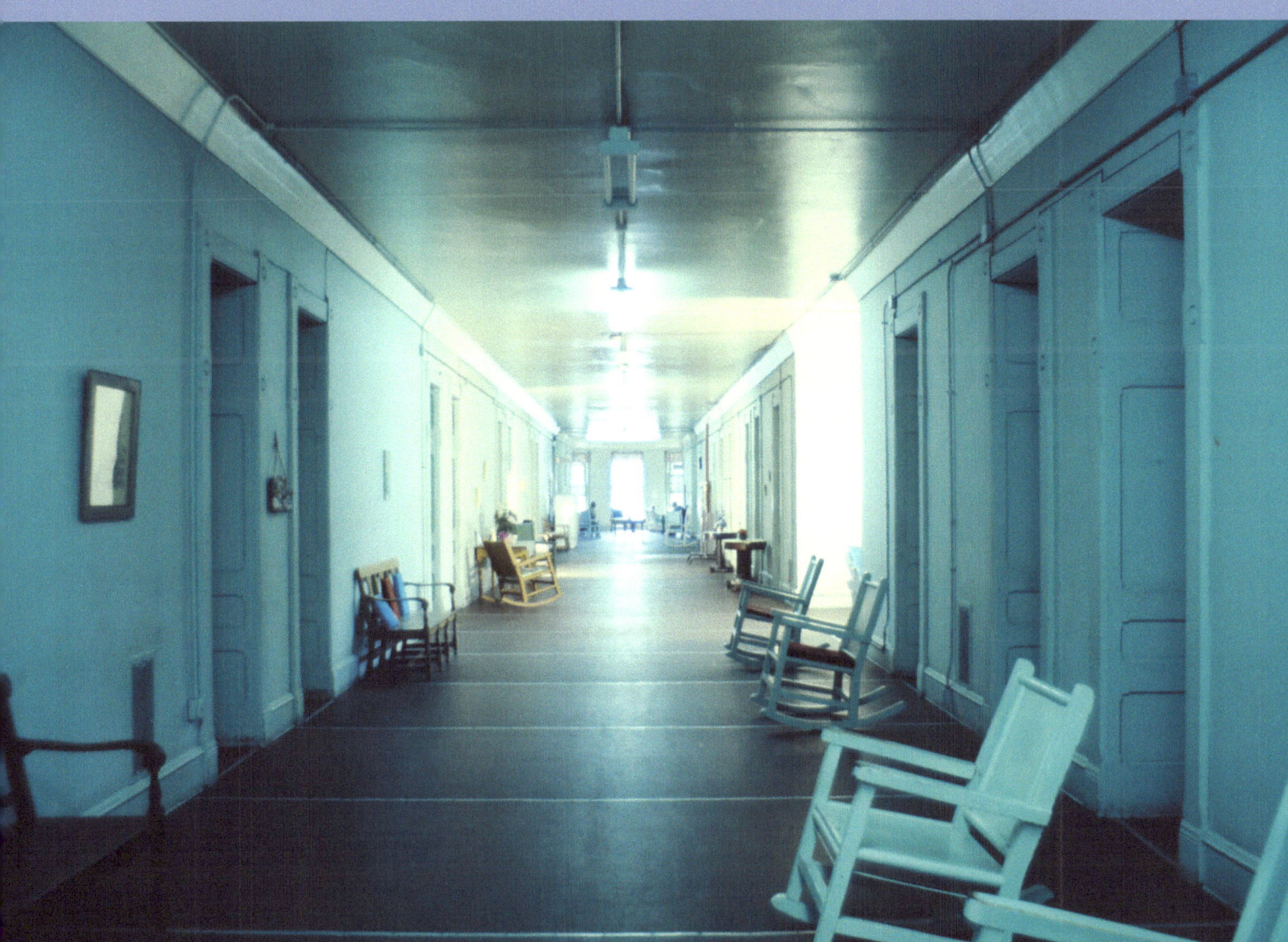

The list contains building numbers from the 1936 and 1956 Sanborn maps. Two numbers were unaccounted for. These numbers may have been Cottages 5 and 6 that were planned, but not built.

BUILDINGS *(according to 1936 and 1956 Sanborn maps)*
1. North Infirmary (Women)
2. North Dining Room (Women)
3. Department for Women (Seven Steeples; Old Main)
4. Sick Hospital
5. South Dining Room (Women)
6. Pathology Department
7. Morgue (Storage)
8. South Infirmary (Women)
9. Bake House
10. Ice House
11. Farm and Garden Barn (not labeled in 1936. It had no name at this time.)
12. Pipe shop
13. Coal Room
14. Boiler House and Power Plant
15. Pipe Shop
16. Store and Supply House
17. Laundry
18. Fire Department (interestingly, "18" was the number of the new station)
19. Mattress factory
20. Carpenter's Shop
21. Storage (also known as Paint Shop)
22. Unknown- not on either map
23. North Dining Room (Men) (also known as Men's Recreation Hall)
24. Kitchen (Men)
25. South Dining Room (Men)
26. Infirmary No 1 (Men)
27. Unknown- not on either map
28. Men's Cottage 3
29. Cornelius Mayer Hall (also known as Mayer Hall)
30. Pump House (east of Mayer Hall)
31. Greenhouses
32. Men's Cottage 2
33. Men's Cottage 1
34. Men's Cottage 4
35. Employee Building ("Administration Building")
36. Men's Cottage 7

Other Non-numbered Buildings

These were either small building that were either not considered necessary to have numbering, were razed before 1936, or were built after 1956.

- Department of Men (cottages)
- Pavilion
- Washhouse
- Deep pump house
- Pump house (north of the coal room)
- Pump house (south of the Department for Men)
- Watch house
- Officer's barn
- Junk Shop
- Garbage Furnace (Refuse Burner)
- Tin Shop
- Refrigeration
- Canning plant
- Motel/Employee Housing
- Doctor Housing
- Kitchen/Dining room
- Bahr Building
- Bolton Building
- Evans Building
- Oil House
- Car Storage
- Gas House
- Body Shop
- Car Wash
- Artificial lake
- New Power Plant
- Paint Shop (aka Laundry)
- Exit House

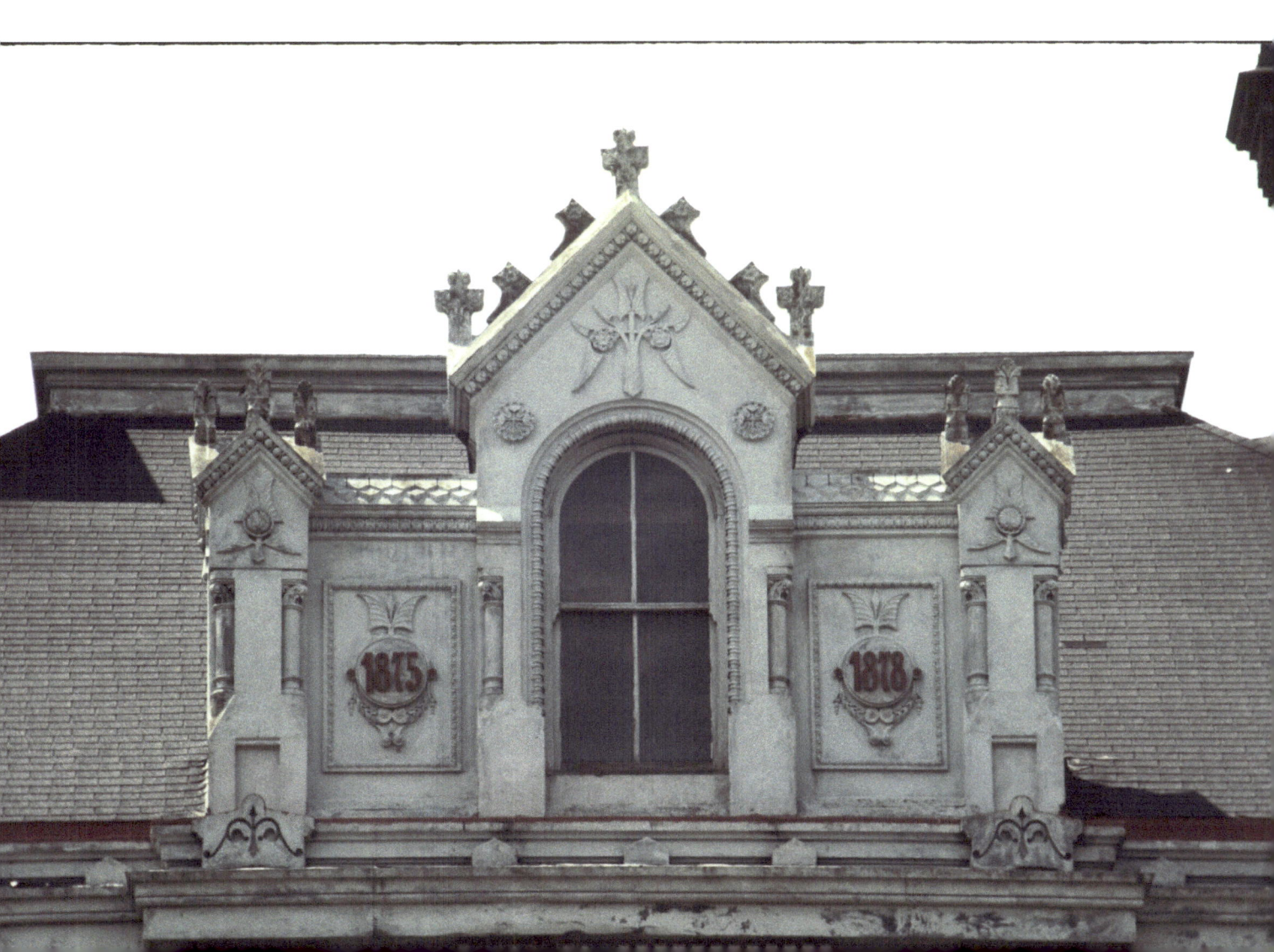

DEPARTMENT FOR MEN
WARDS: Q.T.W.Z.
WARDS: P.S.V.Y.
WARDS: O.R.U.X.
WARDS: M.G.F.T.
WARDS: A.D.C.K.
WARDS: B.E.H.L.
DINING ROOM
KITCHEN
STORAGE
LAUNDRY
DRY RM.
CARP'R SHOP
BENCH WORK
PLANING MILL
OFFICE
MATTRESS FACTY
FIRE DEPT.
SLEEPING RMS.
OFFICERS STABLE
JUNK SHOP
STORAGE
"THE STORE"
DIRECTORS RMS.
TREAS. OFFC.
CORNELIUS MAYER HALL
CHAPEL
GREEN HOUSES
GLASS ROOFS
CORR. IRON ON STEEL TRUSS ROOF
CEMENT FLOOR
10"W. PIPE (CITY)
8"W. PIPE (PRIVATE)
8"W. PIPE (CITY)
12"W. PIPE
4"W. PIPE
6"W. PIPE
14"W. PIPE
4"N. PIPE
TUNNEL
CISTERN
500 BBLS.
SHED
PIPE SHOP

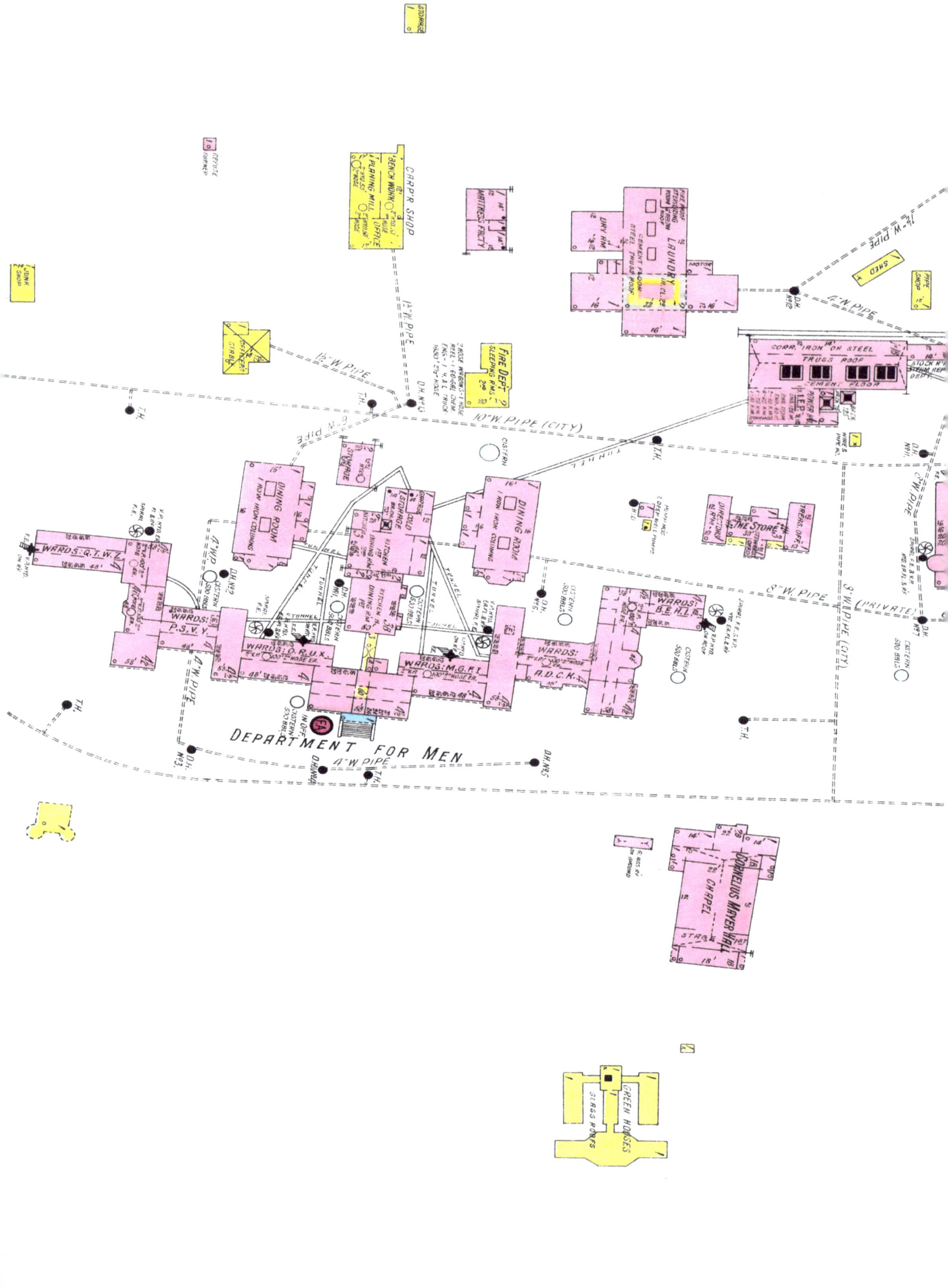

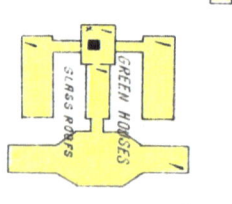

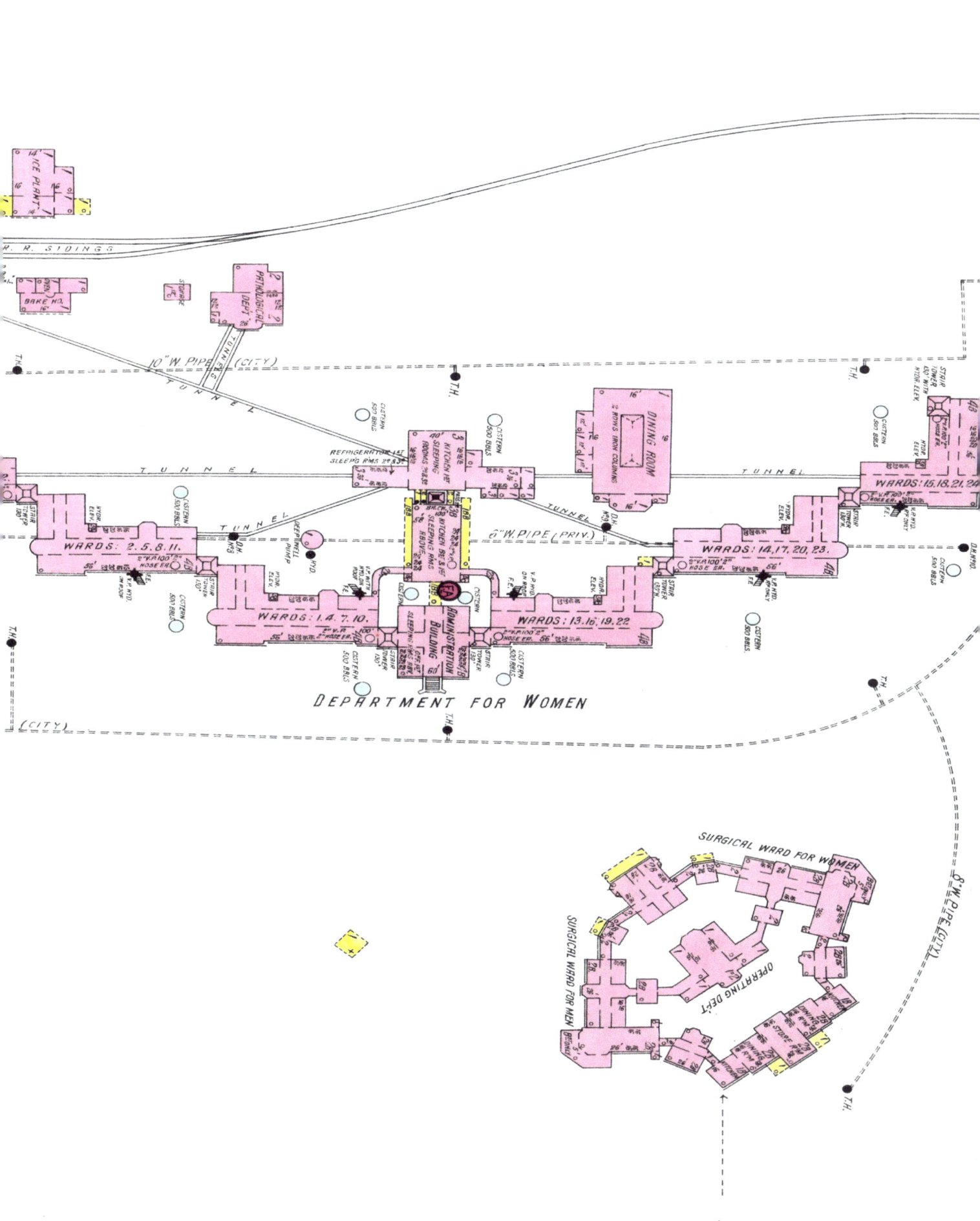

Original Central State Building (aka the Department for Men)
Built: 1845-1870
Razed: 1930s

Originally, the hospital's first building was used for men and women. The hospital planned to have wings for women and men but in the very early days of the hospital women and men were housed in the same area but separated as best as possible. The superintendent recommended the wings be finished as quickly as possible because of the "excessive talking and physical communication" going on between the men and women. Once the wings were built, the north wing was for women and the south wing for men.

The south wing was completed in 1853 and opened on March 1, 1855. The north wing opened in 1870. The reason the south wing took a year and a half to open was that in 1853, there was no appropriation for the hospital. When an appropriation was made in 1854, there were other pressing items which took place over furnishing the wing. The original cost for the wings, $35,000 was exceeded because labor and materials were in deep demand and more expensive. The foundation had to be put in twice as deep at twice the cost. During this time, the hospital administration indicated they had to pick and choose who could be admitted based on the likelihood of being cured. Other insane people who were considered incurable or dangerous were housed in jails. The superintendent's report stated in 1852, "These things ought not to exist in a Christian community. They will not long exist in Indiana."

The building was four stories tall with a basement. It was built on a "straight block system" versus the Kirkbride Plan, which began in 1852 (see the section on Kirkbride in this book). The building contained over 600 rooms, 206,341 square feet, and 2,269,751 cubic feet to heat. The attic contained 100 gallon tanks for holding the running water for the indoor plumbing. This water was forced into the tanks through steam pumps, and gravity pushed the water down.

Shortly after the building opened, the administration asked for part of the building be set aside for the "furiously sick", meaning the noisy and violently insane. These rooms were created as small areas with thick brick walls between them to keep the noise level lower and to keep the patients and others safe. The wall thicknesses throughout the building were 16 to 20 inches. Based on maps and some patient recollections, it is believed these wards were the basement and first floors of the "back wards", meaning the northern most and southern most areas of the north and south wings.

The building seemed to need repairs quite often and the hospital needed outside upgrades to function. In 1853 while going through a budget shortfall (the State had made no appropriation for the hospital), the superintendent said that just five short years after the hospital opened, the heating needed repaired. Additionally, the hospital sewers filtered raw sewage into Eagle Creek. As a result, the current wells were contaminated and a new well needed to be drilled eight feet in diameter below the level of Eagle Creek. The contractor used lead pipes, which didn't dispel the bad sewer gas well enough but they were constructed big enough that they administration noted that the rats that enjoyed making homes in the pipes.

Additionally, the floors in the upper part of the building were unable to support the 100 gallon water tanks. As a result, the floors were damaged. To solve the problem, the tank was suspended from the roof rafters so as to not damage the floor and the bathrooms were completely redone.

In the early days, Pinel Chapel (named for Philippe Pinel) was just a small part of the original building used for services. The central part of building had hospital offices. In the back center of the building was a kitchen, a dining room, staff sleeping for men and a separate sleeping area for women. Behind this was a store room.

The superintendent lived in the middle section of the building. According to the 1853 report, Superintendent Richard Patterson left, and as the hospital administration claimed he furnished the apartment himself, he took the items in the apartment with him. However, records show he installed a piano ($250), and bought a buggy ($50) and medical books ($124) - all of which were charged to the hospital.

A small building behind the main building contained a furnace and boiler. The engine house had the motors for the boiler also served as the laundry, ironing and drying rooms and the bakery. However, as the hospital grew and the south wing was completed, the boiler and engines were not sufficient for the hospital and the hospital proposed turning the old boiler room into a space for the boiler, laundry, sewing, bakery and sleeping quarters for staff, eliminating the need for these services to be in the engine room.

The hospital also proposed a 3 story building with a slate roof. On the first floor were apartments, five boilers and a hot water tank. The second floor also had a boiler and a machine room. The third floor would be for sleeping rooms.

Before they could implement this plan, it was found the old boiler couldn't be removed without damaging the building. Three years later, reports indicated that the old boiler house needed to be razed because it was "cracked, useless, and dangerous." The proposal was changed to include a separate bake house, wash house, sewing room, chapel, library and cellar for cold storage. By providing this place, the patients could work (as a precursor to occupational therapy) in these areas.

In 1878 when the Department for Women was opened, the original building became the Department for Men. For another 62 years, the men were cared for here. As the building had three sections: the middle, north and south wings, so it was razed. When the new men's cottages were built in the 1930s male patients were moved into them. In 1941 the Department of Men was razed. The only trace left of the building is the original circular drive to the main entrance, which became the drive and parking lot of the Administration building.

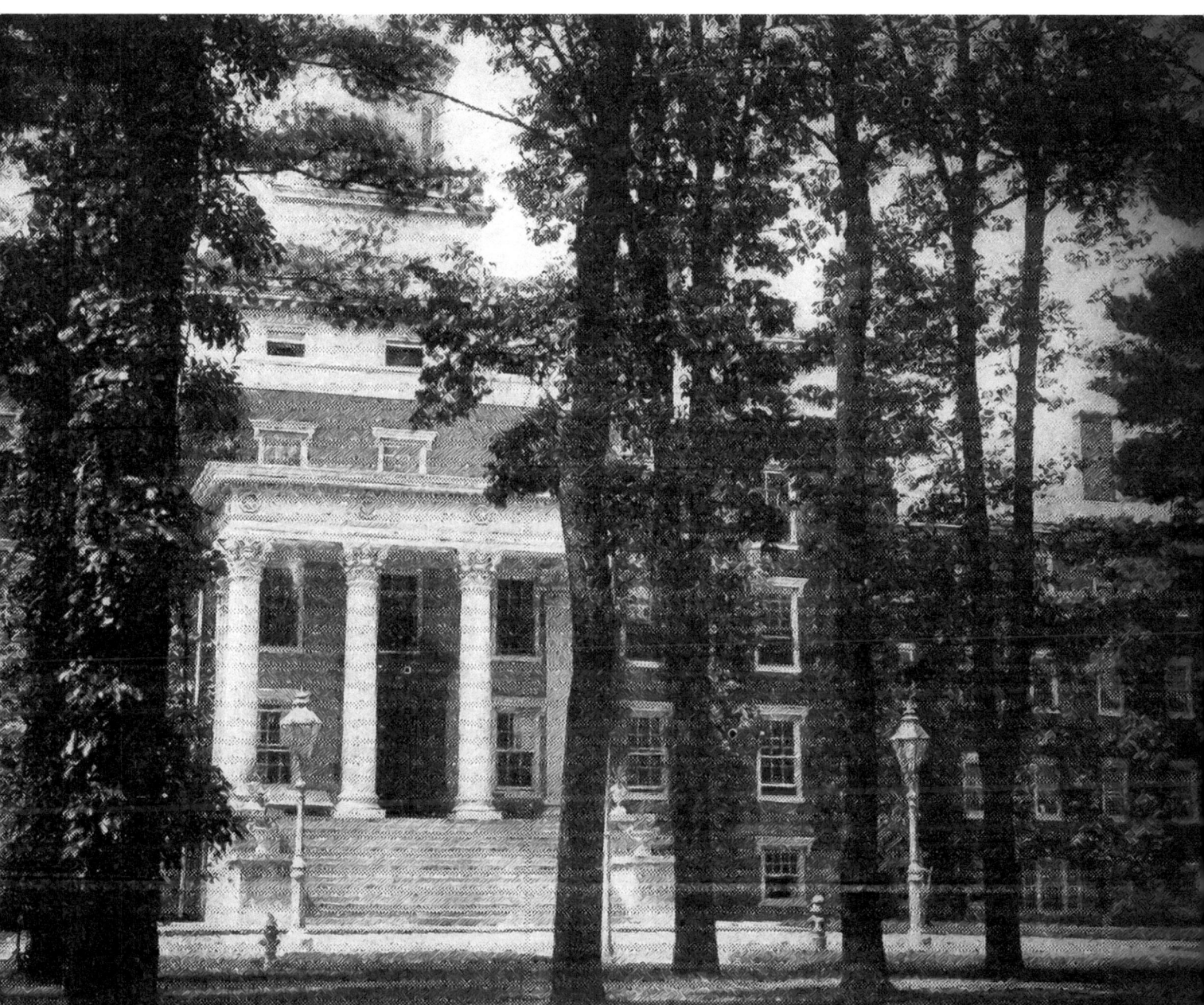

Department for Women
(also known as "Old Main" and "Seven Steeples")
Built: 1875-1878
Razed: 1974 with the opening of the Evans and Bolton Buildings

This building was built on The Kirkbride plan. It consisted of four and a half stories and a basement and had

7.7 massive acres under its roof. There were 65 miles of steam lines, ten miles of water and gas lines, 1,142 rooms, 1,970 windows, 79,000 panes of glass, ten elevators, 11 water heaters, 68 miles of heating system, 12 miles of plumbing and gas system. It was 337,234 square feet, contained 2,500,000 bricks and it boasted a 175 foot smoke stack made with 85,000 bricks and stone. It had over 45,000,000 feet of lumber in it and cost about $800,000 ($15,700,000 in 2014 money). This building was one third bigger than the Department for Men.

    The Department for Women building also had a system of tunnels and cisterns for the steam heat and its walls that were between 16 and 50 inches thick. The building was made as fireproof as possible and in the 1880s, outdoor metal fire escapes were added to each ward. During its construction, 25 year old Edward Meyers, a well digger for Charles Krauss, was suffocated in the well.

    The center section of the building contained offices, living rooms and a sewing room. The middle of this part also contained a kitchen and sleeping rooms on the lower level as well as a chapel. In the back center of the building was another kitchen and there were sleeping rooms on the second and third floors. South of this kitchen was a large refrigerated section. The building also contained hydraulic elevators to the 130 feet tall towers.

    The Department for Women was nicknamed "Seven Steeples" because although it had eight majestic steeples, only seven could be seen from any one vantage point. It was also known as "Old Main", possibly because it was the oldest building left on the grounds for a time, and because the Administration of the hospital was headquartered there for a few years.

    By 1936 the building still had Administrative offices in the front. Sleeping quarters were made on other floors and in the middle section of the building. In 1939 the steeples were scheduled to be taken down because they were "flues for fire".

    By 1950 the building was considered a "scandal". It lacked adequate bathrooms facilities, proper air conditioning or sufficient fire protection. Even the press called it a "tinderbox". One legislator asked that the building be replaced in the 1958 assembly, but Dr. Clifford Williams, Superintendent at this time, believed that it was fourth in priority- behind finishing the Bahr Treatment Building.

    Only a year later the Women's building was officially called a fire hazard by the Fire Marshall. The hospital

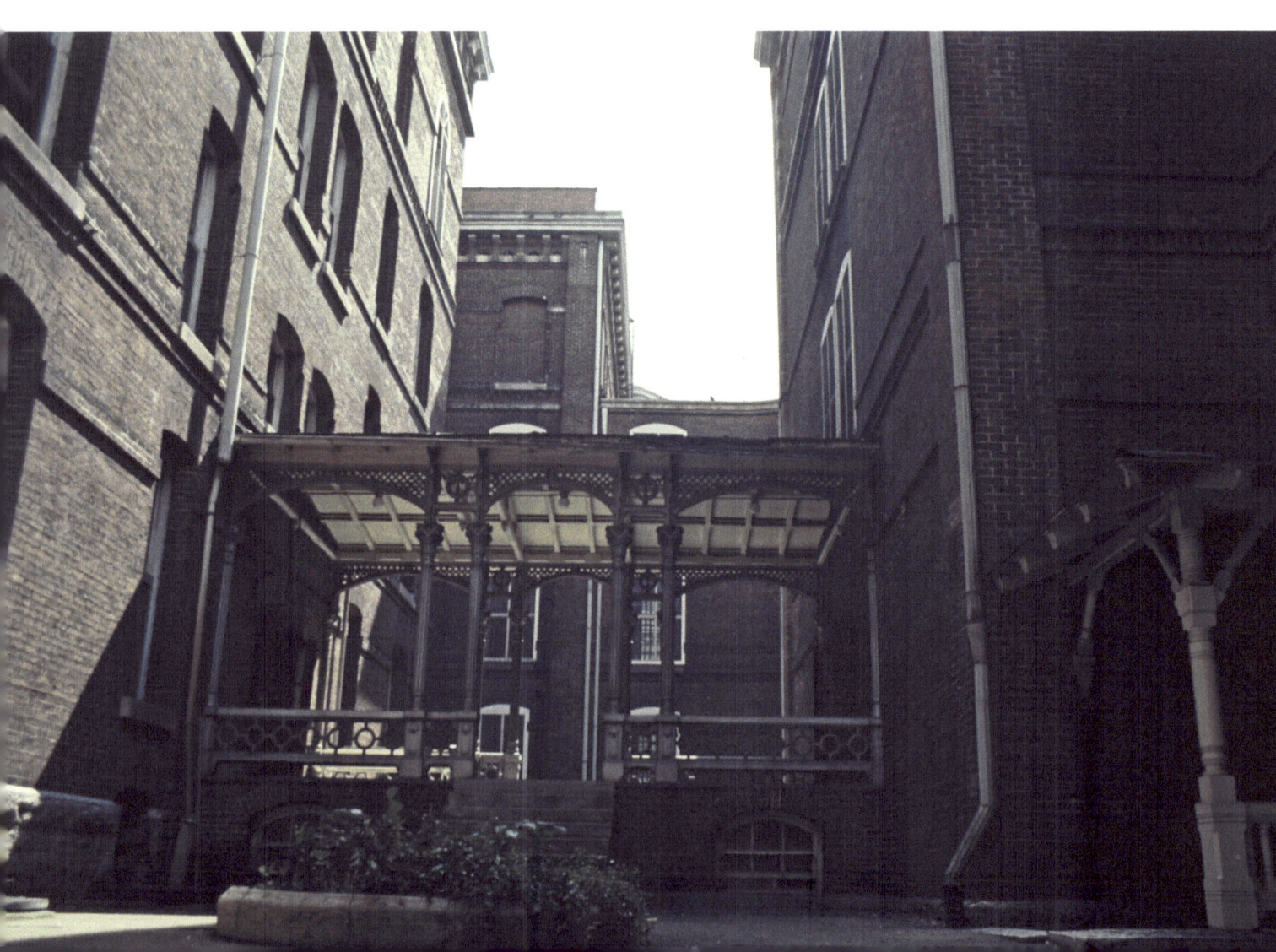

fixed the issues it could and the building passed inspection. The hospital administration developed fire safety plans including:

- Wards were to be evacuated in six to ten minutes.
- The bedridden patients were placed on the first floor and the younger patients on the upper floors.
- Renovations included a modern sprinkler system, newly plastered walls, fire resistant paint, and updated tubular fire escapes. All wood floors were covered with linoleum.
- Once a room was vacated it was to be locked by an attendant.

As the patient population declined and more patients were being treated as outpatients, the need for such an aged building diminished. In 1973 Seven Steeples was replaced by the Evans and Bolton buildings, and razed in 1974 after the transition. By the time it was torn down, many of the windows were broken and not functioning, the floors were in dangerous condition and even areas that were fire damaged and not repaired were still being used to house patients. Some of the ornate woodwork was removed, and was planned to be installed in the governor's mansion.

Fire Departments
Original Fire station No 18
Physical Description: Two-story, 20-inch thick walls. ; 5540 square feet
Location: Northwest of central section of Department of Men, next to gas meter
Other: Sleeping rooms on second floor, 2 horse wagons, 1 hose reel, one 60 gallon chemical engine, one hook and ladder truck, 1,650 feet of 2.5 inch hose, two house wagons, 650 feet of 2.5-inch hose (each hose real 350), 3,000 feet of 1-inch hose; 8 250 gallon, 93 5 gallon and 104 3-gallon chemical tanks; fire alarm by whistle, two city fire alarm boxes on grounds (behind Administration Building in the women's ward and by the front steps on the south side of the men's dept.) By 1936, the hospital had a watchman (no punch clock), electricity, steam heat fueled by coal, two hose carts, 10,000 feet of 2.5-inch hose, one 60 gallon chemical cart and chemical extinguishers.
Built: 1894
Razed: Unknown

Station 18
Physical Description: Two-stories, wood and brick
Location: Southwest corner of property (Tibbs Avenue and Washington Street)
Other: Built especially for the hospital and per the 1936 report, it was under city control.
Built: 1936
Razed: Still standing

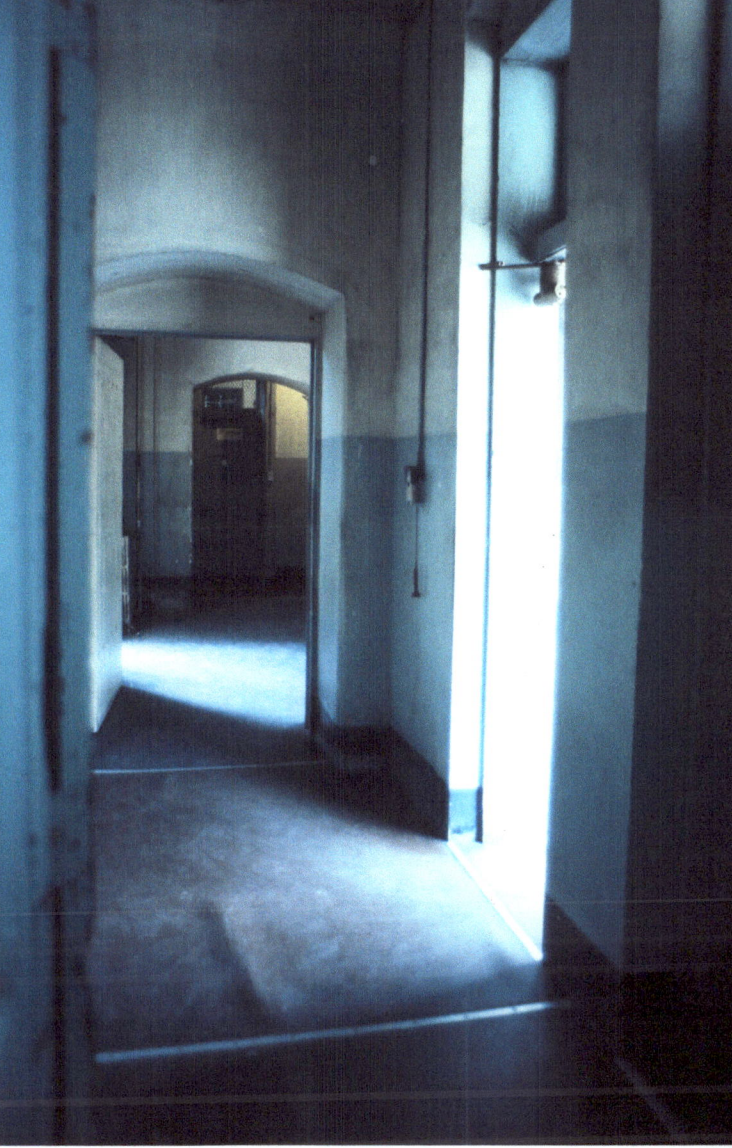

Opposite: view of airing court.
Above: view of corridor.
See the front cover for picture of the building.

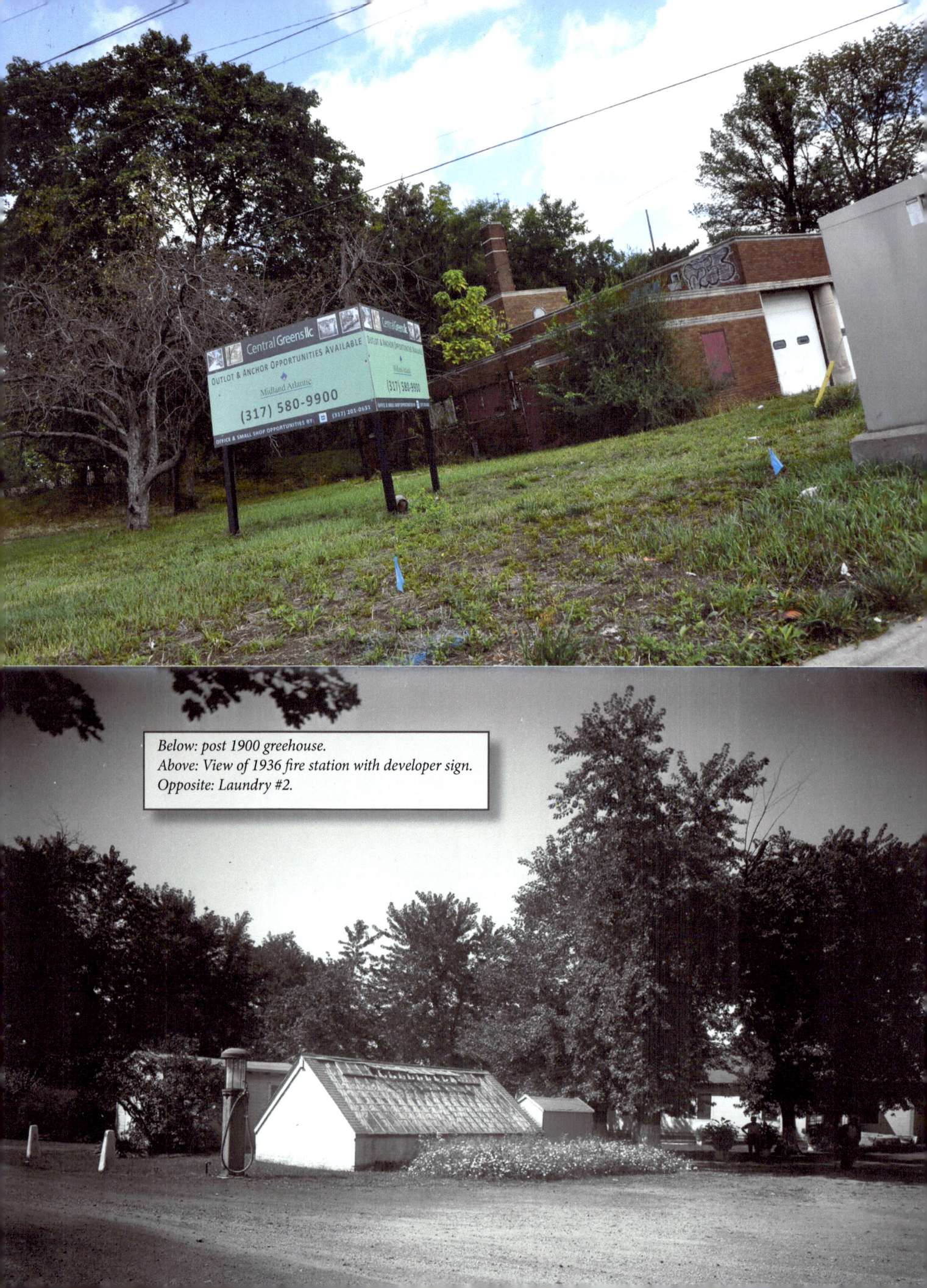

Below: post 1900 greehouse.
Above: View of 1936 fire station with developer sign.
Opposite: Laundry #2.

Station 18 *(New)*
Physical Description: Brick
Location: Southeast corner of grounds (Warman Avenue and Washington Street)
Other: This is the third Station 18.
Built: 1994 to replace old fire station on Tibbs Avenue and Washington Street
Razed: Still standing

Greenhouses (Conservatory)
Physical Description: one-story, wood, steel, five rooms, interconnected
Location: In front of the Department for Men; SE of Cornelius Hall
Built: Early ones built after hospital opened and demolished by 1898. The new ones were built in 1899.
Razed: After 1956, presumably to make room for the Bahr Treatment Center

Laundries
Laundry #1
Physical Description: wood
Location: west of carpenters shop
Other: Was a coal shed, later turned into paint shop
Built: Unknown
Razed: shortly after 1888.

Laundry#2
Physical Description: Part of the building was one-story/part was two-story, brick and wood, ventilated with side lights and skylights. 14,940- square feet
Location: Northwest of first Fire Department
Other:. It had one galvanized iron sterilizer, three centrifugal extractors, one 1/100 inch mangle, five ironing machines, one starcher and kettle, one all metal drying room, one dampening room, two soap kettles, one tumbler, one water heater, 24 ironing tables with electric irons, accessories. It was all electric.
Built: 1894-1895
Razed: still standing

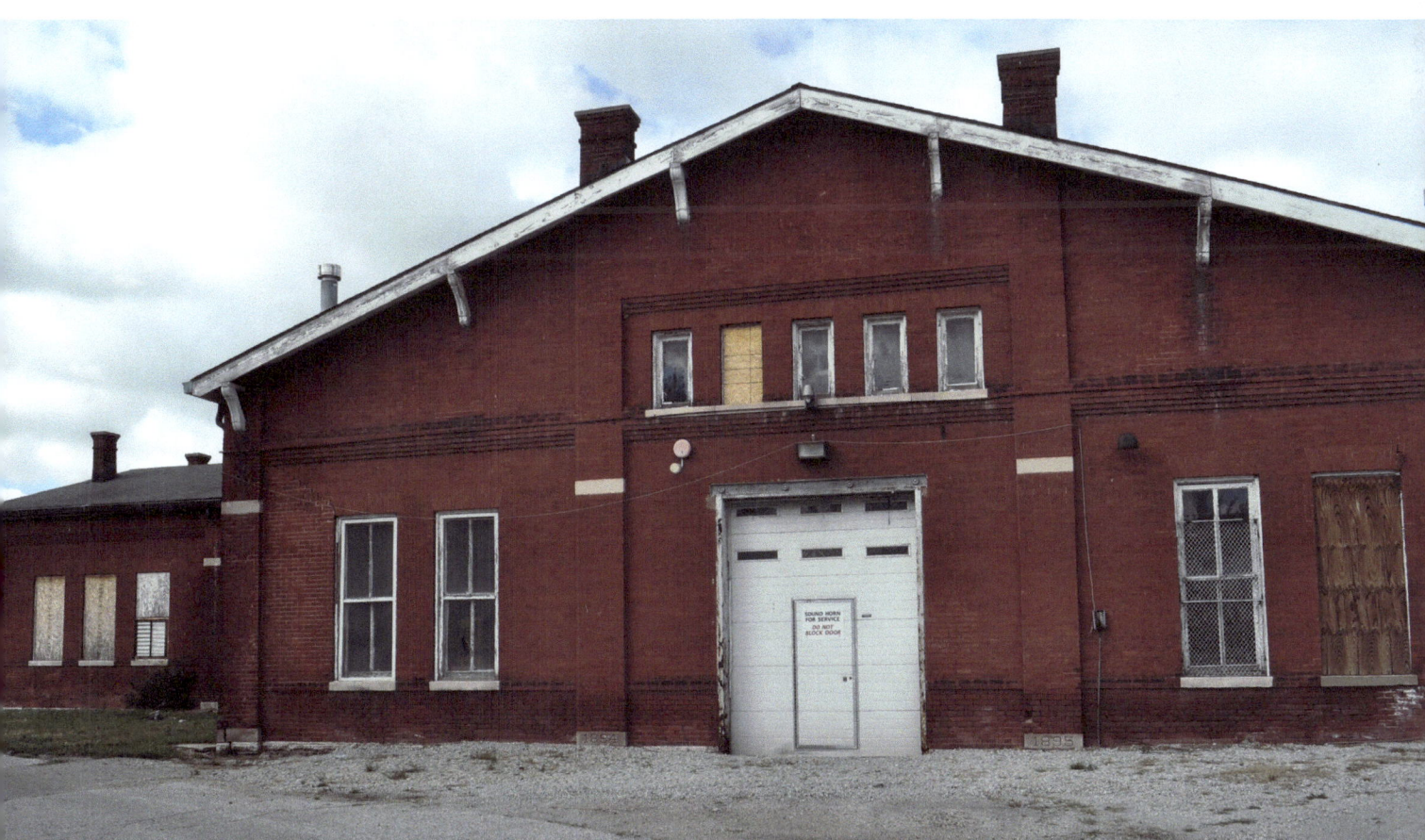

Coal Room / Power House

Physical Description: 2-stories with a basement, some areas were taller. 12-inch walls, brick. Powerhouse 3,308 square feet, engineers department/machine shop 1,824 square feet, boiler house 8,835 square feet, engineer repair shop 960 square feet
Location: West of the Store and Supply House; Next to power house
Other: Connected to Indianapolis Electric Power. Had a natural gas regulator next to it. To the north was a pump room. By 1936 this had become the "Building House" with an attached power house to the east of it. At one time it contained eight Stirling boilers, eight Roney stockers, four Stilwell boiler feed pumps and one Webster feed water eater, and accessories. A coal crushing machine was also installed. It was connected to, but separate from, the Engineer's building and Machine Shop. The building housed general stock for this department as well as lathes, drills, forge pipe-cutter, etc.
Built: 1886 with additions in 1892, 1897 and 1939.
Razed: still standing

Pipe Room

Physical Description: 12-inch walls, wood
Location: Northwest behind the coal room.
Other: This building is where all the pipes needed for plumbing and other needs were stored and created. A second pipe shop was built behind it (no number). A third pipe shop was built as No 15 Pipe shop in front of the Coal Room.
Built: Before 1898
Razed: still standing

Below: view of old power plant, coal and pipe rooms. Opposite: view inside power plant.

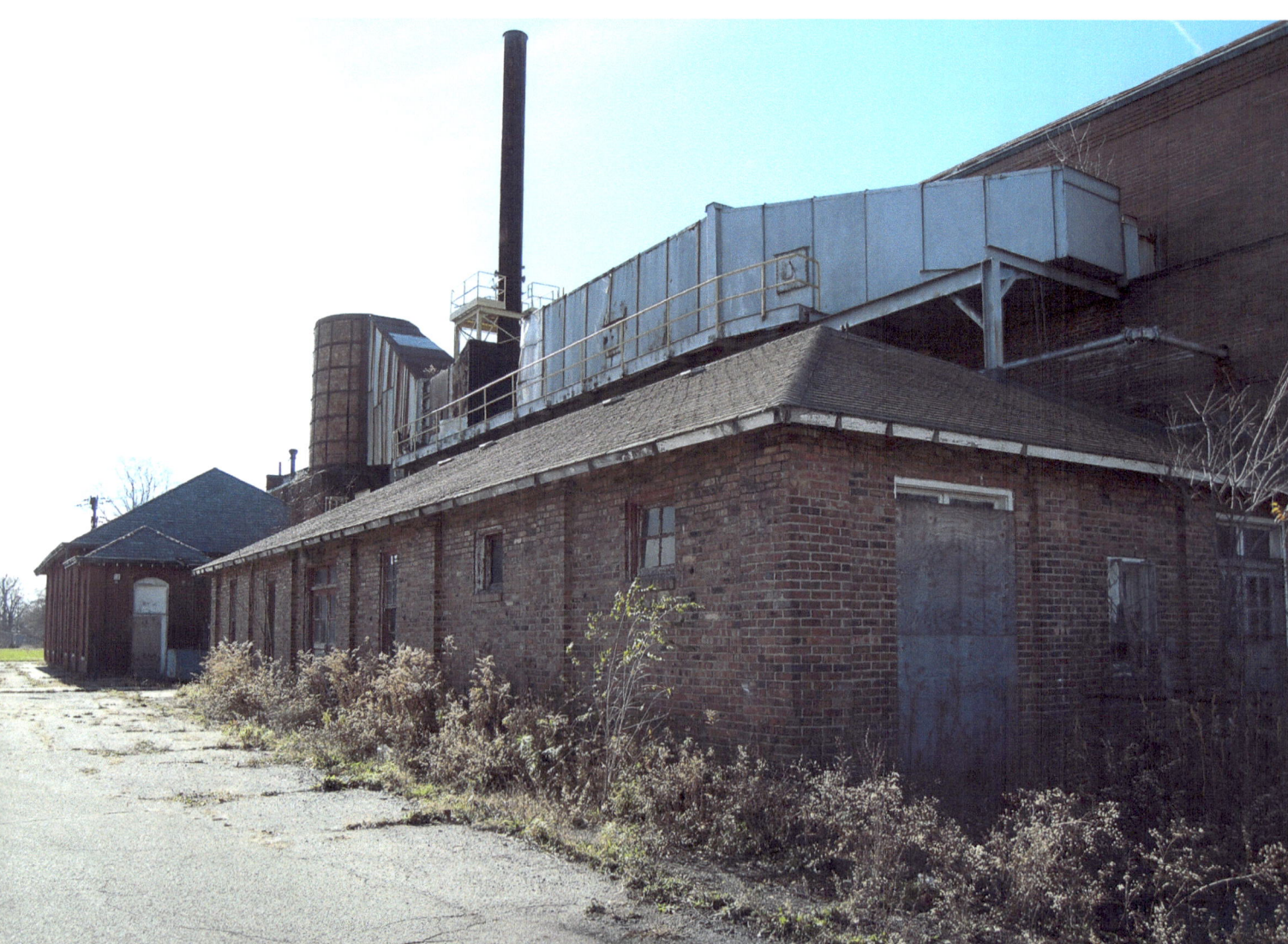

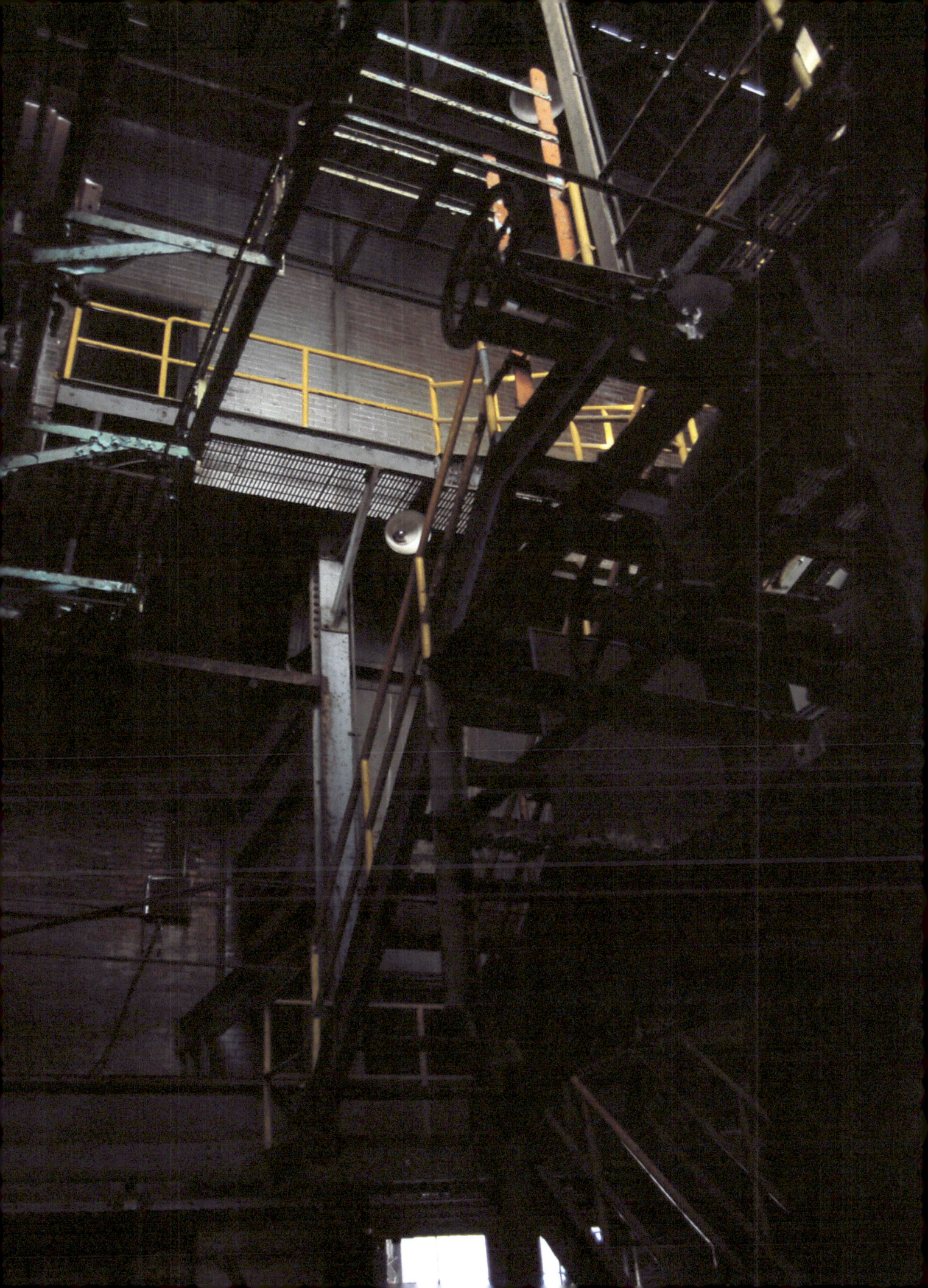

Sick Hospital

Physical Description: one- and two- story, brick, 16=inch thick walls, some 26-inch thick. Several areas on building (mostly porches, that are wood.) some parts have a basement

Location: Northeast of Department for Women

Other: In 1899 $110,000 was appropriated for the construction of the Hospital for the Sick Insane. It was constructed with a window in every room, and access to the outdoors. The administration section separated the men and women's wards. It had separate kitchen and dining for men and women. In 1936 the hospital had a surgical ward for women; kitchen and dining for separate sexes, and operating department. The administration part of the hospital seemed to no longer be a part of the hospital and had moved elsewhere, presumably to the Women's Department. This section seems to be patient rooms. Store room between the dining rooms. Each ward had its own sitting room, dorms, ten bedrooms, nurses. day room, clothing room, linen and supply rooms, lavatory and bathrooms for patients and separate ones for attendants and nurses Operating had general diagnosis, anesthetizing and instrument rooms. Also rooms for sterilizing, drugs, supplies and bandages.

General dining rooms, storage rooms, sculleries, dish rooms, linen rooms and kitchen to the back. Because of the corridor cross ventilation, the odors from the kitchen do not reach the ward. Second floor sleeping rooms for attendants. Basement eight feet tall was under the whole building. Concrete foundation inner; outer is limestone. Inside walls brick.

Outside of entire structure is brick, and oolitic stone. Hollow construction ventilated from basement to the roof. Bathrooms and lavatories lined with enameled brick. Wired for electric incandescent light with iron armored conduits. Plumbing and ventilating modern sanitary methods. Forced air heating. Faces southwest for good light exposure. Airing roofs allow patients to be outside whenever possible.

The Evans Building was constructed in its place.

Built: 1899-1901
Razed: 1971

Opposite top: Main Entrance
Bottom: Sick Hospital

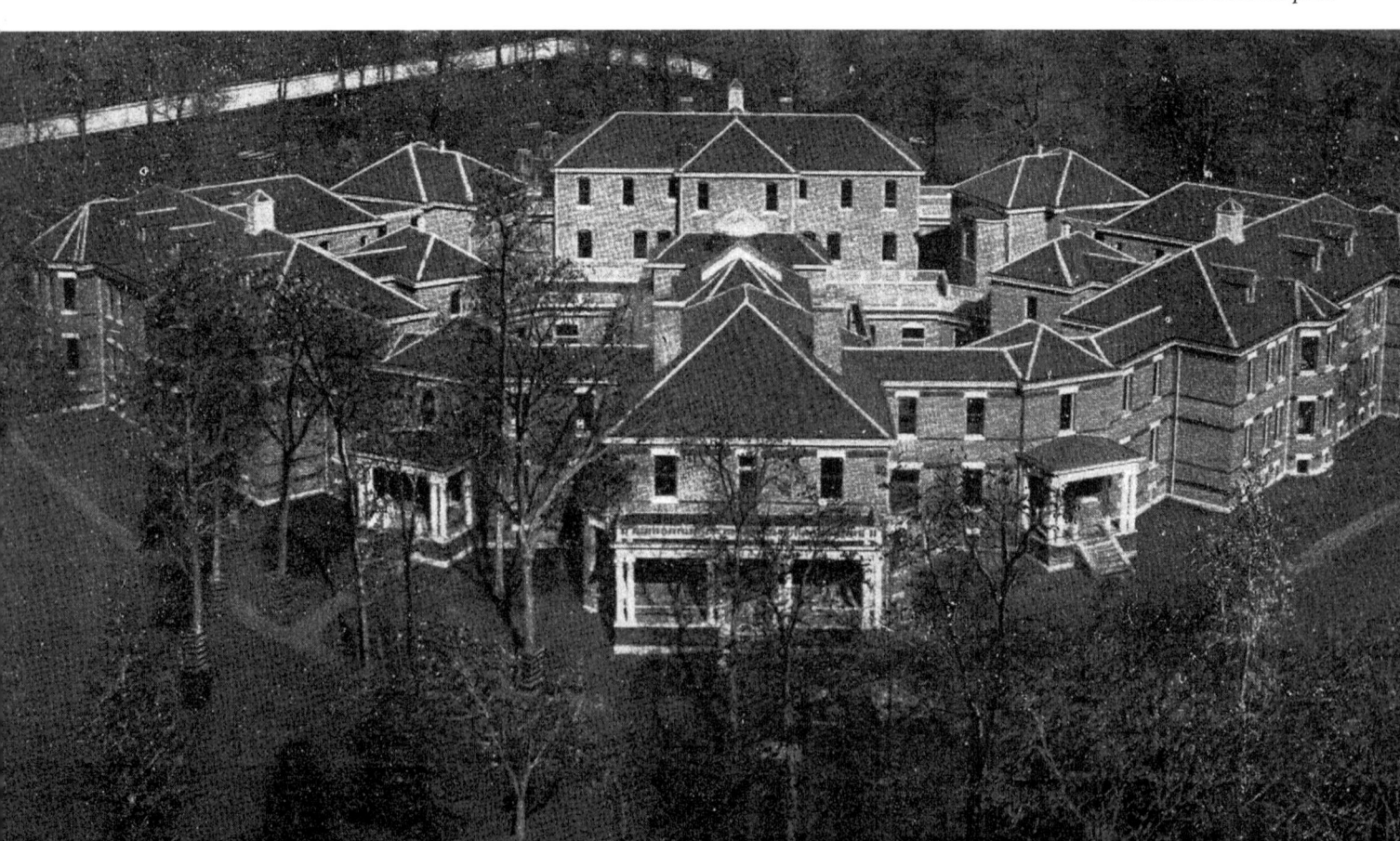

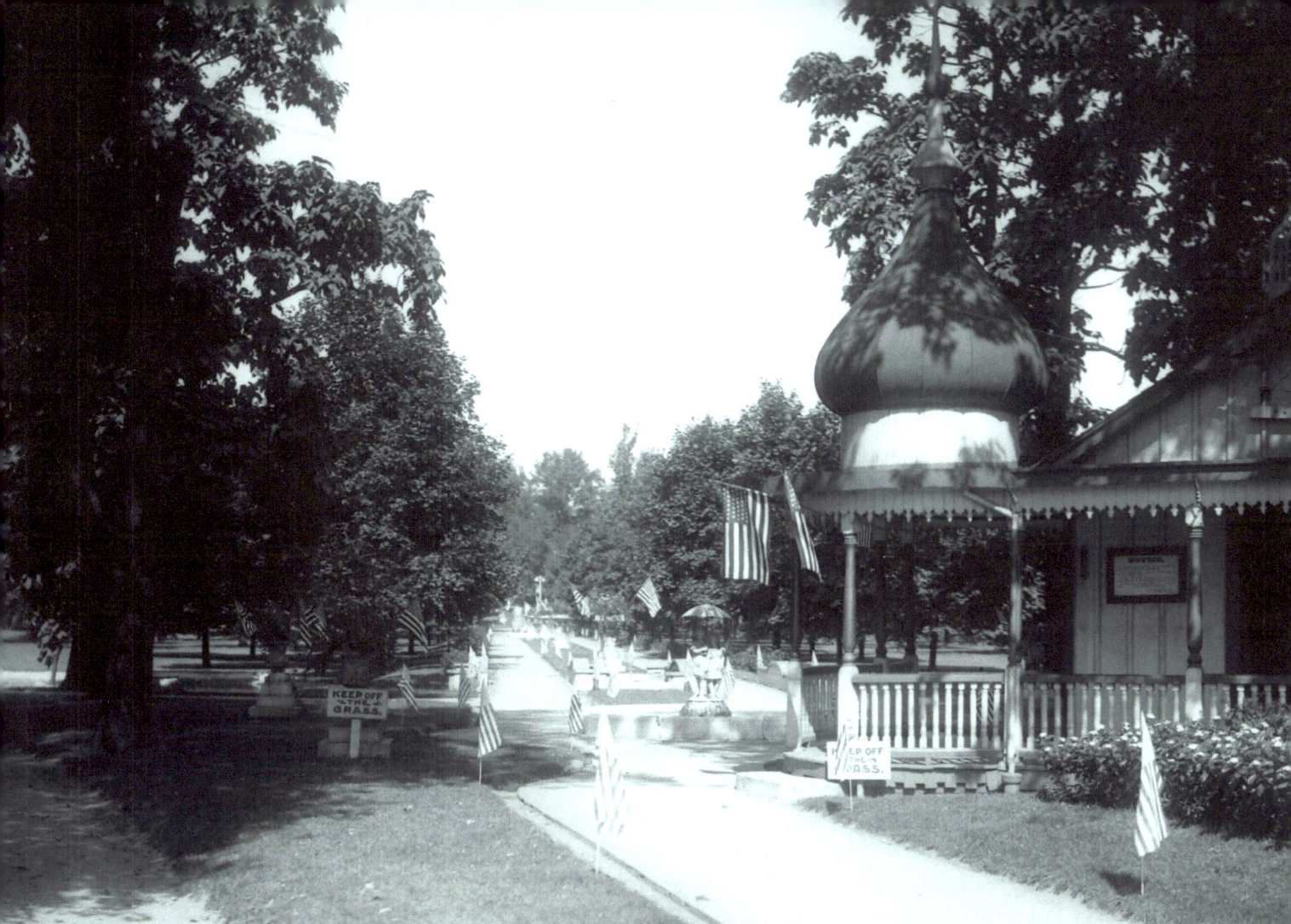

The Main Entrance

Physical Description: cement, five iron vases, two fountains
Location: From Washington Street to the Department of Women
Other: At the entrance, the watch house had a stove, a clock and a lamp for people waiting for the streetcar. In 1901 two lakes were added. The first ran under the double sidewalk requiring the addition of two bridges. The second sat to the west. Both were the hospital's backup water for fire protection.
Built: 1893
Razed: Gravel walkways replaced by cement in 1900. Gradually removed by 1915, the only remnant is part of the fountain base which now has trees and brush growing in it.

Cornelius Mayer Hall
Physical Description: one-story brick building. 13 rooms, stage, chapel
Location: North of Employee building
Other: named for Cornelius Mayer, secretary at Central State Hospital for 30 years
Built: 1915
Razed: After 1956

Employee Building *(also known as Administration Building)*
Physical Description: 12 -32 inch walls, 2.5 stories plus basement, stone building, three sections. 88 feet by 177feet, 35,000 square feet
Location: South of Mayer Hall
Other: This is what contemporary people remember as the Administration Building. It was an employee home first for staff and officers. Contained office space for doctors and dentists as well.. Meant to house 100 people. Third floor for unmarried male employees and had 20 double rooms. Plastered walls and ceilings with neutral colors. Double bedrooms and one bath were also in the plan. Furniture was made of solid maple with a dark cherry finish. East half of the first floor was for officers. Large lounge and library with paneled walls of red birch. Office space for doctors and dentist will be in building.

West half of the first floor was five two room suites for doctor and dentist offices, consultation room and medical library. Each had oak office furniture.

Center part of the first floor was the lobby, information desk and clerk's office. Fire flashed tile floors and tile wainscoting in buff with rose tinted plaster walls with dark cherry furniture. The basement contained the dining rooms, kitchens and equipment for ventilation. The corridors had Terrazzo floors.
Built: 1939
Razed: still standing

Dining Room *(aka Men's Recreation Building)*
Physical Description: one-story, 16-inch thick walls, iron columns, brick, 9,458 square feet
Location: north wing of men's building
Other: Later turned into the Recreation hall for men and even later for women. In 1990 the building was to be torn down, but it would have cost $25,000 so it wasn't. It was eligible for the State Register of Historic Sites and Structures because of its architecture and that it was on historic grounds. Steve Leonard, physical plant director at CSH, said he hadn't been able to get estimates on restoration because the money just wasn't there. Tall one story with a gabled roof and parapet end walls. Two skylights atop the slate room provide extra light to the interior. Used for the therapeutic care of patients.
Built: 1899
Razed: still standing

New Men's Cottages and Buildings
Cottage Plan
The Cottage Plan movement had four types of cottages. Early cottages were very similar to the Kirkbride plan but on a smaller scale. The Utilitarian cottage plan (which is the closest in similarity to Central State Hospital's Men's Cottages) housed hundreds of patients in dormitories. The Metropolitan Plan included sleeker smaller buildings designed to house many patients in smaller groups. These hospitals became sprawling and very few exist today. The Post Drug Cottage Plan went back to some of Kirkbride's thoughts and were made sometimes more decorative and interesting. They were meant to hold smaller groups of people. Central State Hospital's 1970s buildings are similar to these, although they were not decorative and were more utilitarian in design.

Cottages were meant to be arranged in a park like setting where they were a mini neighborhood. They typically had dormitories for patients ranging from 6 patients or more, had separate dining and infirmary services. Sometimes each building or a group of buildings housed patients that were part of a specific industrial therapy or disease group. The buildings were simpler than Kirkbride's, but had the comforts of nice architecture and may trees, shrubs and

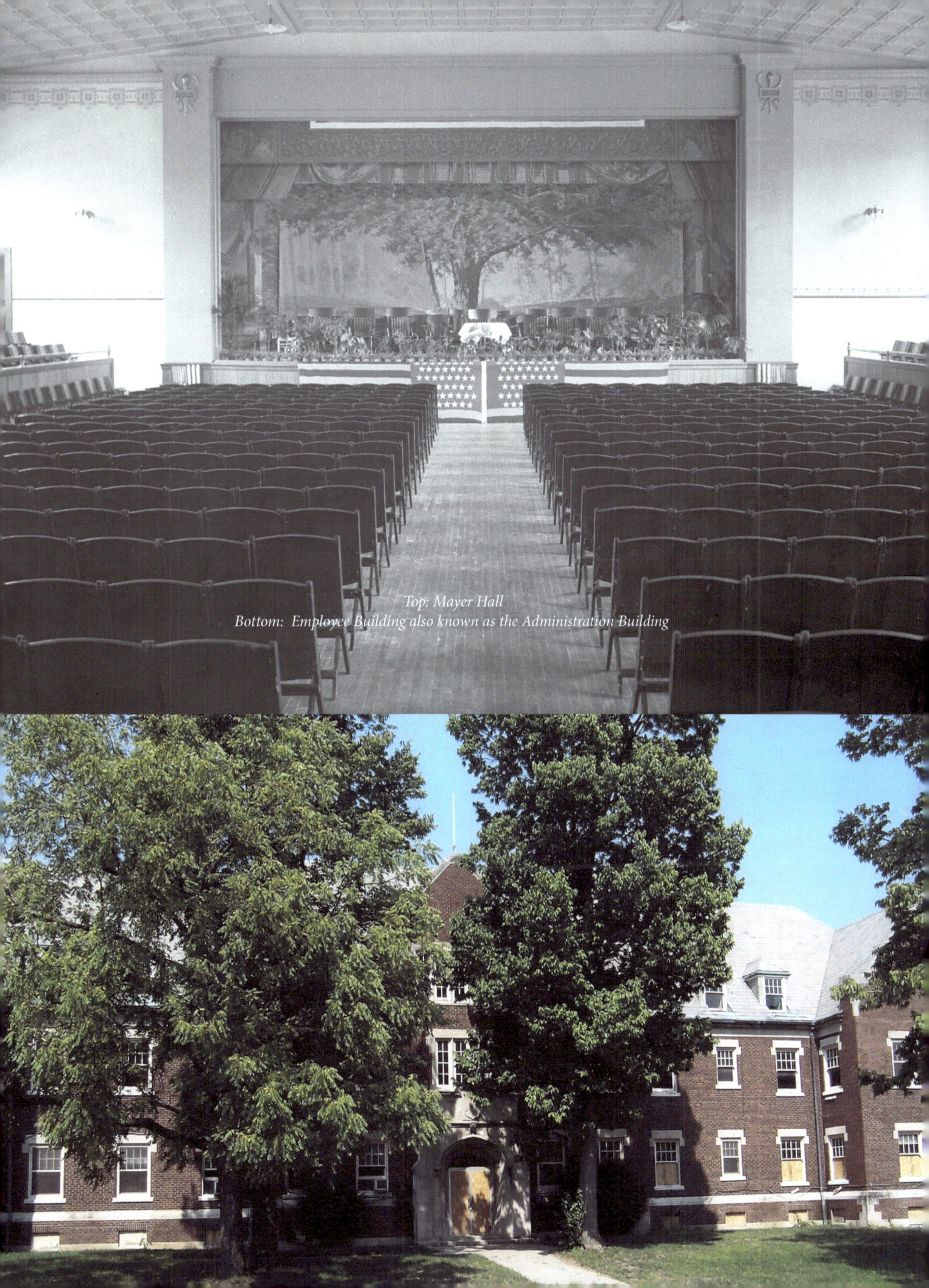

Top: Mayer Hall
Bottom: Employee Building also known as the Administration Building

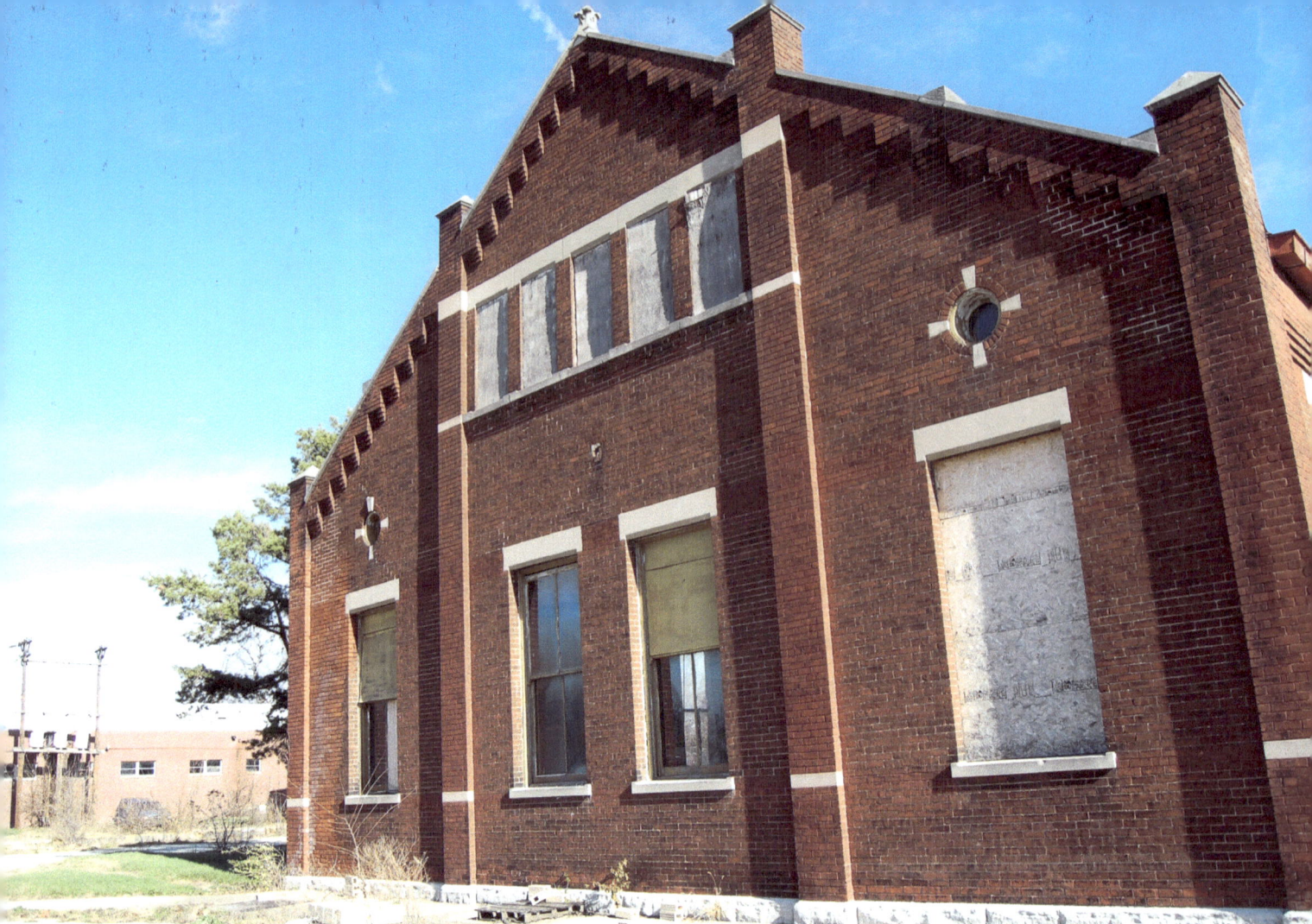

Above: Men's Recreation Building.

flowers. This made living at the hospital more home like. While the Indiana Village for Epileptics embraced the village like atmosphere, treating one disease, Central State Hospital built cottages on the grounds and kept the men more integrated into the whole hospital.

- Cottage 1 (1931): East and connected to Cottages 2 and 3
- Cottage 2 (1937): South and connected to Cottages 1 and 3 (no 32)
- Cottage 3 (1931): West and connected to Cottages 1 and 2 and the infirmary
- Cottage 4 (1938): North of cottage 3 and connected to Cottage 3
- A barber shop and sewing room was in the basement of Cottage 4
- Cottage 7 (1939): West of 3 and 4 (and the infirmary)
- Infirmary No 1 (1931): East of Cottage 7 connected to Cottage 3

Physical Description: brick, wood roof, basements
Location: South of and on the Department for Men land
Other: Each had two wings and aback section. Each had 2 stories plus attic space and a basement. Cost of $169,231 (under a budget of $175.000)   First two floors were for patients with two wings of 13 single rooms, dormitory, day room, porch, mattress room, linen room, toilet bath and lavatory, clothing, utility rooms, fire stairs, refuse and soiled clothing chutes; third for staff with sleeping room for eight people plus a living room, bath and toilet; basement has chamber for piping and plumbing and passage to underground tunnels used by patients to reach the men's dining room during inclement weather. Architect McGuire and Shook.

Cottages 5 and 6 were planned. They were to go where the Department of Men stood. However, due to funding, they were never realized. The last time they were mentioned was in 1943.
Razed: razed, unknown date

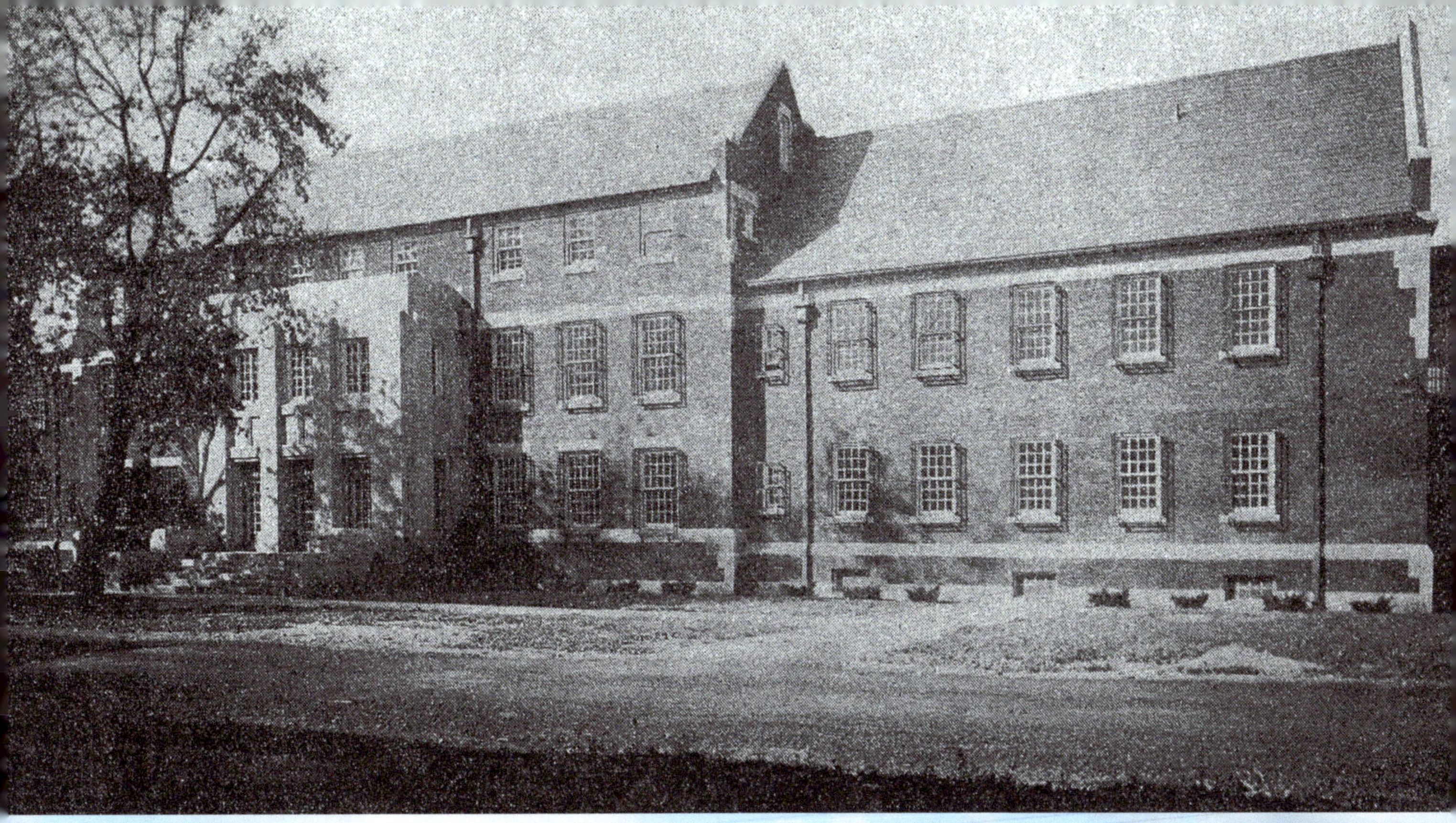

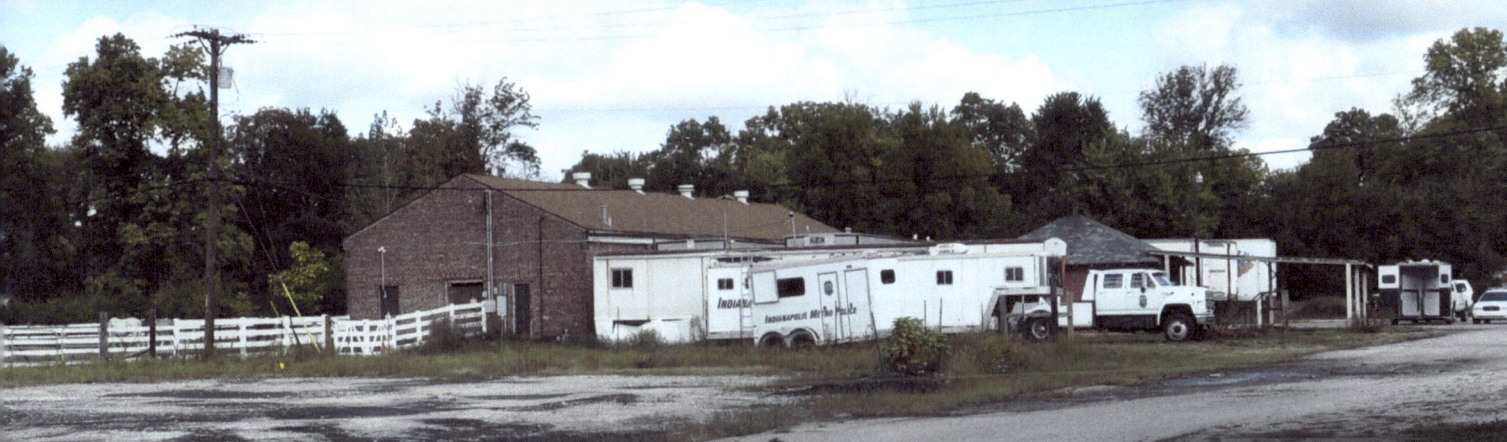

Above top: Men's Cottage 7
Above bottom: Canning Plant

Canning Plant 1947
Physical Description: Brick with frame section to north, 14-inch this walls. 40 feet by 130 feet
Location: Behind the west most pipe shop was a canning plant.
Other: two rooms; created from old bricks from other structures.
Built: 1947
Razed: still standing, police use it

Kitchen/Dining Room
Physical Description: brick, 14,500 square feet
Location: Where "The Store" used to sit, north of Men's Recreation Hall
Other: New kitchen $668,000 in 1955 and completed in 1958. Won an award in 1959 Meal cost $.32 – the savings was attributed to the new kitchen and portion control measures. Miss Arelene Wilson consulting dietitian for the Department of Health. John Fleck from Fleck, Quebe and Reid designed it.
Built: 1955-1958
Razed: still standing

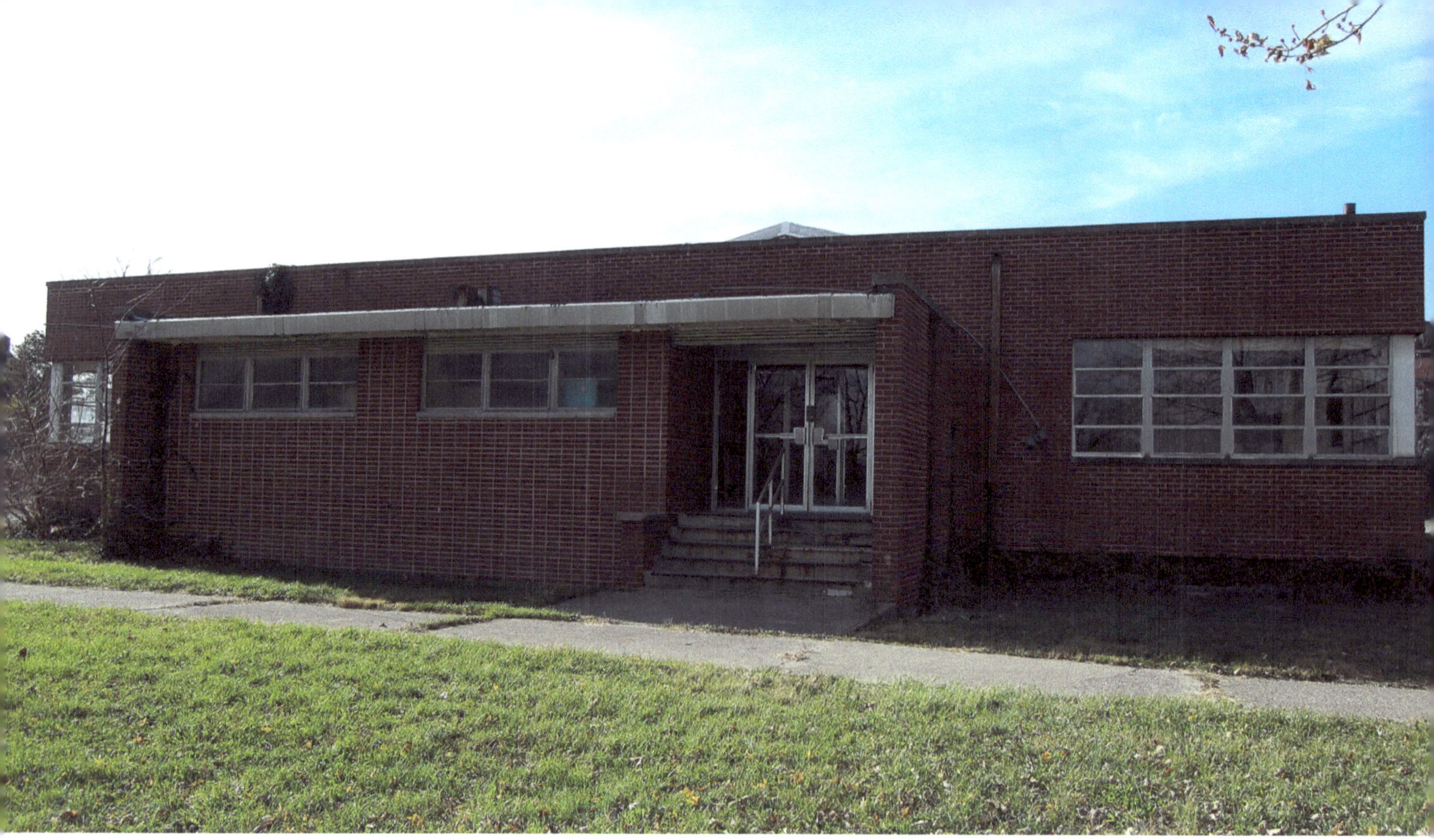

Above: 1950s dining room.
Below: Dining room later used as a carpenter's shop.
Opposite top: View of the 1950s dining room interior.
Opposite bottom: View of the South Dining room (later used as a carpenter's shop).

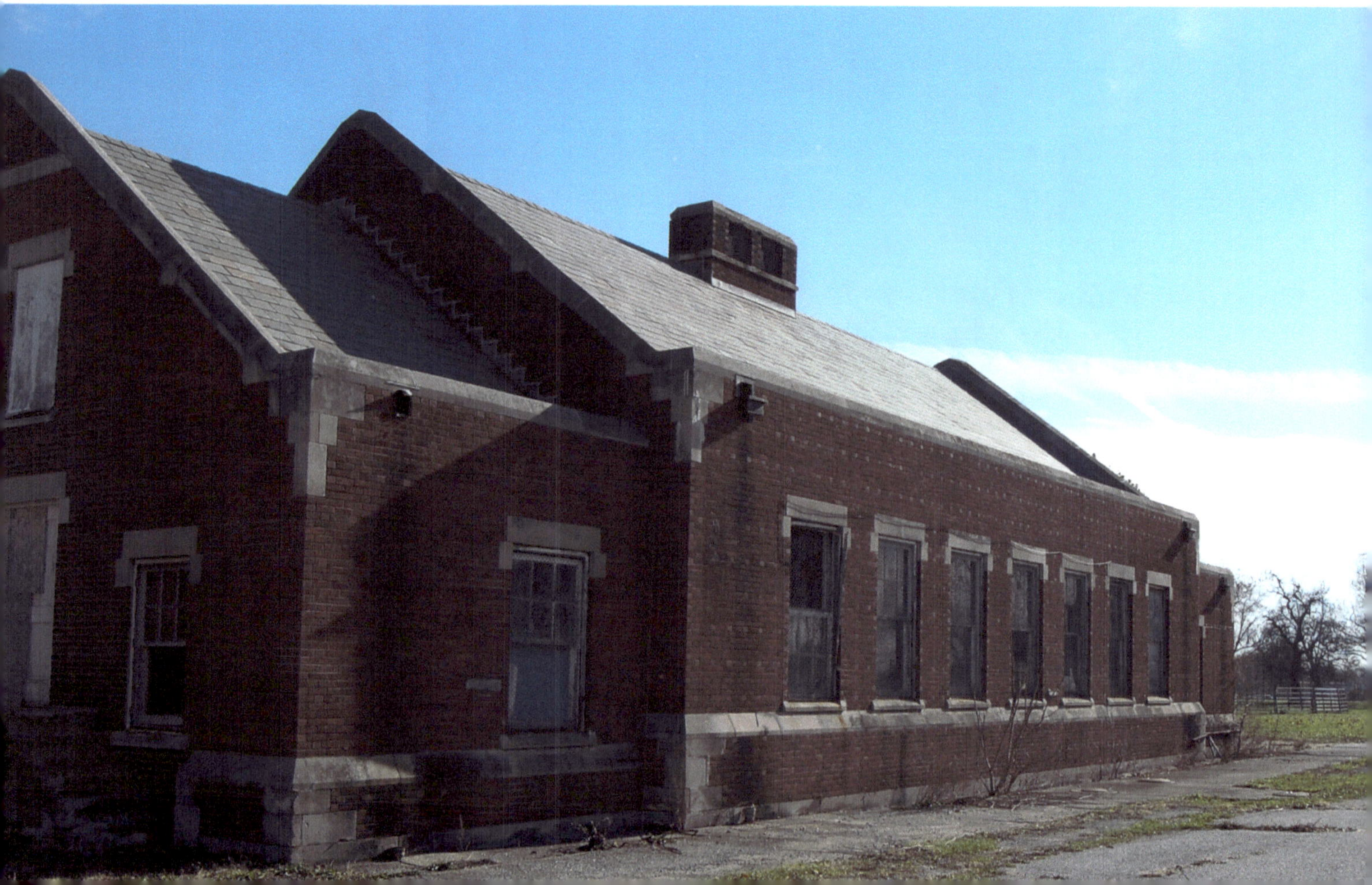

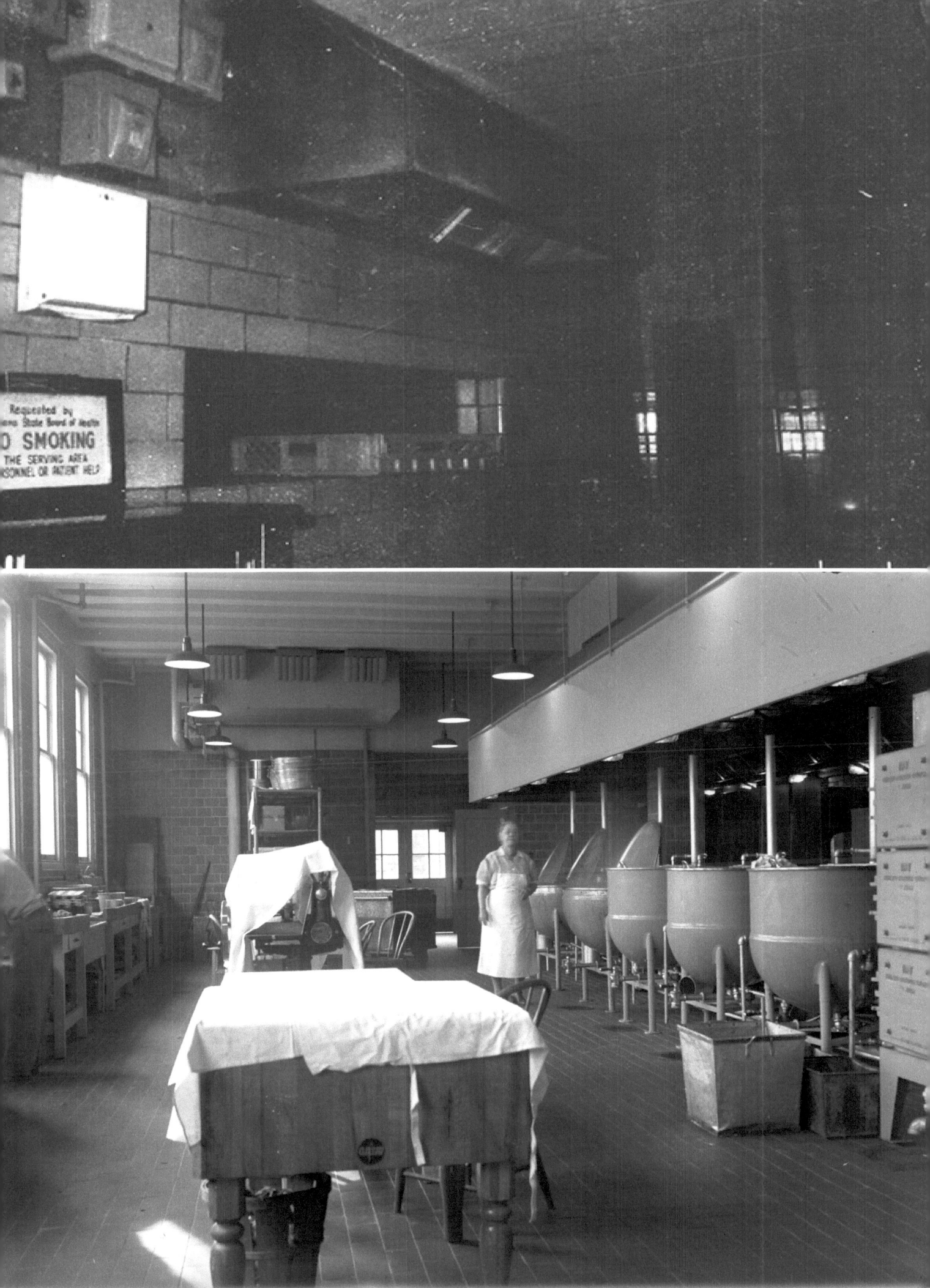

SOUTH DINING ROOM
Physical Description: one-story, 12- and 16- inch thick walls
Location: South of Men's Recreation Building
Other: was also used for carpentry and storage
Built: 1930s
Razed: still there

MOTEL/EMPLOYEE HOUSING
Physical Description: brick, wood
Location: Northwest corner of property next to first hospital cemetery
Built: 1960s
Razed: Still standing

DOCTOR HOUSING *(aka Veterans Housing)*
Physical Description: wood
Location: East side of grounds on Warman Avenue.
Other: When on call, they used the houses on Warman Avenue. Later used for veterans housing. An exception is Dr. Williams who was said to live on "a corner" of the grounds. It is believed he lived in one of these homes.
Built: Some sources say 1940; others indicate 1950s, but this was not on any Sanborn map before 1956.
Razed: still standing

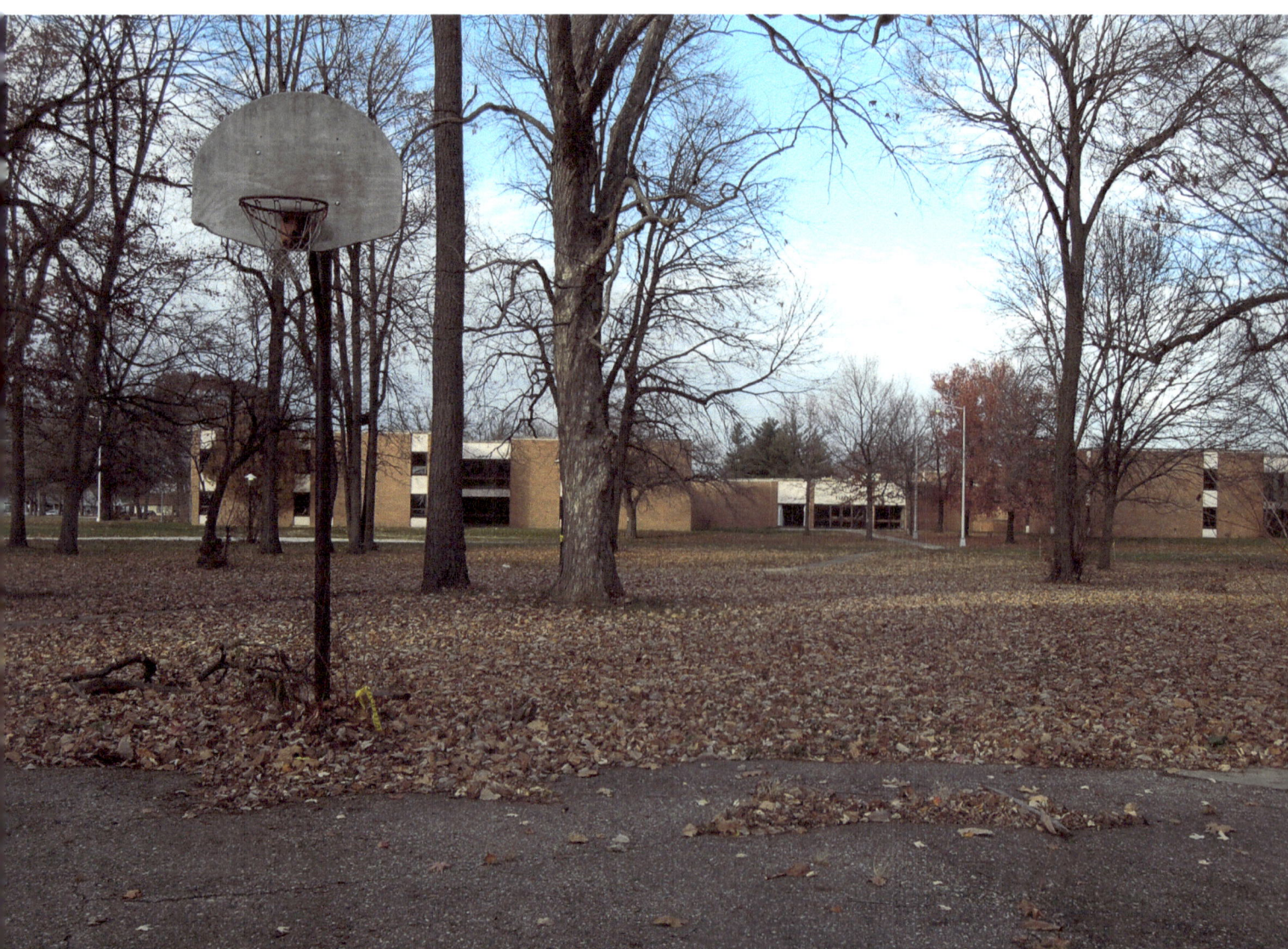

Evans Building *(aka Evans Hall)*
Physical Description: brick, wood, 140,180 square feet
Location: Former site of the Sick Hospital
Other: Named for Dr. John Evans, the first superintendent of Central State Hospital. Governor Edgar Whitcomb said these buildings were landmarks because great strides had been made in mental health in the last three years. Dr. Keating said it was "the most exciting day in the history of Central State Hospital," when the building opened.

This was an adult psychiatric unit for addiction services and developmental disabilities. Green carpet in the lobby and a dining room behind that which was used as a multipurpose room. The wards are pods. Two pods have four bedrooms, one has three bedrooms, one has two bedrooms, and two have one bedroom each. Separate restroom facilities for men and women and closets for each patient. Each area were used by 45 patients with a sitting room. Restrooms have stainless steel sinks, showers and air hand dryers. Laundry and cleaning provided but patients can also use the washers and dryers and irons provided. They have a canteen and kitchenette to prep snacks for themselves. Quiet rooms provided. Rooms for rowdy or tranquilized patients also existed. Air conditioned.
Built: 1973
Razed: in process of being razed

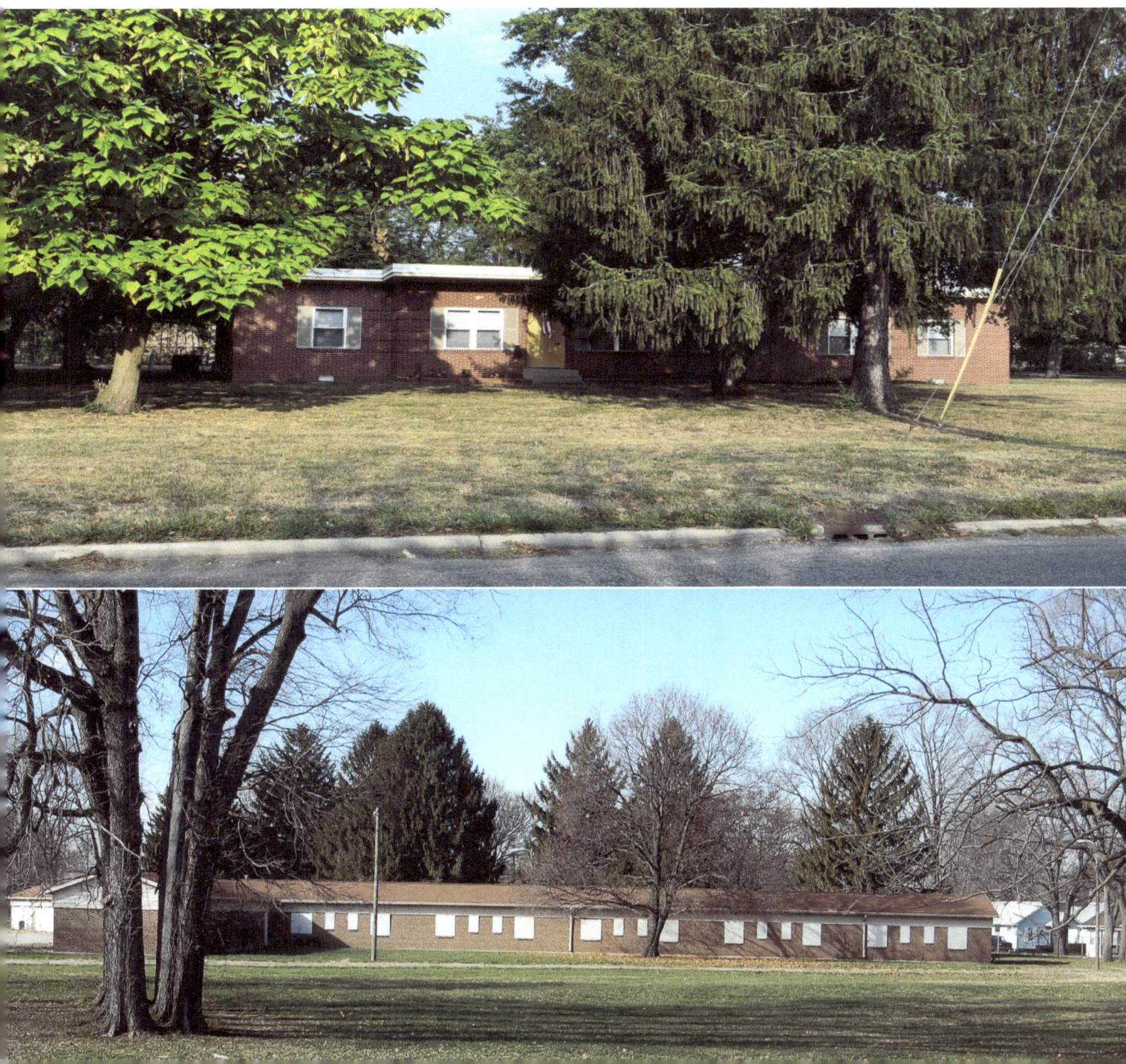

(Sarah T.) Bolton Building
Physical Description: brick, wood, 140,180 square feet
Location: SE of Evans Building; north of Bahr Treatment Building
Other: Same as the Evans building. Named for Sarah Bolton, the wife of the man who sold the state the property for the hospital. Indiana poetess. It was also used for geriatrics.
Built: 1973
Razed: 2013-2014 (Housing, offices and shops now occupy the spot.

Exit House
Physical Description: wood
Location: 212 Warman Ave; North of Veteran houses, east of Bolton Building
Other: Designed for the patient to learn living skills to be placed in community living. Accommodated 12 patients and accepted hospital referrals of patients who are expected to complete a training period that averages 12 weeks. A house manager was available 24 hours a day. Family living, community orientations, individual, family and group therapy, medical and psychiatric services.
Built: 1976
Razed: still standing

Body Shop
Physical Description: wood, 1,200 square feet
Location: West property near old cannery
Other: Used for police
Built: 1990
Razed: still standing

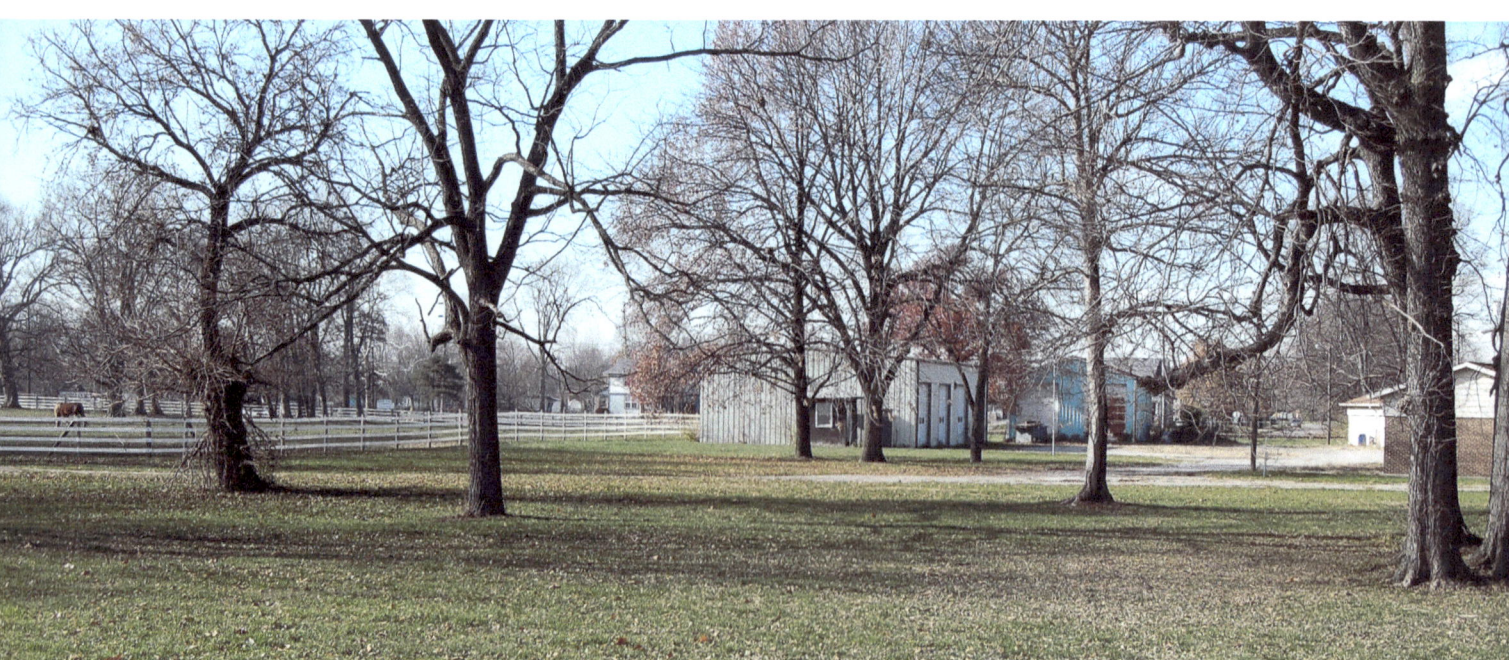

Above: Body Shop; Opposite top: Bolton Building; Opposite bottom: Exit House.

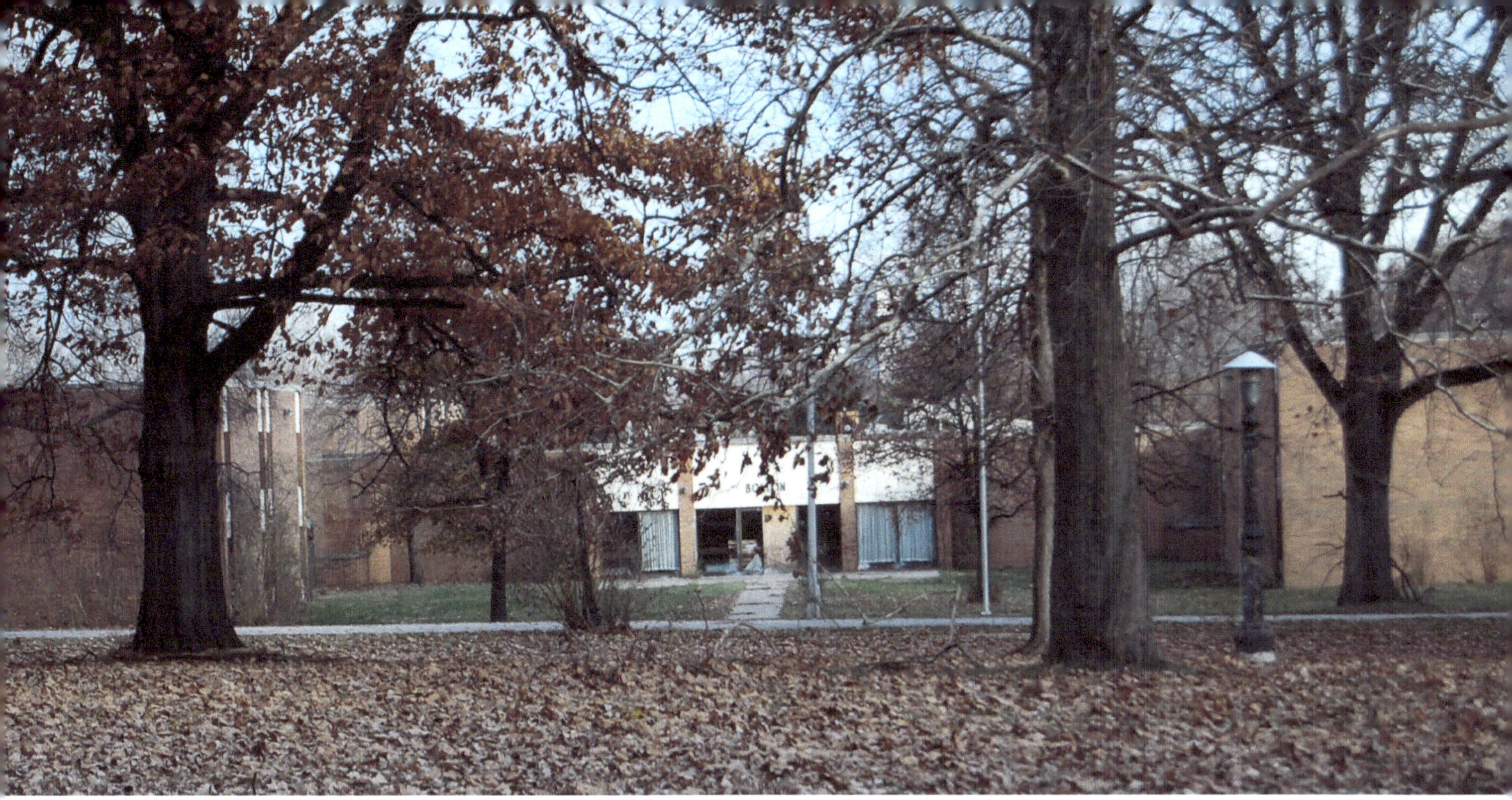

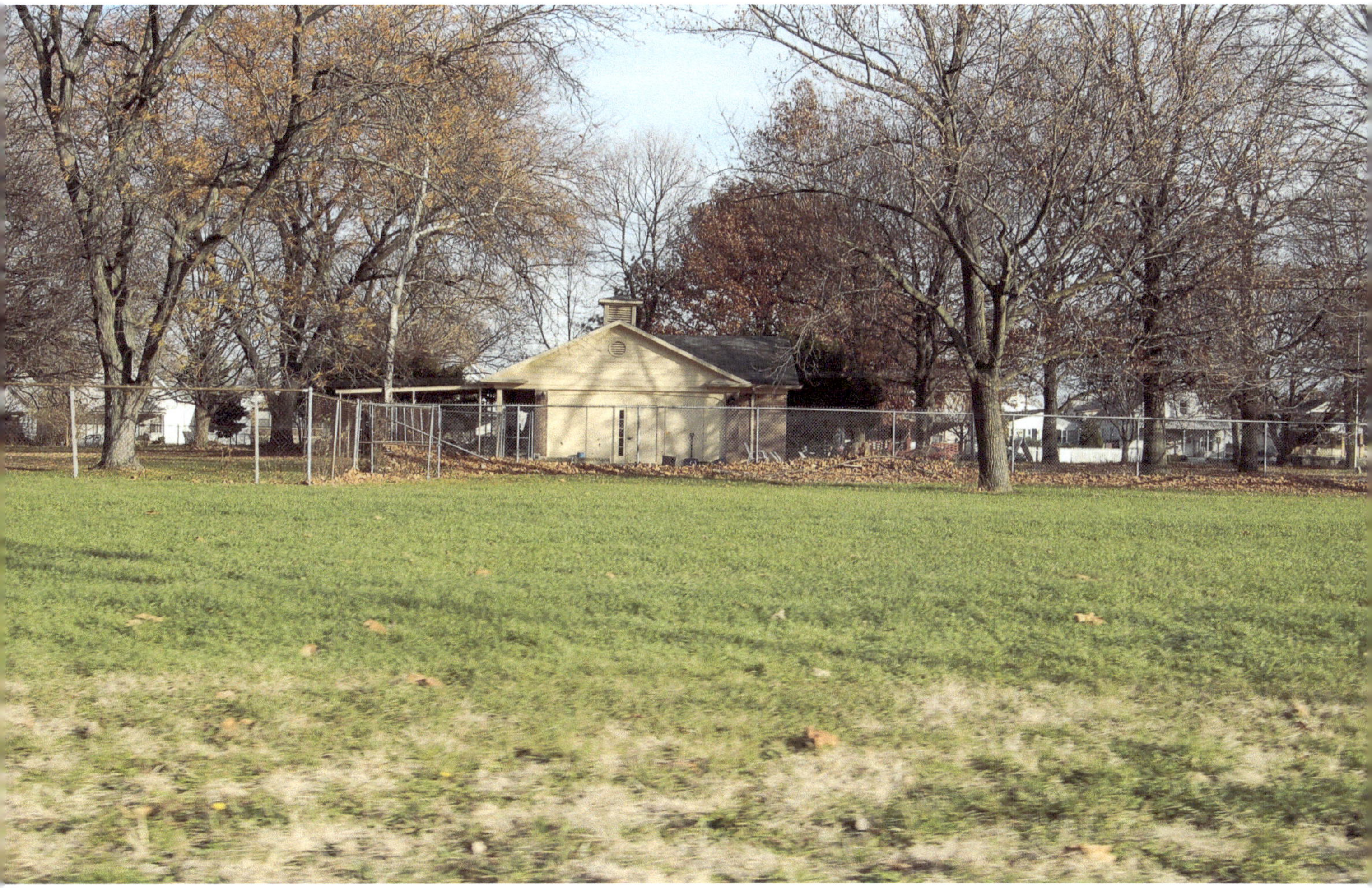

New Power Plant
Physical Description: brick, wood
Location: north of Kitchen, across from old Power Plant
Built: 1989
Razed: still standing

Refrigeration
Physical Description: brick, one-story plus basement
Location: Northwest of Pathology Department
Other: Was used as storage and for the Red Cross
Built: 1953
Razed: still standing

Bahr Treatment Center
Physical Description: Brick, wood, 123,000 square feet
Location: East side of property where greenhouses were, to the west of doctor housing
Other: 1.5 million to build. Doors and floors sprouted cracks before it even opened. It had an eighty-eight patient bed treatment facility with central offices and therapy rooms. 1957 appropriated $1,548,152 and in 1959 $650,000. Hundreds of cracks appeared in the 50,000 square feet of terrazzo floors and doors in the building. John Fleck (Fleck Quebe, and Reid Associates), architect, said the floors would have to be refinished and the doors replaced but said that this would not be done at cost to the state. The flooring underperformed and the floors and doors cured too fast from the intense heat. To cut costs, Fleck used a liquid latex terrazzo flooring which was applied to concrete. Regular terrazzo flooring has a sand base. When the concrete cracked, the terrazzo cracked. The building was empty, waiting on equipment and furniture because money had not been appropriated. The state finally released $150,000 to furnish and equip the facility. At the time, the first patient was scheduled to be in the building in eight weeks. New staff for the building: 39 attendants, one psychiatrist, one dietitian. The furniture was made at the State Reformatory. The building had one and two bed rooms, painted in pink and blue. Special rooms for electric shock and hydrotherapy treatment. An outpatient clinic was provided. Two security wards, special services (patient accounts, pharmacy, dental and other clinics, x-ray, central supply, admissions, and medical records).
Built: 1957-1960
Razed: in process of being razed

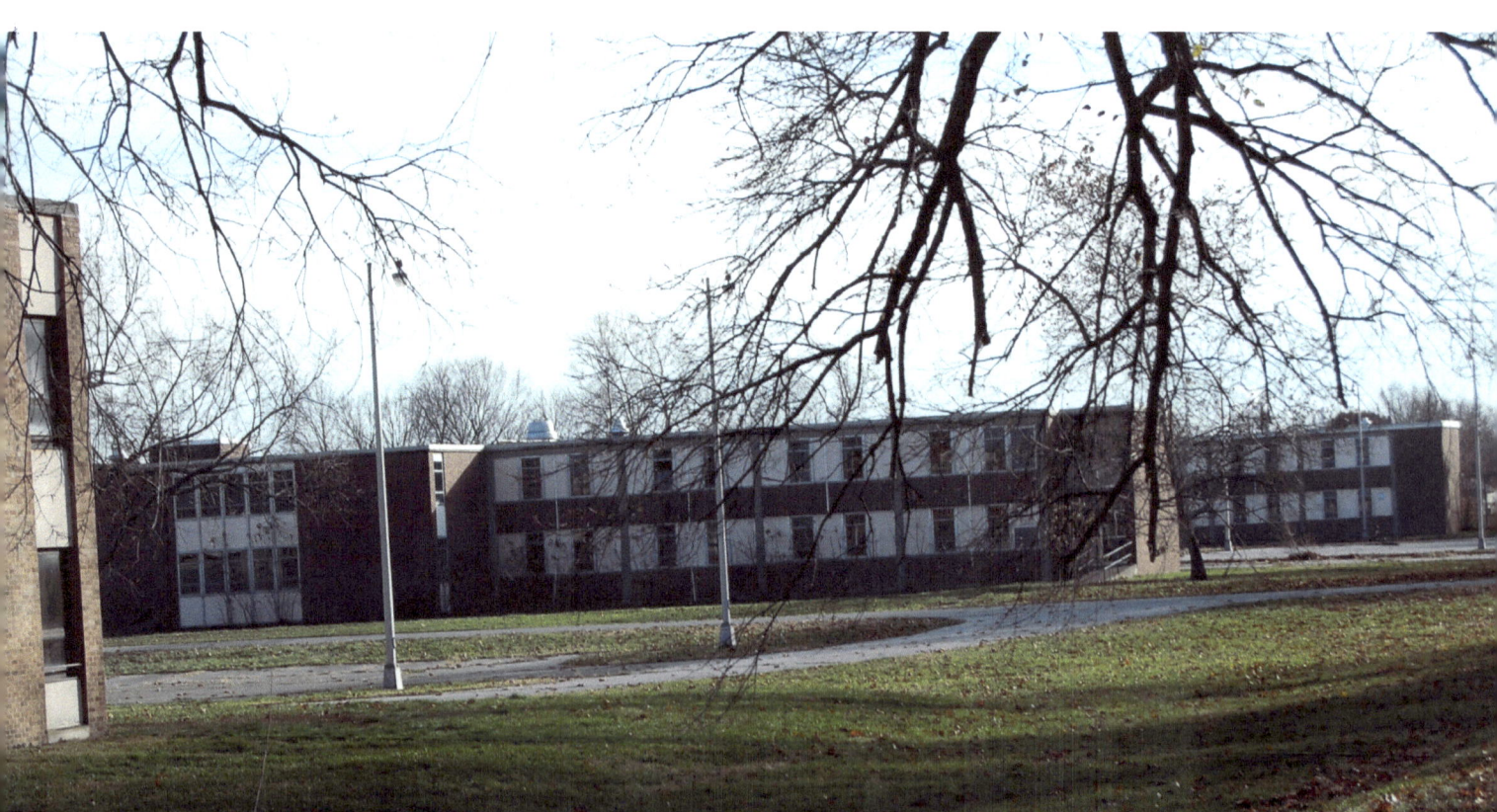

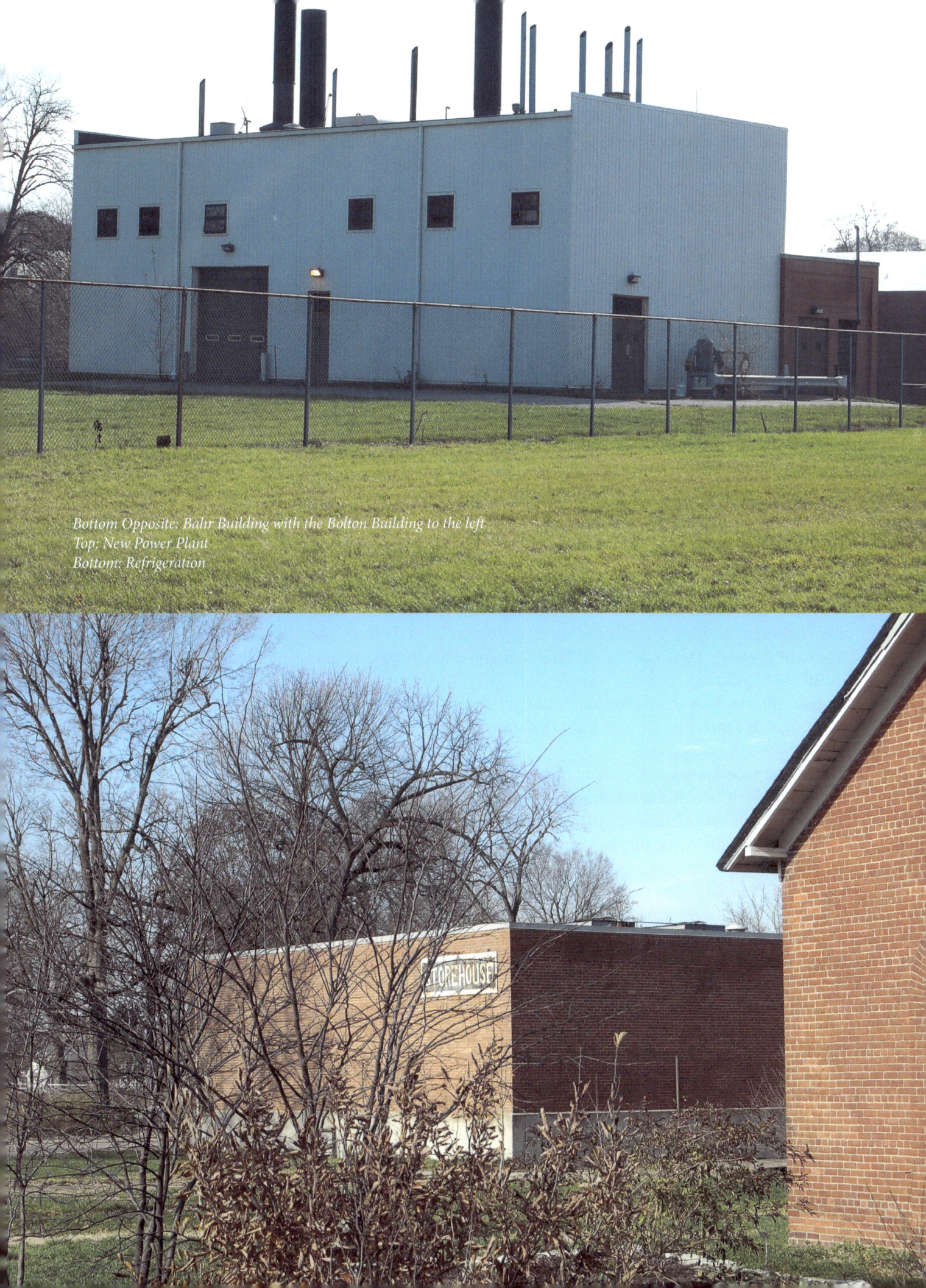

Bottom Opposite: Bahr Building with the Bolton Building to the left
Top: New Power Plant
Bottom: Refrigeration

Pavilion

Physical Description: One-story, frame, 32 feet by 32 feet; 1824 square feet
Location: Southeast of the Department for Men
Other: The annual reports mention more pavilions, but no record of their location exists other than they were "in the Grove". There were three places on the grounds that were considered a "grove": the north west side of the property where the first cemetery is, the north in front of the Employee and Evans buildings, to the south east of the Employee building where the Steeples on Washington apartments currently are.
Built: By 1898
Razed: Razed by 1936, presumably to build the Men's Cottages. Pipe Shop

Carwash

Physical Description: wood, 4,600 square feet
Location: West property near old cannery
Other: Used for police
Built: 1998
Razed: still standing

Pathology Department

Physical Description: brick, two-story, crawlspace, 1-story visitation room, stone foundation, 23 rooms, 5,705 square feet
Location: north of Morgue
Other: Nineteen working rooms, general reception, reception for relatives, viewing, mortuary, dissecting, furnace, supply, chemical laboratory, anatomical and pathological museum, lecture room. One hundred and sixty seats in auditorium. Second floor pathologists study (private), records, photography, accessory, models, charter, diagrams; library and conference, microscopical laboratory, bacteriological laboratory, pathologist's research (private). This building was built to do research in and out of state. $15,000 cost ($362,000 today).
Built: 1895
Razed: still standing. Currently houses the Indiana Medical History Museum
(Note: See the chapter on the Pathology Department for pictures of this location.)

Morgue *(also known as The Dead House)*

Physical Description: brick, one story; 480 square feet
Location: South of Pathology Department
Other: in 1915 labeled as storage. 400 square feet
Built: 1895
Razed: still standing
(Note: See the chapter on the Pathology Department for pictures of this location.)

Gas House

Physical Description: unknown, 180 square feet
Location: Unknown
Built: by 1899
Razed: Unknown

Deep Pump House
Physical Description: Brick, one-story
Location: Behind Ward O
Other: By 1914 razed and part of the South Dining Room (Men) was built in its place
Built: Unknown
Razed: Unknown, by 1914.

Pump House
Physical Description: one-story with basement, brick, 12-inch walls 151 square feet
Location: North of coal room
Other: Was a wire and pipe shop in 1936
Built: Before 1898
Razed: By 1956

Pump House
Physical Description: wood
Location: South of central section of Department for Men
Built: Unknown
Razed: Unknown. Presumably when Department of Men was razed in the 1930s.

Pump House
Physical Description: Unknown
Location: East of Mayer Hall
Other: Unknown
Built: unknown
Razed: unknown

Warehouse
Physical Description: wood, 12-inch thick walls
Location: East of Sick Hospital
Built: Before 1936
Razed: razed, unknown date.

Watch House
Physical Description: wood
Location: East of Department for Women on the Main Entrance
Other: At the entrance, the watch house had a stove, clock and lamp for people waiting for the streetcar.
Built: 1893
Razed: unknown

WARDS

The ward numbers for men were consistent until the 1930s when the Men's Cottages were built. Unlike the earlier Sanborn maps, wards were not mentioned on the 1936 Sanborn map. These cottages were referred to by floor and wing number (e.g. 3A, 3B). The ward numbers listed below for women were consistent until the building was razed in 1974. After that time, there was a massive reorganization and changes in the way mental health was treated. The wards changed into departments with smaller wards with more meaningful names. The sections of the building closest to the middle were low security, the middle parts of the wings were medium security and the "back wards" or the points furthest from the central part of the buildings were where the most challenged patients lived.

Men's Building- North Wing	Men's Building- South Wing
North: B, E, H, L	North: O, R, U, and X
Central A, D, C, K	Central: P, S, V, and Y
South: M, G, F, and I	South: Wards Q, T, W, and Z
	Note: No J ward. Reason unknown.

Women's Building- North Wing	Women's Building- South Wing
North: 15, 18, 21, 24	North: 1, 4, 7, 10
Central: 14, 17, 20, 23	Central: 2, 5, 8, 11
South: 13, 16, 19, 22	South: 3, 6, 9, 12

THE MYTHICAL FIVE MILES OF TUNNELS AND OTHER FANTASTIC STORIES

Central State Hospital has a mystique about its tunnels. Everyone loves a deliciously scary tunnel. Who knows what is lurking around the corner, or just out of sight? In the case of Central State Hospital, it is pipes. Numerous yearly reports attest to this starting in the 1880s. In 1888 the yearly report specifically states: "Tunnel for steam pipe from the boiler house to the women's department should be arched brick tunnel. " Some tunnels were also built for the convenience of transporting food and materials between buildings. Later, staff would use the tunnels as a warm respite from rain, wind and snow. Patients would also be transported through the tunnels as time went on.

One of the widest spread pieces of misinformation about Central State Hospital is that there are over five miles (sometimes exaggerated further to ten miles) of tunnels under the grounds. And all the buildings were connected. This is simply not true.

The tunnels weren't all the same size. Some were five to six feet tall and two to three feet wide. Others were a little taller and six feet wide. Based on Sanborn maps, in 1898, there were approximately 1,600 feet of brick and other tunnels and all pipe chases (i.e. tunnels specifically for pipes) that may or may not have been in a tunnel (versus simply buried underground). This is far below the 5,280 feet needed to make up one mile, let alone the 26,400 feet needed to make up five miles!

In 1915 the tunnels added up to 2,800 feet. Between the 1936 and 1956 Sanborn maps, the number grew to 4,200 feet of tunnels (excluding pipe chases, which by now were labeled as "underground tunnel"). Even if we add the Employee Building tunnel to the Mayer Hall tunnel, the total is still 4,300 feet.

The growth of the hospital between 1956 and 1973 really included razing old buildings and adding three main new buildings (Evans, Bolton and Bahr) as well as the removal of the Department for Women, the Sick Hospital and other smaller buildings (and consequent backfilling of tunnels). They added about another 2,600 feet (being generous), which would only bring the length of the tunnels up to one and a half miles at best, if the tunnels from the buildings that were razed were included.

Nor is it true the tunnels connected all the buildings together. True, they connected the majority of the buildings with patients, patient services and maintenance buildings together. However, they did not connect some outbuildings such as the pipe shops, the carpenters shop, and other small, unmarked, presumably utility, buildings. Many of the early outbuildings were either unheated (e.g. Farm Barn, Officer's Barn, Storage) or had small coal stoves, and were therefore, unconnected by tunnels for heat. It is highly unlikely the State would willingly pay for piped heat for horse stalls and coal bins.

Furthermore, it is not true that patients were kept in the tunnels or secret rooms. The first mention of any tunnel being built was in 1888 when the one from the Department of Women was built as a pipe chase. This was after the time when restraints were used on a large scale at the hospital. In 1885 the superintendent burned all the restraints. There was no need to hide patients who needed to be restrained. They had already been forced to house patients in the basement of the Department of Men and Women due to overcrowding. It was known the backwards, basements and attics housed the patients that the hospital didn't want the public to see and/or the patients that became upset when overstimulated. It was also known that restraints were used until the 1880s. Why would the State of Indiana pay for something so frivolous? The doctors had ultimate control and could have done whatever they wanted in public view of other staff.

Also, there is no evidence of the legendary tunnel that went from the original building (Department of Men) to the city morgue.

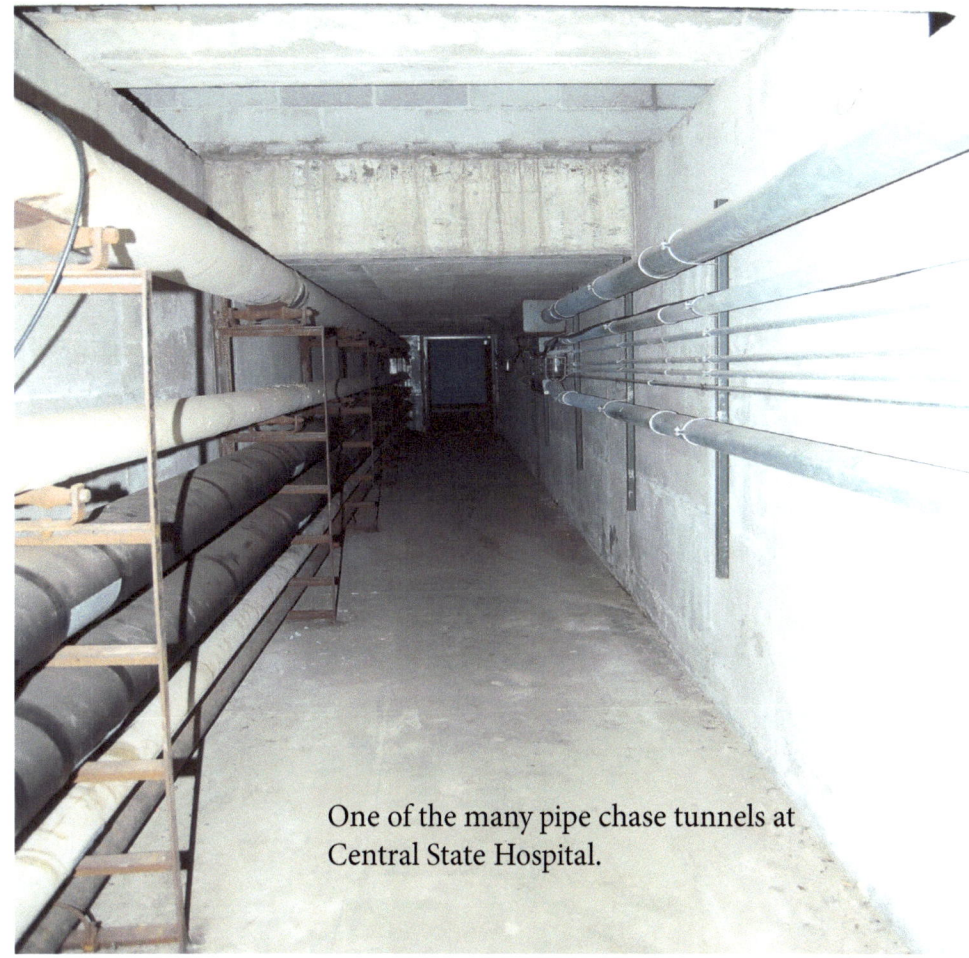

One of the many pipe chase tunnels at Central State Hospital.

Using Sanborn maps, there is no indication of a tunnel that went off site. If one thinks about it, they realize by the time Central State was in the habit of building tunnels -1870s because the hospital had more than one major building by that time- there were houses between the hospital and the City Hospital morgue. It is hard to believe as cash strapped as the hospital and State seemed to be that a tunnel to take bodies to the morgue or other purposes would be built.

Additionally, the 1898 Sanborn map first shows two tunnels from the Pathology Department that connected to a tunnel that went to the coal shed and the kitchen for the Department of Women. The entrance for these tunnels was not fronted by a fabled brass door or any other door. These tunnels, like others, carried steam heat, nothing more. The Pathology Department building is built on a slab and always has been. A former director, who photographed the narrow crawlspace, stated she was "near panic" because the crawl space was so small she was afraid she wouldn't be able to get out.

The original hospital grounds are about one half mile by one half mile square (not including Sections Two, Three and Four of the cemetery or the land sold to the State Highway Department. The only way five miles of tunnels could have been added to the land would have been by winding it like a snake over the property. That would have make it impossible for the ground to support the massive buildings we know existed.

Finally, what is not well known is that the Farm colony was not only a miniature version of Central State with its patient housing, dining rooms, and self-contained town-like feel. It also had service tunnels which connected its buildings with the boiler house. While Central State Hospital wanted the Farm Colony to be self-sustaining, it never reached that point before it was closed.

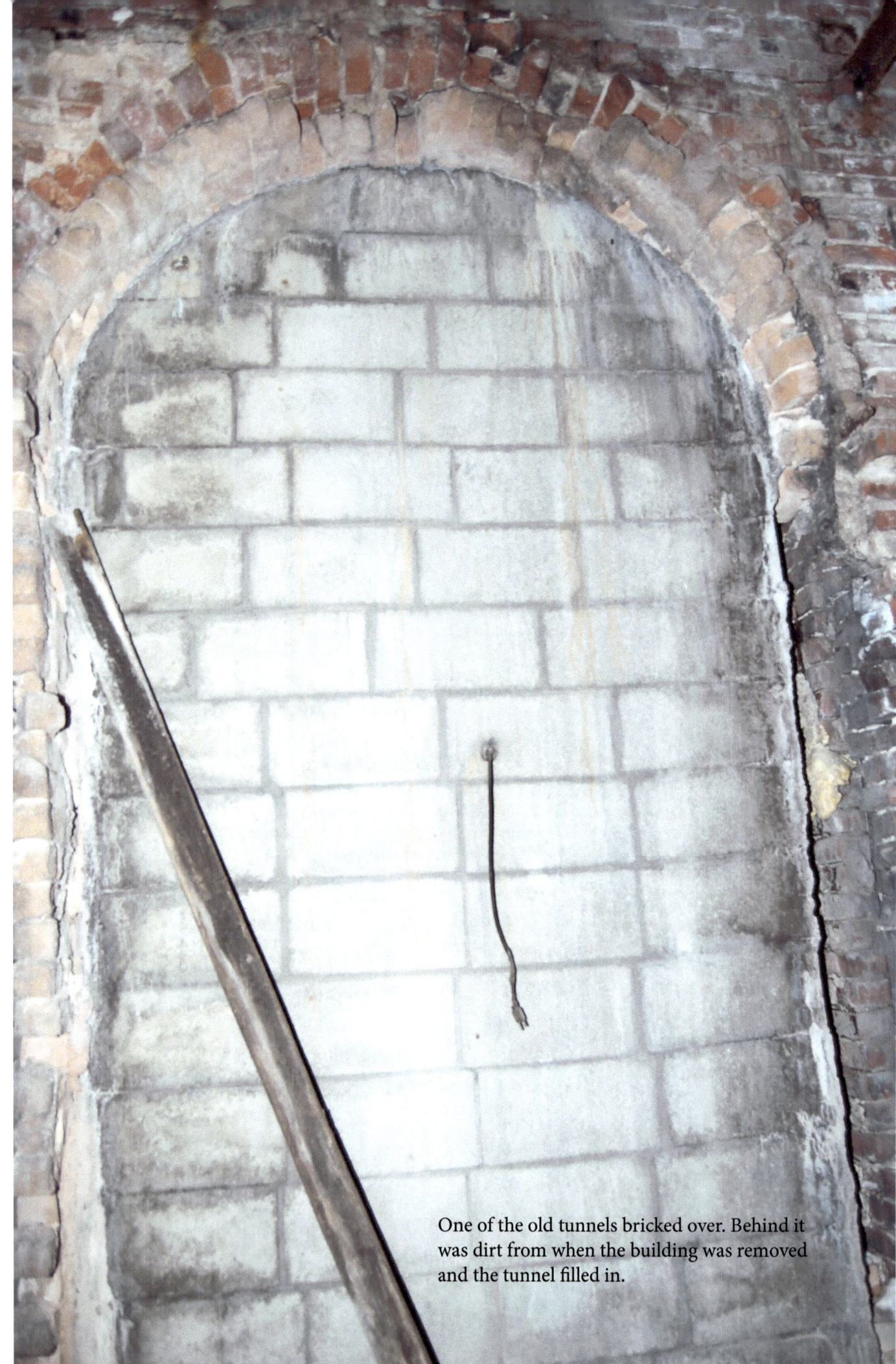

One of the old tunnels bricked over. Behind it was dirt from when the building was removed and the tunnel filled in.

Eleven

FINAL DECLINE AND CLOSURE

Every year since Central State Hospital opened, closure was on the minds of staff and legislators. In the years leading up to the closure, deinstitutionalization was a primary focus, but progress was slow going.

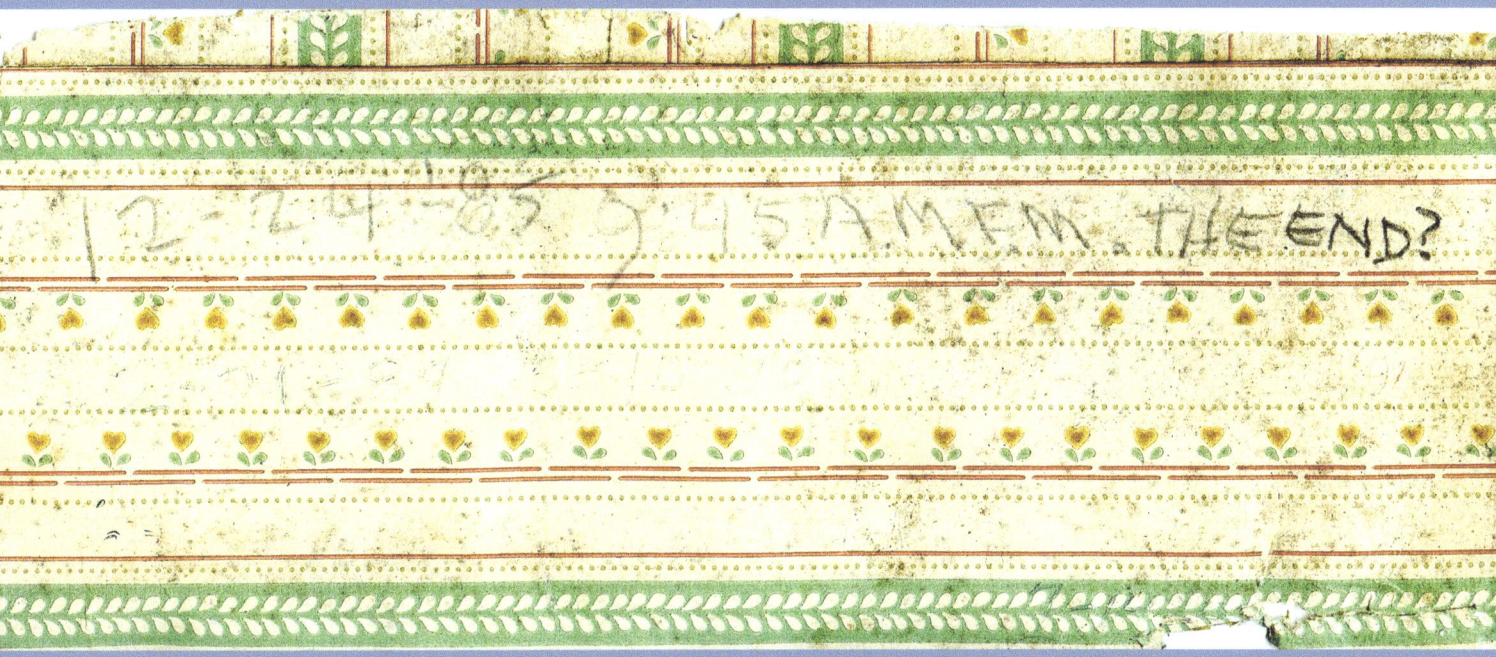

Despite higher resident populations and the aging of materials and institutions, the Indiana Legislature refused to appropriate the necessary funds to keep Central State Hospital's buildings in good repair, furnish them or staff them properly. This did not allow superintendents to implement reforms, conduct repairs or hire adequate staff, and new buildings were costly to build. The administration of the hospital and the way it cared for patients had grown larger than the people it was to treat. Because of its size and the number of duties assigned to the supervisor and the hospital administration structure, it was riddled with abuse and the opportunity for abuse. Despite newer buildings like Bahr, Bolton and Evans built to replace the old, the hospital was on the down slide.

Superintendents sometimes did not figure the budgets correctly, either basing them on inaccurate estimates, or old information. The State of Indiana fixated on yearly costs per patient and sometimes no money was allocated over old amounts despite increasing costs.

Also, the superintendents had no real control over the resident population. Superintendents were able to decide which patients were admitted to the hospital, usually favoring those they felt they could help (versus chronic, violent or repeat cases). Additionally, with more chronically ill in the hospitals and some violent patients admitted as well, they could not discharge patients as quickly or justify additional cost. It also seemed that every time the political party in power changed, focus on reforms changed, money was appropriated differently- if at all- the staff changed and nothing seemed to move forward.

Three dominate therapies in the 1950-1980 period changed the lives of mentally ill patients. First, drugs were the biggest breakthrough to the asylum system. Most were developed through trial and error. The first, Chlorpromazine, was a surgical anesthetic, used because of its calming effect. The use of this drug led to fewer restraints in mental hospitals. This drug led to over 40 other drugs being developed and introduced as patient therapy from the 1950s to the mid-1970s.

Second, cognitive behavioral therapy, which involves talking through patient issues, had solidified itself as a viable form of patient therapy.

Third, modern activities therapy came into existence. The hospital had a department specifically for activity therapy. It included music, recreation, occupational and vocational therapies. Eventually it would also include art therapy. By finding activities that made patients happy, or helped soothe them in times of crisis, patients were able to move forward with their mental health.

The dismantling of the warehouse system was seen with the 1950s introduction of anti-psychotic medication. Drugs equated to doctors and legislators as better treatment and meant more patients could live in the general population, at better health and less risk. Some patients, who a few years before, would have needed 24-hour care were now free to live their lives outside the walls of the hospital. Only acute cases needed immediate attention and fewer patients meant a smaller need for large, costly buildings. Even patients who needed frequent checks were being given group home and assisted but independent living opportunities. This led to declining numbers of patients and the large buildings, which had been built for a different time period, were simply perceived as no longer needed or useful (1).

SOCIAL REFORM FOR PATIENTS

As social reform swept through the 1960s and 1970s, concerns over patients' rights and the influence of movies such as "One Flew Over The Cuckoo's Nest" brought to light inequality and tyranny in old institutions.

In 1961 enrollment in Central State Hospital was 12,905, and serious talk began about downsizing and developing an array of more individualized and cost-effective community-based services. Heath care officials and doctors believed that this would be more humane and lead to better outcomes.

In 1963 the U.S. Congress passed the Community mental Health Centers Act and John F. Kennedy signed it into law. States could now get federal assistance to build community health centers. To qualify for the federal money, the centers had to provide:
- Inpatient Services
- Outpatient Services
- Partial hospitalization
- Emergency services
- Consultation services
- Treatment and research

Unfortunately due to the economic crisis at the time and the Vietnam War, this program never really realized its full potential.

Additionally, during President Jimmy Carter's administration, the Mental Health Systems Act was made into law. It required additional services such as psychiatric screening; children and teen services; rape crisis, alcohol and drug abuse services; and residential and elderly services. However, when the Reagan administration came into power, the act was repealed and the money was given to the state without direction as to its use. The Federal government cut funding for mental health by 30%.

By the early 1980s, the Central State Hospital employed 357 clinical employees. However, due to cutbacks and staffing needs, only 85 of them could be available to take care of over 500 resident patients (there were over 4800 total) at any given time.

"The cuts are beginning to hurt us the worst in the area of direct patient contact," said E. Keith Miller, Assistant Superintendent for Administration.

The hospital was accredited in 1986 by the Joint Commission on Accreditation of Healthcare Organizations (JCAHO). This meant that the hospital followed nationally accepted standards for the care and treatment of patients. It remained accredited from 1986 through its closure.

THE LAST YEARS

By late 1970s the information in yearly reports had become more about what the hospital accomplished in units, and less about what it needed. By 1980s yearly reports made the hospital seem like it was a well-oiled machine, speaking of "reorganization," "chain of communication," improvements, and "building for the future." Despite trying to build this perception, below the surface unrest was brewing. The hospital administration also spoke of staffing being "kept at a minimum." For years, a Band-Aid™ had been placed over the hospital and it was slowly being peeled back. In the early 1990s, it was finally ripped off with frightening finality. The closure documentation for the hospital reveals:

- 1984: Federal, State and Local governments have not developed systematic ways to finance deinstitutionalization
- "…more than 60% of patients studied were inappropriately placed in state hospitals and could benefit from treatment in other kinds of settings.
- "But the main reason mental healthcare has left so many homeless is that funding didn't follow the patients out of the hospitals and into the community

Funding in 1990 was as crunched as ever at Central State Hospital and the Community Mental Health Centers (CMHCs) that were part of the growing services for mental health patients. Lack of funding was a result of several factors. In 1981 CMHC's were funded by federal block grants that were paid directly to the centers. With the Reagan Administration, those funds were given to the state for disbursement. The State of Indiana gave some of the money to the centers and kept a roll-over fund. In 1990, the roll-over money ran out. Additionally, Congress cut Indiana's mental health funds by 30%, from $16 million to $10 million. The hospital's budget for 1990 Indiana was $177,000,000, which was the same as the year before, making repairs, upgrades, replacements and staff funding very tight.

Also in 1990, instead of the 1980s patients wandering around all day and receiving no therapy except drug therapy in excessive amounts, ward-based programming was instituted. When reporters for NUVO, a local news magazine went out to the hospital, they saw a "modern, relatively pleasant facility in which patients seemed decently dressed and groomed." They also witnessed group activities, and other patients who were "hanging out," "chilling" or "chatting."

Still, investigations were becoming commonplace at the hospital. Investigations were prompted by the deaths of the following patients:

- Cynthia J. Stanley, 35 died November 2, 1989 when she accidentally set herself on fire while smoking in a restroom. Her parents, Lee Ann and William Stanley of Kokomo brought suit.
- Charles Brent Barthelemy, 45, died November 28, 1989 of a seizure disorder aggravated by "water intoxication." He was found dead in a bathroom after swallowing massive amounts of water.
- Prentice L. McAnish, 25, died February 21, 1990 after he walked away from the hospital and was struck on Interstate 65.

The investigative panel reported that when one of these patients died, one nurse was responsible for three wards, meaning 80 patients in all. In March 1990, the ratio of staff to patients was 1 to 7.3 instead of the 1 to 1.4 that the Indiana Department of Mental Health deemed as the norm, and although 55 registered nurses were authorized for March 1990, at most only five were caring for patients. The hospital had no uniform procedure to investigate deaths.

Staff with the least training (attendants and volunteers) had the most contact with patients.

Later that year, new guidelines for state mental hospitals were proposed:
- Standardizing internal processes of investigation within hospitals
- Developing uniform protocols for determining "usual" and "unusual" causes of death, and when they should be investigated
- Plans of correction should be filed with the State Department of Mental Health
- Notifying the Indiana Protection and Advocacy Commission within 71 hours (2) of every death within a state mental facility
- Review of death records, investigations and developing correction plans would be done by the Protection and Advocacy Commission
- Expanding training.

In the same year, a shortage of supervised community homes forced 140 patients who were well enough to be placed in such homes, to be left in the hospital. At the same time 146 people were waiting to become patients of the hospital, but couldn't because the hospital had no room. During this period, over 500 mentally ill patients in Indiana had been hospitalized for more than ten years.

The people who were unable to get into the hospital had few choices. They could be cared for by family and friends, or be temporarily housed in other hospitals. Some could use outpatient services at community mental health agencies with varying degrees of success. Some would end up jailed once they committed a petty crime because law enforcement had no other place to send them. It seemed history was repeating itself.

The Public Citizen Health Research Group and the National Alliance for the Mentally Ill conducted a study which stated that Indiana was only one of four states where the care of mentally ill patients was declining. Indiana mental health experts agreed. Litigation against Central State Hospital led to ongoing monitoring of Central State by the United States Department of Justice. The Legal Services Organization brought suit a number of times to force state mental facilities to meet their statutory obligations to provide adequate care. For example, in October 1989 an order was asked for requiring Governor Bayh to provide therapeutic residential treatment for children.

After one such investigation in 1989, the director of nursing services at Central State Hospital, Sheila Mischler, submitted her resignation. She cited her frustration over what she believed was failure by the state to care for its mentally handicapped residents. Mischler said she became a mental health nurse to "help some of society's most vulnerable people. That job is virtually impossible under existing conditions at Central State Hospital."

Insufficient staffing, inadequate funding for programs, lack of commitment by state officials to address problems within the mental health system were all part of the problem. Mischler stated, "I am unwilling to continue jeopardizing my personal integrity and professional reputation in order to work for a system that is unresponsive to the needs of the individuals for which it exists. Legally, I am compromised when I am not allowed to meet the requirements of the Indiana Nurse Practice Act because of unsafe staff ratios which interfere with the nurses' ability to practice nursing. I am also legally accountable for providing a safe staffing level appropriate to patient needs - an impossible task given the current available staffing resources."

Superintendent Ruth Stanley believed at this time about 50% more clinical staff were needed. It was hard to attract nurses especially. Where an RN might garner $28,000 to $30,000 at a job outside the state system, at Central State, starting pay was $24,000. Ward attendants started at $12,000. General staffing was unavailable due to hiring freezes.

Stanley thought the hospital did a great job, especially considering the funding. She and other healthcare providers stated they tried to stay upbeat or otherwise it would be too hard to come to work or lead. Stanley supported the departure of the Director of Nursing, she said that Mischler in some ways "was expecting something that is just never going to be there in any state system."

At the same time, Robert L Dyer, State Mental Health Chief believed Central State Hospital could be saved as long as the "will" was there. He proposed the following actions could save Central State Hospital.

1. Hold each worker accountable for their jobs. Make it "crystal clear" what their responsibilities are.
2. Fire workers who are "incompetent, lazy, or mean and hire more carefully" (Dyer wanted to fire up to 5%).
3. Clarify lines of authority.
4. Force doctors, nurses and social workers to document the time they spent on the wards with patients and in contact with patients' families.
5. Recruit one more level of worker- licensed mental health technicians. Workers with two year degrees were

employed at other mental hospitals in other states. Attendants could aspire to this hiring level of education and pay.
6. Open lines of communications between staff, patients and families.
7. Beef up security and crack down on racial incidents.

However, over the next two years, these actions were not adopted properly or effectively.

CLOSURE

The hospital was plagued by poor care and bad press. On May 21, 1991 Linda Shelby, a patient, died of a heart attack due to over medication. On November 4, 1991 June Christy Highsaw died. She'd been admitted in 1970 when she was 14 years old. Her conditions included schizophrenia, bilateral cataracts, mild mental retardation, and seizures. It was determined she of hypothermia when freezing air blew in her window. Witnesses said that the window had been non-functioning for a long time and she died of hypothermia when the wind blew in but also because it blew in on her soiled, wet bed linen.

The last straw for Central State's troubled past was on March 20, 1992 when Linda Heine drowned in a bathroom while the attendants were playing cards. Two former employees, Susan M. Sneed and Sharon Jett were charged with reckless homicide, neglect of a dependent and obstruction of justice.

Superintendent Ruth Stanley resigned March 4, 1992, giving a month's notice, but she was fired March 23, 1992 a few days after Heine's death (and before her term of notice concluded) for insubordination and refusing to cooperate in conjunction with Heine's case. A nurse, psychiatric attendant supervisor and five attendants were fired. One of the attorneys for the group stated that he felt some of the parties were "scapegoating lower level workers". Healthcare advocates said firing and lawsuits weren't going to fix the problem. For them it was the system that was at fault. They said the hospitals were "starved for money, staff and attention." (3)

By the time 1992 rolled around and Governor Bayh called for the closure, there were only 389 patients left. Governor Bayh believed that closing the hospital "will guarantee safer, more compassionate care for patients, and the most cost-effective use of taxpayer dollars." Bayh ordered a comprehensive study on the future of Central State but later decided to close it. "We need to take dramatic action, and closing Central State will guarantee safer, more compassionate care for the patients and the most cost-effective use of taxpayer dollars," Bayh said. Joanne Barreno who had mentally ill children in Central State Hospital hoped Bayh would keep his promise by providing "good care in the community. Our children must have good care."

In May of 1993, two employees were indicted on charges of rape and sexual battery, but the hospital Medical Director, Dr. James Donahue and the former Superintendent Ruth Stanley, were cleared of any wrongdoing in these and Shelby and Heine's deaths.

The Central State Closure Plan update on June 2,1993 state that all mentally ill and/or people suffering disabilities should be served in local communities. The patient and the caregivers should be part of the treatment design process. Services should support the bridge between care and community. Funding needs were to follow the patients, meaning the money should be consumer driven and in the communities, versus at a state level. Provider creativity, streamlining the process. And abandoning "prohibitive, unnecessary rules" should be encouraged.

Many people agreed but some people were concerned for not only the welfare of the more able-bodied patients, but also what would happen to the most violent patients or those least able to take care of her/himself.

On the day of the closure announcement patients were visited by member of the Central State Hospital management to advise them and let them know the next steps. Then, on June 25, each ward was revisited to reassure patients and answer questions. The families were sent a letter by the Department of Families and Social Services (FSSA) briefly explaining the decision and invited them to info meetings conducted by Jeff Richardson, head of Family and Social Services (FSSA) and Robert Dyer, State Mental Health Chief and other State representatives.

A closure process was implemented including closing quickly and efficiently, insuring that no patient was moved until she or he was "clinically" ready, ensuring the mental health centers were put in place as case managers, and that the money for the patients followed them to the community. A key to the closure was obtaining Medicaid money when possible for the patients to offset costs of care. Patients were to be given appropriate residential programs and that patients that could not be in a residential setting were to be kept in safe and secure environments. The State studied the specialization of state psychiatric hospitals, such as hospital for only children and specialized programs at other facilities was the outcome. The State also prepared recommendations for changes in licensing of residential facilities. Central State Hospital was to work with the State to transition personnel and develop policies and procedures to make the downsizing go smoothly.

The transition of patients to community based care included steps which allowed time to reflect and decide if this was the correct path for each patient, or if a new direction needed to be taken.

Each patient was assessed in order to:
- Create a CMHC wide plan of community based care
- CMHC plans are reviewed for funding by the Community Mental Health Transition Fund
- Central State Hospital patients were to be reviewed and compared to healthcare funding proposals.

Specific plans for placement were to be made.
- Patients would be moved and their care would be monitored.
- New groups of patients repeated the process with other state operated facilities.
- Review the process as it progressed.

Patients with developmental disabilities were also assessed
- Identify and select providers
- Providers arranged community based services
- Providers designed services to meet patient needs
- Providers initiated patient placement
- Patients were monitored and followed after placement

Several organizations were responsible for planning care for the Central State Hospital patients.

Each center had a separate plan to accommodate the patients referred to them.
- Adult and child mental health center (Marion and Johnson Counties)
- Comprehensive Mental Health Services of E Central Indiana (Delaware, Henry and Jay Counties)
- Cummins Mental Health Center (Hendricks and Putnam Counties)
- Gallahue Mental Health Center (Hancock, Marion and Shelby Counties)
- Howard Community Hospital Psychiatric Services (Howard, Clinton and Tipton Counties)
- Integrated Field Services (which treated individuals with developmental disability throughout state)
- Midtown Community Mental Health Center (Marion County)

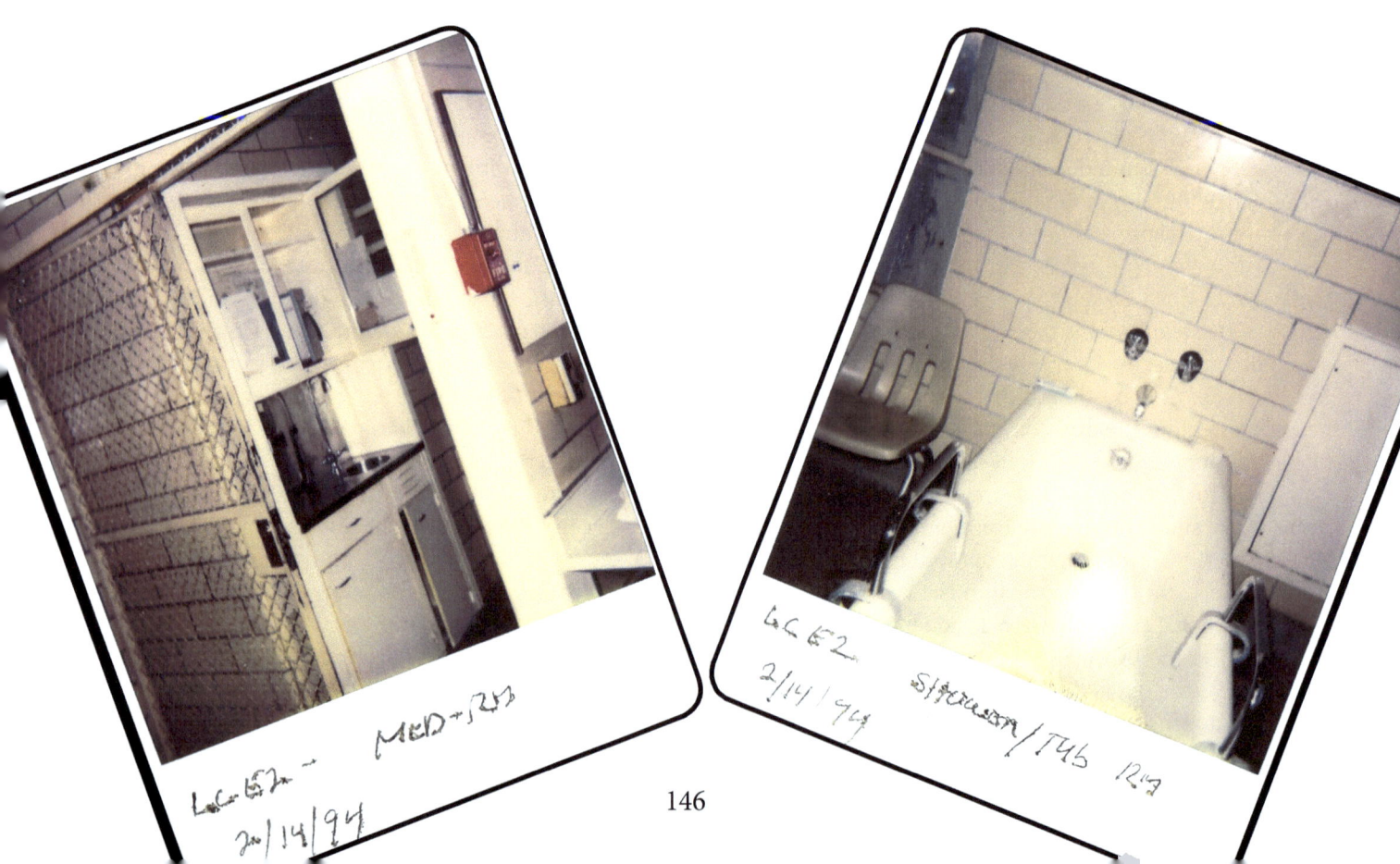

- Porter Starke Services Inc (Porter and Starke Counties)
- Tri-City Comprehensive Mental Health Center (Lake County)
- Tri County Mental Health Center (Boone, Hamilton and Marion County)
- Wabash Valley Hospital Incorporated (Benton, Carroll, Fountain, Jasper, Montgomery, Newton, Tippecanoe, and White Counties)

The closure was slow. In the first seven months over 122 patients were to be moved. At the end of the deadline only six had been moved.

Finances and Continued Improvements

Financing the move was a challenge. First, funding from Central State Hospital came from the Indiana's General Fund and from third party reimbursements to the Mental Health Fund. The General Fund was used to fund the community placements. The money that was sent to the Mental Health Fund was now to be collected by the community-based caregivers.

Interestingly, on January 23, 1993, just 17 months from the closure, Central State received a near perfect score from inspectors who surveyed the facility. The only issues were 15 minor points such as sweeping up rubbish, or reminding patients to wear their glasses. The following week the Joint Commission on Accreditation of Healthcare Organizations assessed the hospital but found serious problems such as hiring more nurses, the need to keep better records and documenting the criteria for hiring psychiatrists; to provide better treatment plans for the addiction patients and to repair the always-run-down Bahr Building. The hospital was praised for excelling in the dietary department and for controlling infectious disease.

During this time, projects to improve patient safety and comfort were completed. This included glass replacement, power plant removal, furnishing chairs and other items for patient areas, and hot water heater (Bahr) and electrical switch gear replacements. Additionally, security was scaled up to include officers at the patient buildings and making changes to the lock and key systems.

In March 1993, $2,200,000 was spent on new beds, paint, couches, shower curtains, mirrors, tables and ceiling lights. Parking lots and sidewalks were repaved. The administration stated patients deserved a "safe and cheerful environment" until the closure. Other projects such as new phone systems, renovating the laundry and another $3,600,000 in projects were scrapped. Still, after the closing was ordered, the Central State Hospital conference center underwent

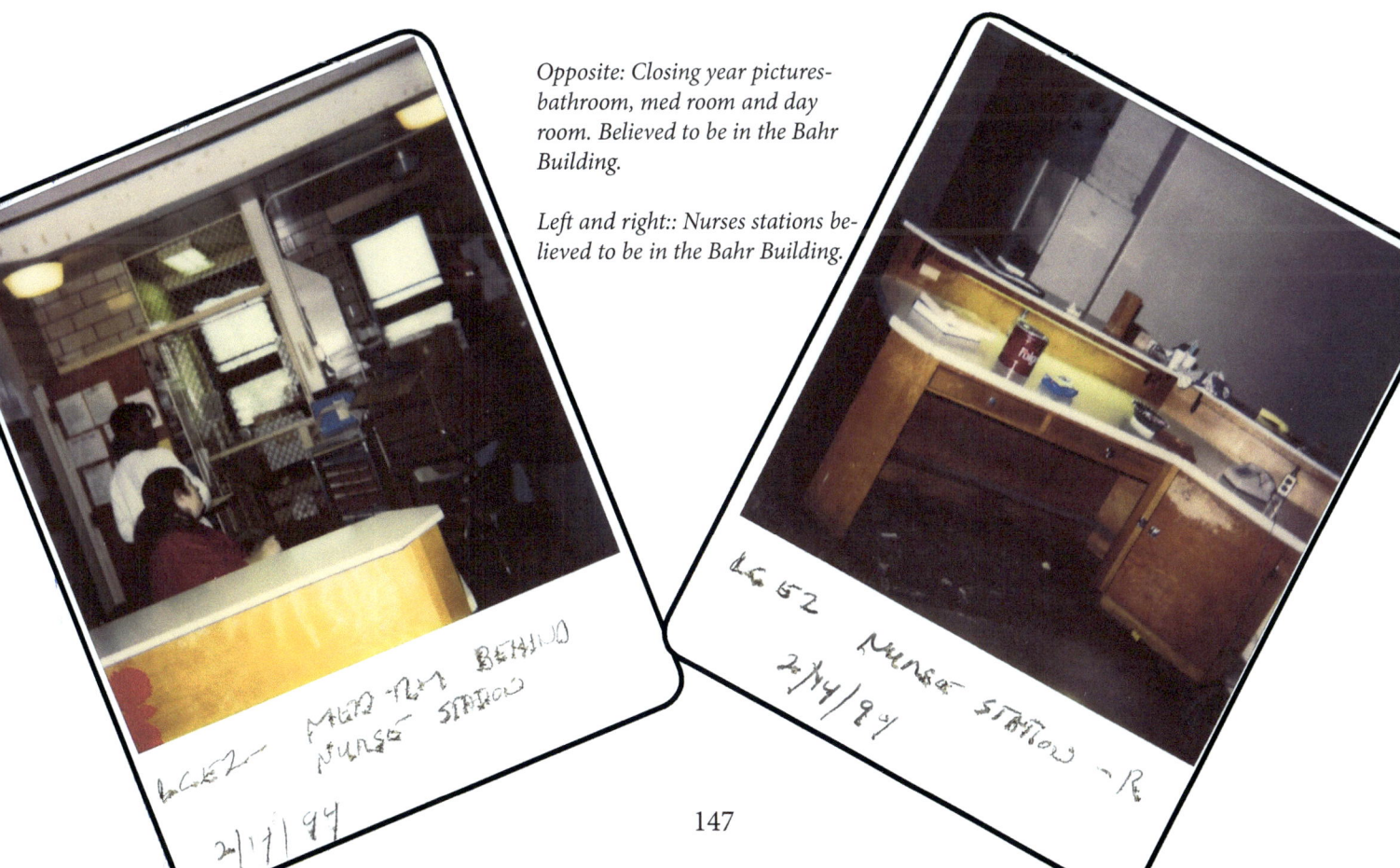

Opposite: Closing year pictures- bathroom, med room and day room. Believed to be in the Bahr Building.

Left and right:: Nurses stations believed to be in the Bahr Building.

BoLToN Bldg
Window's Check List

		Phone #	Time Call	Window's open
WARD 25	Fisher	3760	7:52 AM	118-107
WARD 26		3770	7:56 AM	237-222-221-214-212-211-20?
WARD 22			7:30 AM	Check and is OK
WARD 28			7:34 AM	Check and is OK
WARD 23		3786	7:36 AM	Check and is OK
WARD 24	Magers	3789	7:39 AM	233-232-225-223-222
WARD 21	Smith	3789	7:59	-134-
WARD 22				209-223-230

A window checklist post-Linda Highsaw's death.

Wm M. Taylor
Carpenter Foreman
Bolton Bldg
6-29-92

renovation. With improvements in the ever-plagued Bahr Building, Albert McCray, who worked in the locked wards there, said that he felt it was "so much better….It used to be like a dungeon." Patients were able to choose the color for their rooms. Former patient Kevin McGill said he wanted white because it was "cheerful-looking."

Other improvements included at $25,000 computerization of the pharmacy department to reduce misinterpretation of handwriting. A mechanical gate around maintenance buildings to keep patients from hiding and not partaking in therapeutic activities.

Patient, Family, and Staff Reaction

Patients, families and staff also had an opinion.

Two studies were completed pre- and post- closure. In the pre-closure study, 65.4% of patients and 39.8 % of families agreed on the closure, that it was good, but only 27.8% of the public thought it was a good idea. And only 10.4% of the staff believed it was good. More than two-thirds of the public and 48.7% of the workers disagreed with the decision. In fact, over half the patients, over three quarters of the family, and even more workers, as well as over 95% of the public involved in the survey, thought Central State Hospital should have been overhauled and kept open. The family, workers and the public cited the reason that patients would be homeless as a huge factor in their answers.

As the pre-closure study continued, patients generally became more positive about the closure, the chance for a better life, and the chances they would not become homeless. Workers were less optimistic about the patients' quality of life post closure. They also believed less that closing CSH was a good thing and that more patients would be homeless.

In the post closure study about a third of the public believed closure was a good thing. The number of people who thought Central State Hospital should have stayed open dropped by 20%.

The attendants were concerned as well. Attendant Rowley had 30 patients who were so severely ill that none of them were able to go home. Attendant Catherine Reynolds said that staff was "like family" to the patients, and that a lot of them loved the patients and wanted to stay with them. She thought when the closure happened that all of them would suffer, staff and patients alike. Reynolds was so disappointed" for herself and more for the patients. She was convinced it would take a long time for them to trust new caregivers.

However, not everyone thought that it was a family or home. Joann Owens, a Central State Hospital nurse said, 'They are outcasts. Out of sight, out of mind."

Several patients went to court to stop their transfer to more restrictive facilities, or to facilities far away from family and friends.

- Judge Eichholtz ruled that "W.T." didn't have to go to any facility because he posed no risk to himself or others. W.T. would have been transferred to Madison State Hospital.
- Eichholtz also overruled a decision that would have sent "R.F." to Evansville State Hospital". The patient was to remain at Central State Hospital until a community based treatment plan could be developed for him in Marion County.
- Eichholtz also heard an appeal for "J.B." who was to be transferred to Evansville State Hospital. The move would have cut "J.B." off from his family.

Community mental health centers spoke as well. They were over-strained and under-funded. When $3,000,000 from the Medicaid Rehabilitation option was allocated for the first 150 patients to leave Central State Hospital, Jim Jones, executive director of the Indiana Council of Community Mental Health Centers said, "The good news is that we gain a little relief. The bad news is that it isn't enough to resolve the pressures facing the centers." Jones went on to say that some centers were so strapped for money that they had to fire workers.

Missions asked how many former patients would show up. The sheriff wanted to know who was responsible when patients who were moved ended up in the morgue. Bayh, who had promised "safer more compassionate care" for the patients said that he was satisfied the plan was working. Jeff Dyer pointed out that people in community programs had a choice to participate or not because it was their "civil right."

Families were pressed to express their thoughts after the closure announcement. Many families were afraid and angry. Feeling left out of the decision process, there was a grassroots effort to protest and make the Governor change his mind. The families and others looked to the Indiana Alliance for the Mentally Ill (IAMI, now the National Alliance for the Mentally Ill- Indiana) for help. This advocacy organization was divided on the issue of closure and its issues. Instead of taking a stand, they focused on "broader contextual issues, including "Fragmented care, poor housing, insufficient professional caregivers, unstable funding, and lack of client choice in services." As time went on, the families resigned themselves to the inevitable.

Still, there was a larger concern of how much of the patient care would fall to independent caregivers and organizations instead of the State. In a 1995 survey conducted that monitored this, 69.9% of caregivers did not feel burdened. In fact, the amount of time spent with the patient outside of the hospital setting went down after the closure. It dropped from 37% weekly to 28% and 12% daily contact to 6.5%, but the monthly visits increased from 31% to 37%. The number of caregivers who visited less than once a month rose from 15.2% to 23.9%. Even parents with once a week contact dropped from 51% to 46.4% after the closure of the hospital. Additionally, the face-to-face contact dropped from 57.6% to 45.6% and phone contact became more common. The contact with the mental health professionals also rose from 39.1% of caregivers who did have contact 55.4%. According to the study, "In this regard, the changes in frequency and nature of contact families have with the patients should be viewed with caution as a potential unintended negative consequence of the closing."

Families and caregivers who responded to a survey believed that "the problems at Central State Hospital should have been fixed so that it could stay open." (80.4%). "Overall people from CSH are better off being cared for in the community (53.3%), "The quality of the lives of the people discharged from CSH is better when they are treated in the community (52.2%). The decision to close CSH was a good one. (40.2%) Clearly, they had mixed feelings about the move.

Some parents who had longer drive times- 70 miles or more- to see their children, were not happy because of the drive time. However, parents thought their relatives were in a good, safe place. Wilma Wallace, a sibling, was distraught, wondering what would become of her brother. He'd been put in a group home "and the group home didn't want him. So he was shipped back…"

Wade Stewart III had a mother in Central State. He asked representatives from the State to meet with him before his mother was placed. In response to his concerns, representatives said that "they were trying to find the best match for the patient."

Hazel Bumgardner didn't know what she was going to do if she couldn't see her son every day, "No mother on Earth loves her son more than I do."

James H Martin didn't want to hear any of it. They didn't "fool" him. It was about "Republicans and Democrats and money." He charged that they could have "put that money" in the hospital and made it "operate more efficiently…. But you didn't."

One patient, "Dave" said that it was "scary to start over." Another patient, Jeff Russell wanted to know where all the patients would go. He said, "The governor could care less about us. This is not compassion, this is too much politics." He could have gone home to be with his mother, but didn't want to "make things hard on her."

Dan McGinnis was ready to leave. He remembers saying, "I'm like a stallion. I'll be the first out the door. Let me out and I'm gone." He ended up in a nursing home.

Kenneth Daugherty wasn't sure. He thought there could be "worse places" than Central State Hospital.

Ministers wanted Central State Hospital to stay open. They felt the system was overburdened and this would just "exacerbate the problem. Many will end up homeless or dead."

> "More agile and personalized systems of long-term supports are needed that embrace community inclusion, personal choice and independence… Resources should be shifted away from institutional settings to community based supports. Policies should be geared toward assisting individuals to move into the community."

Plans

Once Governor Bayh made the decision to close the hospital, transition plans and future use plans were developed. A budget analysis was done for the closure, including what upkeep would cost for buildings and materials during the final years of Central State. On June 12, 1992, a report was submitted to Don Perry, the director for the Public Works Division, by Joseph Raper, President of the Cooler Group (now Cooler Design), which specializes in healthcare facility architecture and design). It quoted over $8,000,000 worth of repair, demolition, asbestos removal, and safety changes- many of which did happen including upgrades to the Bahr Treatment Center, and remodeled bathrooms, nurse's stations and paint in the Evans and Bolton Buildings.

One of the early plans for the vacant hospital was to make it a prison. However, security mechanisms simply didn't exist, and the upgrades would have been too costly. In addition, the people in the neighborhood were not open to it.

Another proposal recommended that the hospital raze the patient housing and make ten to 12 "suburban type homes" that could house 144 children in treatment programs. This option was led by former Mayor Stephen Goldsmith, Juvenile Division Judge James Payne, and the State. Part of the problem with this proposal occurred when Governor Evan Bayh promised the neighborhood that only non-violent children would be sent there.

The proposal was further complicated when the people involved turned the proposal into a state wide comprehensive plan (rather than a Marion County plan) for the treatment of children, which to many in power, seemed no better than what was going on at Central State Hospital at the present time.

Proponents of the plan argued that the children would be in a family campus for short term treatment. A separate non-profit agency would standardize processes for handling the cases, including treatment plans and discharge. The emphasis was on keeping the children in a home setting, with parents or a foster family. Jim Killen, the executive director of the Indiana Youth Services Association, thought using Central State Hospital was a bad idea calling it a "cesspool" stating decisions were being driven by finances. Cheryl Sullivan, Secretary of the Indiana Family and Social Services Administration said that these fears were misplaced. Eventually, the plan fell through.

Other plans for the former hospital grounds included using it as training facilities for police and SWAT practice.

After the hospital closed, Larue D. Carter Memorial Hospital took on the long term patients. as well as continuing its focus on being a teaching hospital. These long-term patients were considered to have been patients that "destabilized" in the community based living centers. At the time of the hospital closure 30 community mental health centers treated 95% of all patients through public mental health programs.

Costs

In 1993, just Central State was costing the State and taxpayers $23,000,000 plus $12,000,000 for repairs (4). By contrast, the 30 smaller mental health facilities that serviced the whole state cost $74,000,000. While it may have been easy to justify the closing of a facility that cost so much money to run and was outdated, jobs were at stake, as was the care of the 370 patients left at the hospital.

Employee and mental health union leaders decried this move alleging the state was being "insensitive" to the patients mental health needs. But state officials swore this was a win-win for everyone. The state saw a savings of millions of dollars, and patients were "freed from chronically negligent and dehumanizing care that is virtually synonymous with mid-scale instructional treatment."

Others decried this as political action. State Representative Brad Baylif (R- Kokomo) stated that Governor Bayh wanted to "close the door on an embarrassing political situation. This decision doesn't deal with the systemic problems facing our mentally ill and mentally retarded." However, experts in the state believed the money that is saved by closing the hospital and others like it needed to follow the patients back into the communities and mental health centers.

During the last two years of the hospital, the hospital's executive committee displayed the following Vision Statement in the Administration Building: "The employees of Central State Hospital will provide a safe, clean and healthy environment and a quality program based upon the principle of positive engagement directed toward client reintegration with community and family. Every day the employees of Central State Hospital will lead with pride, and will leave with dignity."

As of April 6, 1994 Robert Dyer, the State Mental Health Chief, was "dumbfounded" at how well the process of moving patients had gone. Out of the patients moved, ten died, seven were in jail, but 134 were now "living richer lives in communities across Indiana" in nursing homes, supervised group homes and apartments, and with family members. The hospital was reduced from 18 to seven wards. Many of the employees were moved to other jobs within the mental health community.

One of the patients, Michael Hudson, 36, died of heart trouble in March at Community Hospital while waiting for a bed in the Madison State Hospital in southern Indiana. He was admitted to Community Hospital because his mental condition worsened and he couldn't live independently anymore.

Another patient, Arleen Curry, 53, was found in her home, where the temperature was well over 100 degrees. (Mentally ill people do not always feel heat and cold.)

When two patients moved went missing, Robert Dyer said none of that could be "counted against our move toward community based care."

Still, some positivity came from the move. In April 1994 Gateways, a group home for the severely and chronically mentally ill, housed six Central State Hospital patients. The patients there practiced everyday skills so they could return to their own homes. It cost $61 per day versus $180 at Central State Hospital. The problem was that group homes were expensive and some neighborhoods didn't want them. People wanted reform but didn't want it in their neighborhood. For example, St Joseph neighborhood protested a group home for 12 of the patients.

In 1994 two of the most instrumental people who had written a blueprint for Indiana's mental health care reform and helped get Central State closed, resigned- Jeff Richardson, secretary of Indiana's Family and Social Services Administration (FSSA) and Robert Dyer. When they left, five former employees had just been indicted on rape and reckless homicide, among other charges. Richardson and Dyer said their resignation had nothing to do with this.

STAFFING

The years up to Central State Hospital's closing had an effect on staffing. Morale was low. One poster that circulated through the wards stated, "Don't tell my mother I work at Central State. She thinks I play piano at a whorehouse." Psychiatric attendants worked double shifts out of work and financial necessity. Nurses were in charge of two to three wards. A 1990 study showed that the attendants, who had the most contact with patients, had the least skills and training. In 1992 attendants made the lowest wages ranging from $12,787 to $17,732 per year. Psychiatrists were making on average $103,264 per year. Turnover was constant.

Just as the State prepared a plan for the patients, so it did for the employees. Despite Superintendent Leo Dillon wanting the hospital to be a "quality facility until the very last day", 50 employees left within seven months of the closure notice. New people were hired to replace those lost by turnover. These newer employees stayed less time than the current employees, leaving 622 people to continue to care for the 304 patients.

Superintendent Dillon, called "Saint Leo" by some because he was a strong patient and staff advocate, was moved from the position of Central State Superintendent to a finance post in the state's Division of Mental health. Diana Haugh, Superintendent of Larue D. Carter Memorial Hospital supervised both hospitals till Central State Hospital closure. The reasoning was that many of the leftover employees would be transferred to Larue Carter Memorial Hospital after the closure.

Staffing was gradually stepped down. Transition principles and actions included open and frequently communication, using attrition to reduce staff, placing some employees into the community-based system, communication regarding open positions within the state, and skill and training opportunities.

The plan to reduce staffing was to cut between 90 and 137 positions over several quarters. As of January 1993 several employee workshops on job banks, insurance, and career counseling were done, with more scheduled. The Department of Workforce Development attended some of these sessions to talk with employees about job training. The Central State task force met with Unity Team and United way and the Central State Hospital employee assistance program staff to enhance services to employees, including training as peer counselors. The employees of the Adolescent program were transferred with the program to Larue Carter Memorial Hospital. A job fair was held by the community health centers. State facilities were requested to consider hiring Central State Hospital employees first.

"We can provide better care in the community. We can help more people in the community. We can harvest more dollars in the community. This is the right thing to do for the mentally ill of central Indiana."

~Robert L Dyer, State Mental Health Chief

Due to "bumping rights" or seniority, some of the newly placed Central State Hospital people bumped others at state facilities into different roles or out of jobs. The money saved by terminating staff was to be used to build community based programs.

Ten thousand dollars were set aside for employees for tuition reimbursement. The decision to award money to an employee was based on "the degree to which employees' present skills lack marketability either within State Government or in the private sector."

Dr. Elizabeth Bowman, President of the Indiana Psychiatric Society, wrote a letter to the governor. She wrote "One issue at Central Sate was the competence of care on some wards. Well, if those employees come to Larue Carter, are we solving the problem or just moving the problem?"

Steve Fantauzzo, the local head of the American Federation of State, County and Municipal Employees, said, "If the state does move forward with massive layoffs, there is no doubt in my mind that the quality of patient care will suffer." He also said, "The community based system is so overburdened, you'd have to be a clown or an idiot to believe this is going to work."

Closing Numbers

The loss of Central State Hospital meant a loss of 600 jobs, but with the expansion of the community mental health centers, many of the jobs were transferred to these smaller facilities. As the then Director of the Indiana Council of Community Mental Health Centers said, "Indiana's government must take a new role in mental health in which it becomes a buyer, not a provider of care for most patients…the challenge is to be a buyer that makes sure its patients get the least restrictive, most appropriate level of care in their own communities."

At the time of closing the costs were very high at Central State Hospital. The table below shows the cost for Central State Hospital to care for patients and the cost for patients to be placed in the community mental health system.

Type	Central State Hospital	Community Placement
Mentally Ill	$14,708,040	$11,017,399
Developmentally Disabled	$3,689,274 (after Medicaid payments)	$4,008,795 (before Medicaid payments)
Patient populations outside mentally ill and developmentally disabled	$1,583,550 (with no Medicaid allowance)	$796,000 (through the Salvation Army; not Medicaid reimbursable)

As the patients were transitioned, the Indiana FSSA funded a study on their on-going care (5). At the time of the closure in 1993 a review of patients found that 54% had schizophrenia, 29% had schizo affective disorder, 22% had developmental disabilities, 5% had a personality disorder, 6% have organic personality disorders, and 4% had drug/alcohol disorders.

Of all the patients transferred out of Central State Hospital, 51% had regular family contact, 32% periodic contact, and 17% had no family contact.

The patients average length of stay:
- Less than 1 year   15%
- 2 to 5 years   30%
- 5 to 10 years   23%
- 10 to 15 years   16%
- 15 to 20 years   7%
- 20 to 25 years   5%
- 35 to 30 years   2%
- Greater than 30 years 2%

The median length of stay for people with developmental disabilities was 847 days; 140 for mental illness; 48 days for addictions.

Most patients were between the ages of 23 and 50 with only one third under 21 or over 50. Less than 1% were over 65 or under 21. Most patients came from Marion, Hamilton, Howard, and Hendricks counties. There were twice as many men as women.

AFTER CLOSURE

When the last patient was moved, a tracking study was conducted by the Indiana Consortium for Mental Health Services Research Institute for Social Research at Indiana University. The following is a breakdown of the status of the 389 patients moved from Central State beginning on March 23, 1992 as of July 25, 1994.

- Room and board assistance: 10
- General hospital: 2
- Home/private residence 26
- Nursing home: 7
- Semi-independent living programs (supported living): 84 total (including sites in Beech Grove, Elkhart, Greenwood, Indianapolis (67), Kokomo, Lafayette, Lebanon, new Castle, Noblesville and Plainfield
- Supervised Group Home : 119 (including Brownsburg, Cayuga, Danville, Franklin, Gary, Greencastle, Indianapolis (86), Kokomo, Lebanon, Merrillville, Shelbyville
- State Operated Facility: 110 (Including Evansville (9), Ft Wayne (8), Indianapolis (22), Logansport (27), Madison (9), New Castle, Richmond (33), Out of state (2)
- Correctional facility: 4
- Deceased: 14
- Unlocatable/missing 3

By August 1994 the only staff on site was for maintenance and security.

Long patients were tracked for ten years after the closure by the Indiana Consortium for Mental Health Services Research Institute for Social Research at Indiana University. It found the patients were in the following placement situations:

- General hospital .3%
- Private residence 17%
- Nursing home 4.4%
- Correctional facility 2.1%
- VA Hospital .5%
- Supervised group living 9.5%
- Semi-independent Living Program 23.1%
- State Operated Facilities 7.5%
- Room and Board Assisted Living 2.1%
- Homeless shelter .5%

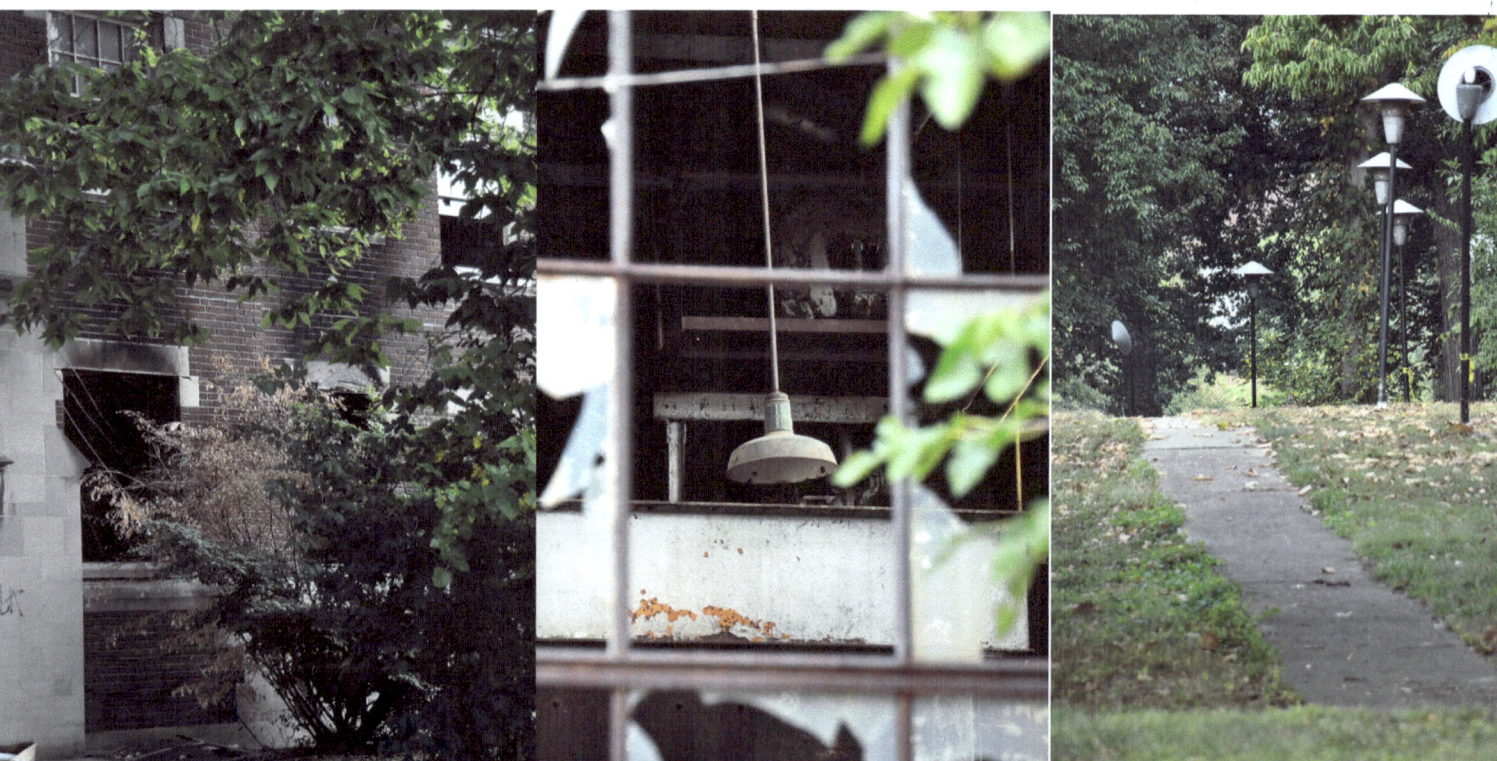

- Medicare waiver home .3%
- Out of state 1.5%
- Missing 6.9%
- Deceased 24.4%

While it would be easy to be shocked at the deceased number or the missing, the exact ages and conditions of the patients at the time they left Central State Hospital or at the time of the report in 2005 were not given.

"A Brief Review on Outcomes of Closing State Hospitals," indicated that it appeared after the closure that quality of life and levels of functioning were improved across all ages and ethnic groups. Another study, "The Closing of Central State Hospital: Long-Term Outcomes for Persons with Severe Mental Illness stated that three features which made the closing successful: forming a closure transition committee with representatives from the receiving mental health centers, the Division of Mental Health and hospital social work staff and administration was formed to help plan the closure. Second, transition funding was provided to "tailor" services to the patients. Third, every patient was required to have a monthly tracking report to force "providers to more closely monitor and treat" these patients.

The goal of closing Central State Hospital was to do no harm and to improve quality of life (QOL) and Level of Functioning (LOF),however a report about long-term outcomes for the closure of Central State Hospital concluded that despite the promise of better care in the community, data has been slow in coming. "Much of the literature on deinstitutionalization remains anecdotal or polemical and there is a relative dearth of well-constructed outcome studies to support or refute the validity of current policies."   The same study stated that
- Quality of life: improved for the patients as compared with living at Central State Hospital.
- Level of Functioning (LOF): increased but may be related to available sources in the community. LOF were neutral to dissatisfied after 12 months. Also, the study noted a failure to find adverse impacts of discharging the patients from Central State Hospital. After 24 months of the closing 1.3% were in jail, 2.6% missing, And 2.6% missing were homeless.

In a study that focused on predicting the community costs of closing psychiatric hospitals, the study argued that by placing the patients in network hospitals or intensive inpatient care facilities, these patients were "transinstitutionalized" rather than deinstitutionalized.

By the time the last tracking report was completed by IUPUI in 2005, (using 2004 data), 2.1% were in jail, 6.9% were missing and 24.4% died, with the most common reasons for death being cardiovascular disease, heart problems, cancer and respiratory ailments. The average age for death was 57 years old

After closure, the staff that had transitioned out of Central State Hospital had "more work conflicts"and a "more pessimistic outlook" on their future. However, they also had more positive attitudes about the closure of the hospital. Former patient mental health was much better. They had less depression and stress, and they used more coping strategies.

Over 21 years after the last building was erected, the hospital closed.

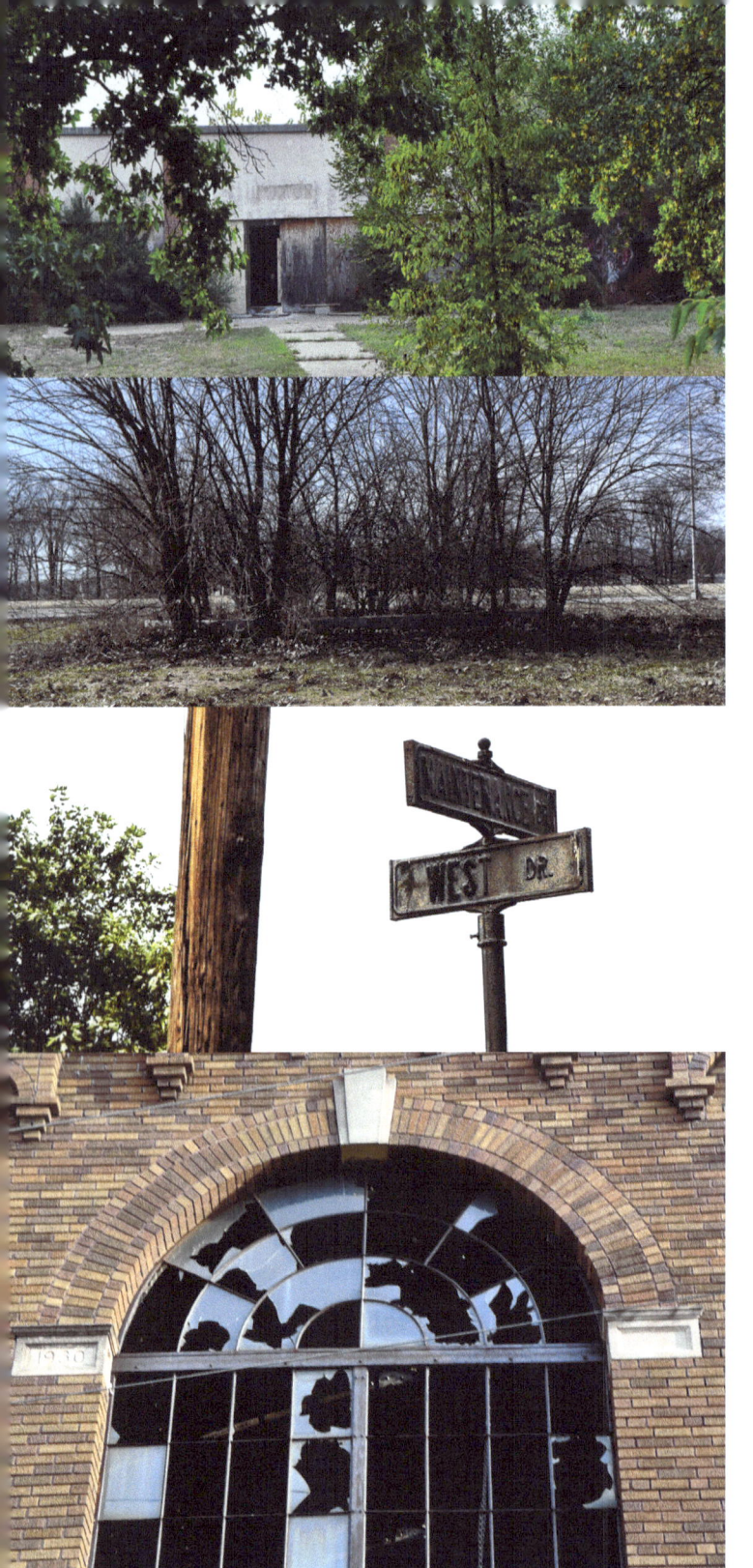

Closing Day Quotes

Blas Davila, a psychologist said that the time had been "stressful…but it worked."

Attendant Earlene Floyd: "I only stayed because I loved the patients."

Patient Mary Harmon, 74: "I don't want to go. I'll just stay here." Central State Hospital was the only place she'd known for 40 years.

David D. Richardson, wanted to stay in his locked ward and "fight and defend this place like the Alamo."

James Johnson, 26: "I'm outta here. I'm going to a group home with a bunny rabbit in the backyard. A man said the bunny could be our pet. I want to go to the State Fair. I want to ride a bicycle. I've been here a long time. Now I want to see the outside."

Right: The burned remnants of the Employee Building (also known as the Administration Building). Now called the Central State Mansion. Center: A time capsule of broken windows and industrial art in the old Power House building. The sad walkway into another grove. Patients used to relax, play games, shoot hoops and have therapy here.

Above: Boarded up Evans Building due to vandalism. A clue to the past- the old fountain base in front of Seven Steeples. Sign near the Powerhouse. The 1930s Powerhouse main natural light source.

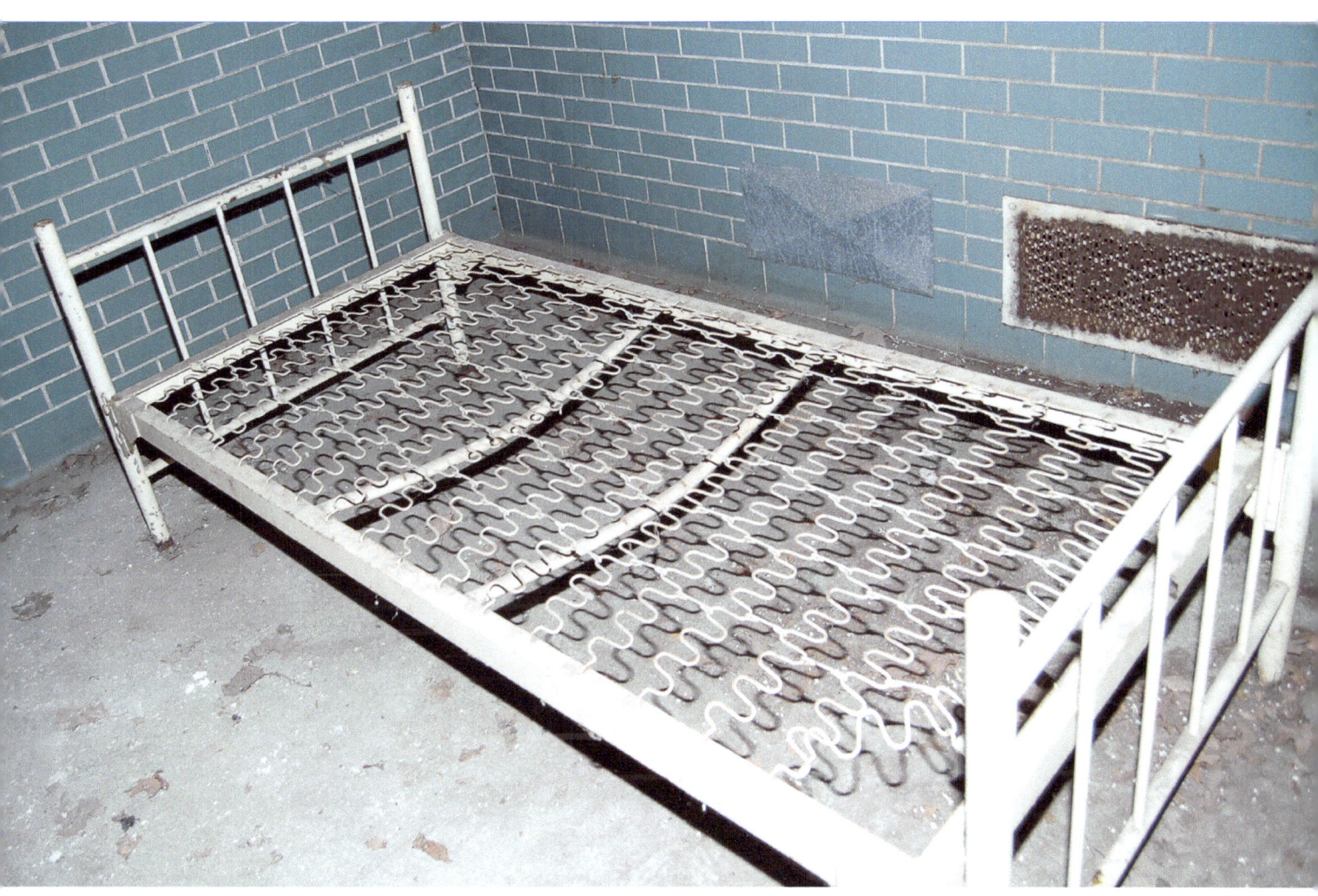

Above: Bed frame in Bahr Building

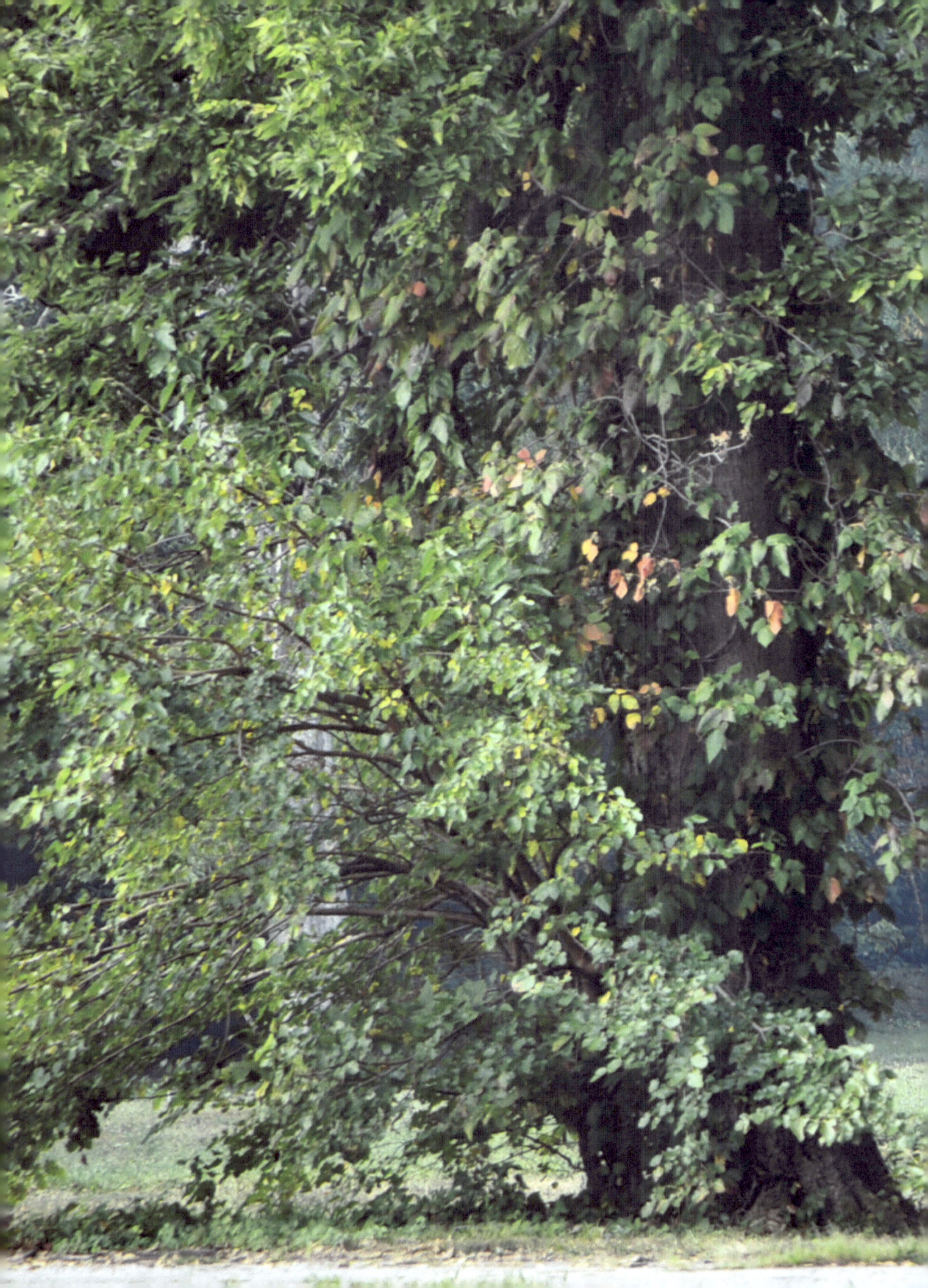

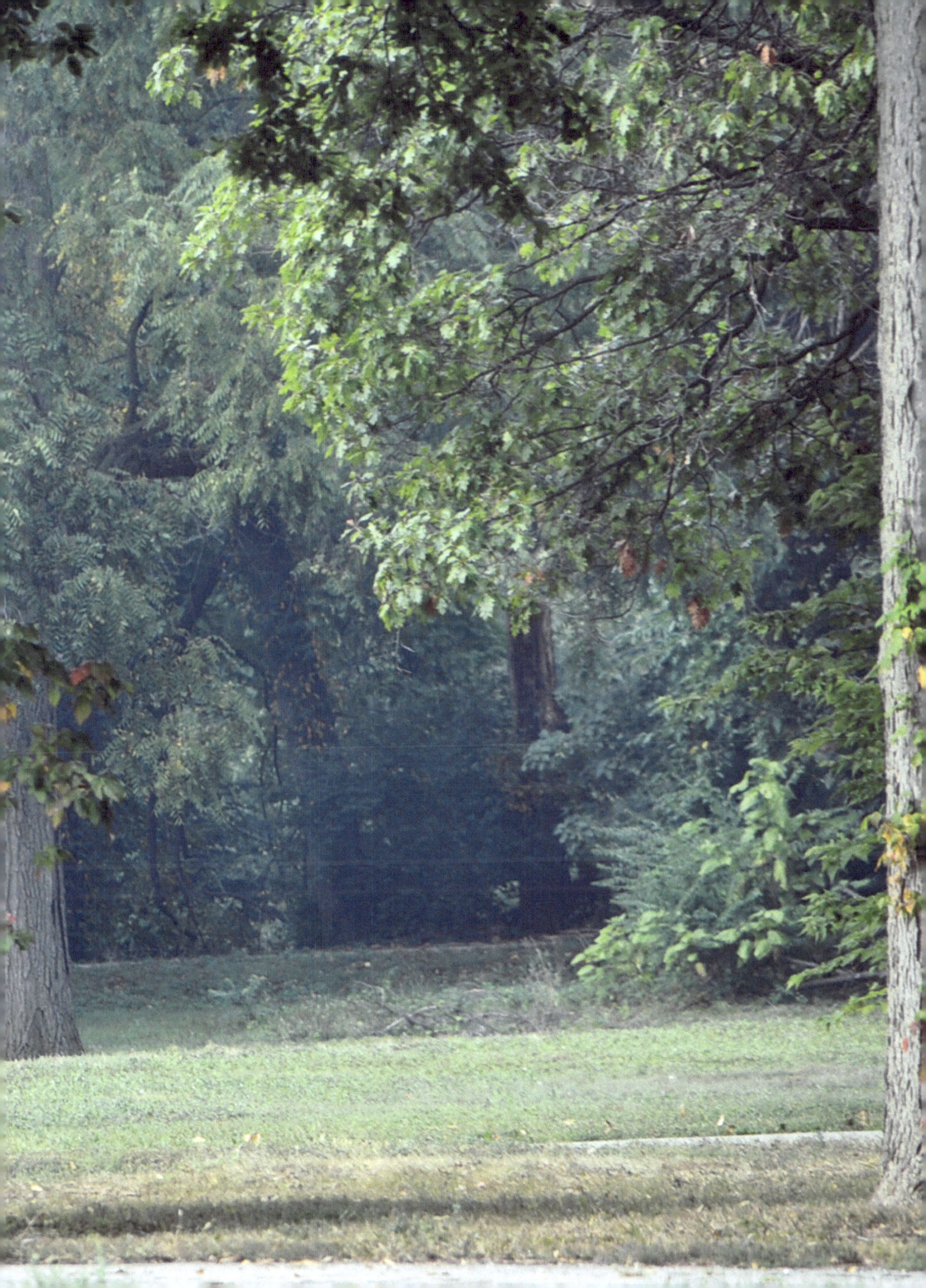

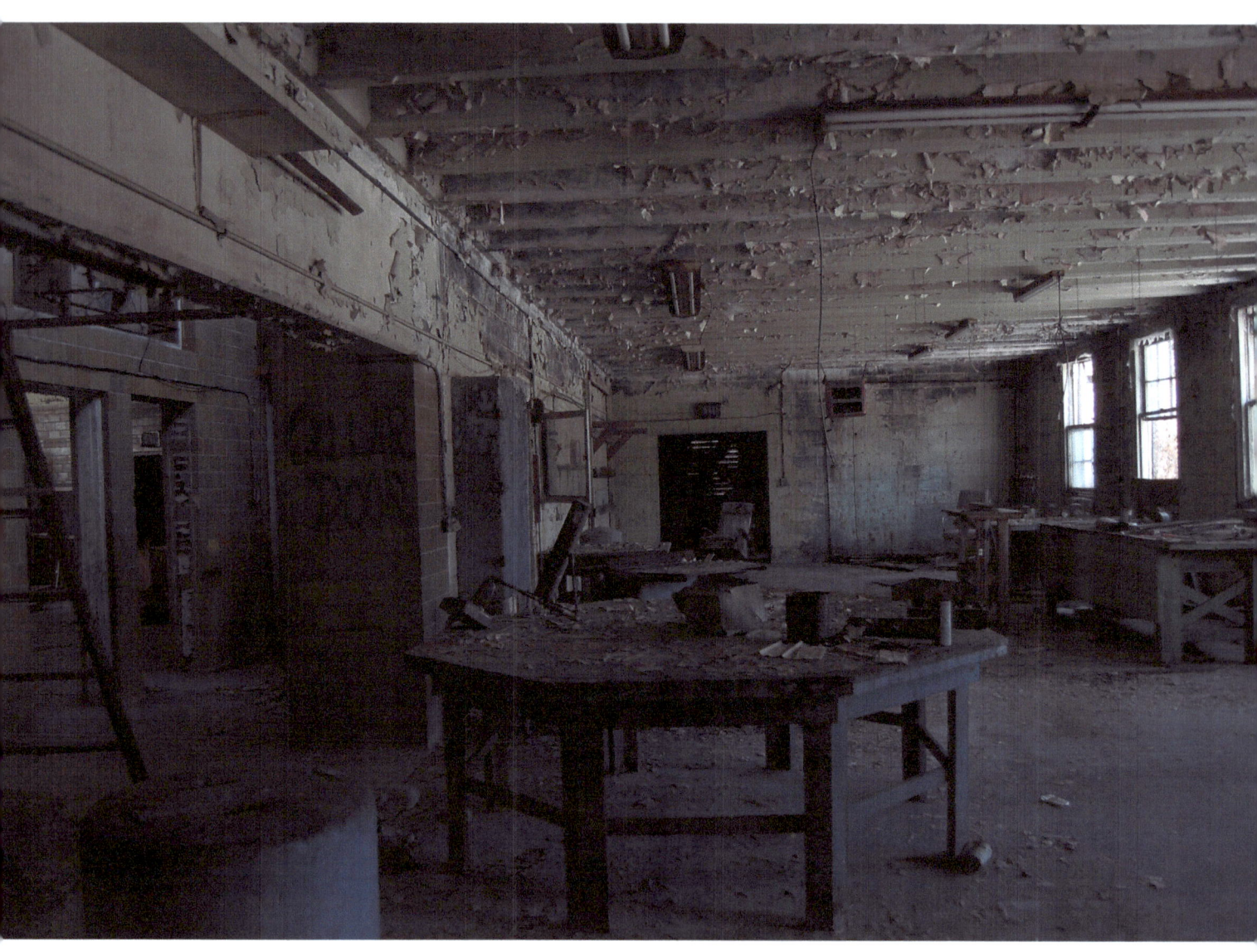
Abandoned tools and tables in the former dining room/carpenter's shop.

Twelve

Interviews

Central State Hospital has been closed for many years. The people who worked at or were associated with it are growing fewer as time goes on. To some, this hospital was a place of family and life. For others, it was a place of sorrow and a place of discard. The hospital was truly a place onto itself.

Below: the guard shack from the 1970s close to Warman St.

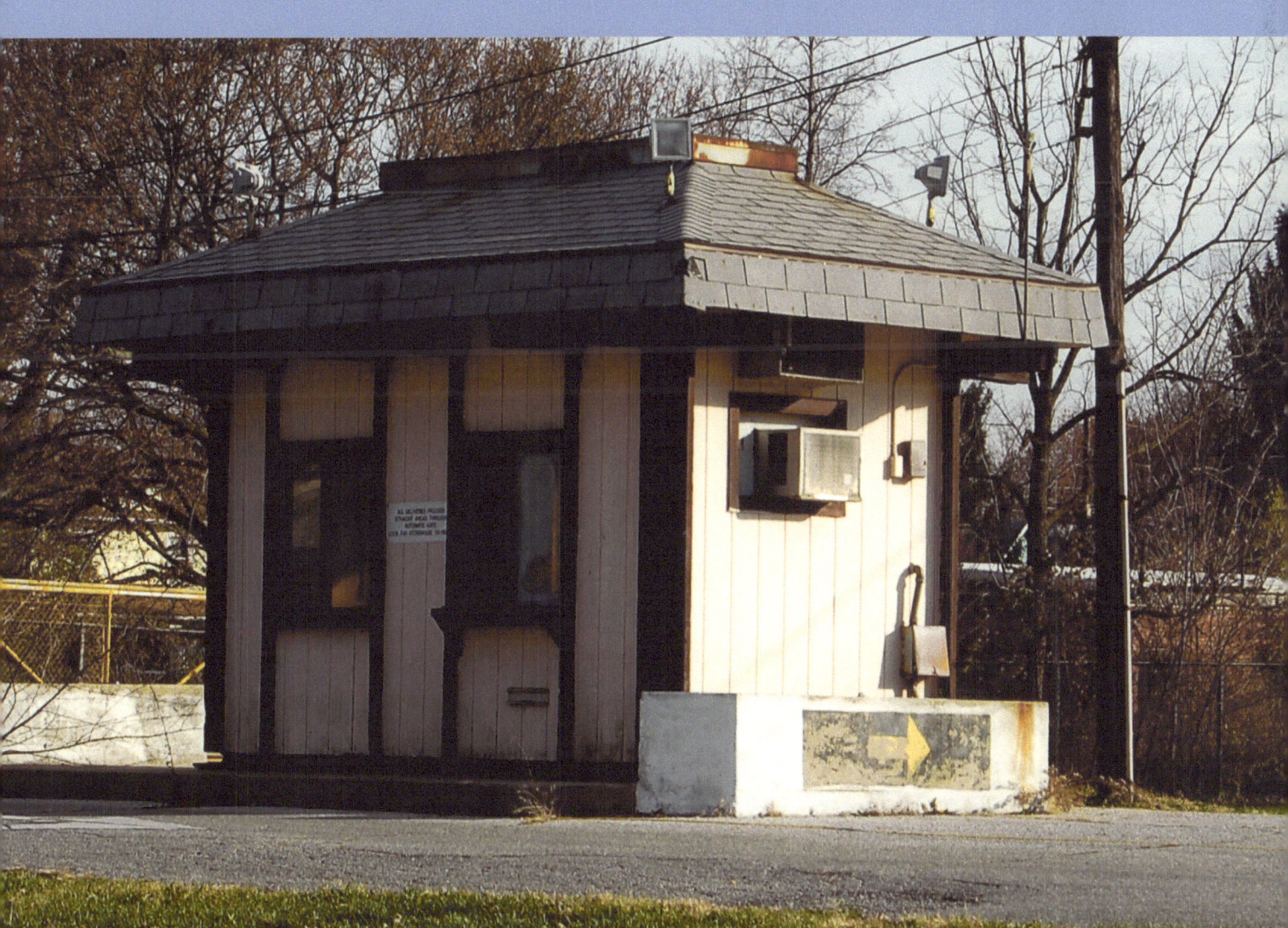

I Felt It Was Hopeless

Tonya Niccum Hicks, now retired, worked as an attendant in the late 60s. She believed the hospital was filled with the energy of the patients and their mental health issues.

For Tonya, it was a "strange place". She was able to get a job through her mother in law, who was the head nurse on a locked wards. Working the day shift, Tonya worked on a locked ward. In the beginning, she went to an orientation which gave her a basic overview on how to work with the patients. She helped patients if they needed something, would make sure they attended meals, lined up for medications, comforted those who were upset, and escort them to and from their rooms. Nursing staff was behind locked doors and glass, away from patients.

Tonya's mother-in-law, Mary Myler Chapel, loved working with people and was used to the working conditions. She told Tonya, "You're going to talk with people here and believe their stories." After working for a while with Chapel, Tonya agreed.

One female patient Tonya cared for had been there since she was 10 or 12 years old. When Tonya worked at Central State, the patient was between 40 and 50 years old. The woman almost had Tonya believing the story she told, because it was unfailingly similar every time. The patient stated that she was a spy and when she came to the hospital it was a retreat. Tonya believed everything because it sounded real. She wouldn't have believed anything was wrong with the female patient, who was schizophrenic.

During her eight hour days, Tonya was not allowed to walk the grounds during her shift. She took breaks, but they were on the floor. If someone needed to smoke they could go downstairs and outside, but otherwise, they remained on the floor for their shift. Patients did not leave the ward except to go to therapy. "I couldn't get used to being unable to get out of there. "

The treatments were also unnerving. Tonya recalled one older woman who was sent to a different building every week. Inside the building they took her to a hydrotherapy room. It consisted of a tub with ice in it. The patient's clothes were removed and she was put into the ice bath. The tub was covered with a thick rubber covering, which allowed the patient's head to remain out. "She screamed and screamed and screamed the whole time she was in there." This woman went through this treatment for many weeks.

Doctors were very much in control of the patients and their care. Tonya worked during a time when nurses couldn't give medication without permission. "You couldn't even get an aspirin without permission. They didn't want to tell you everything going on with the patients unless it was someone who could flip out and hurt you. We did have some

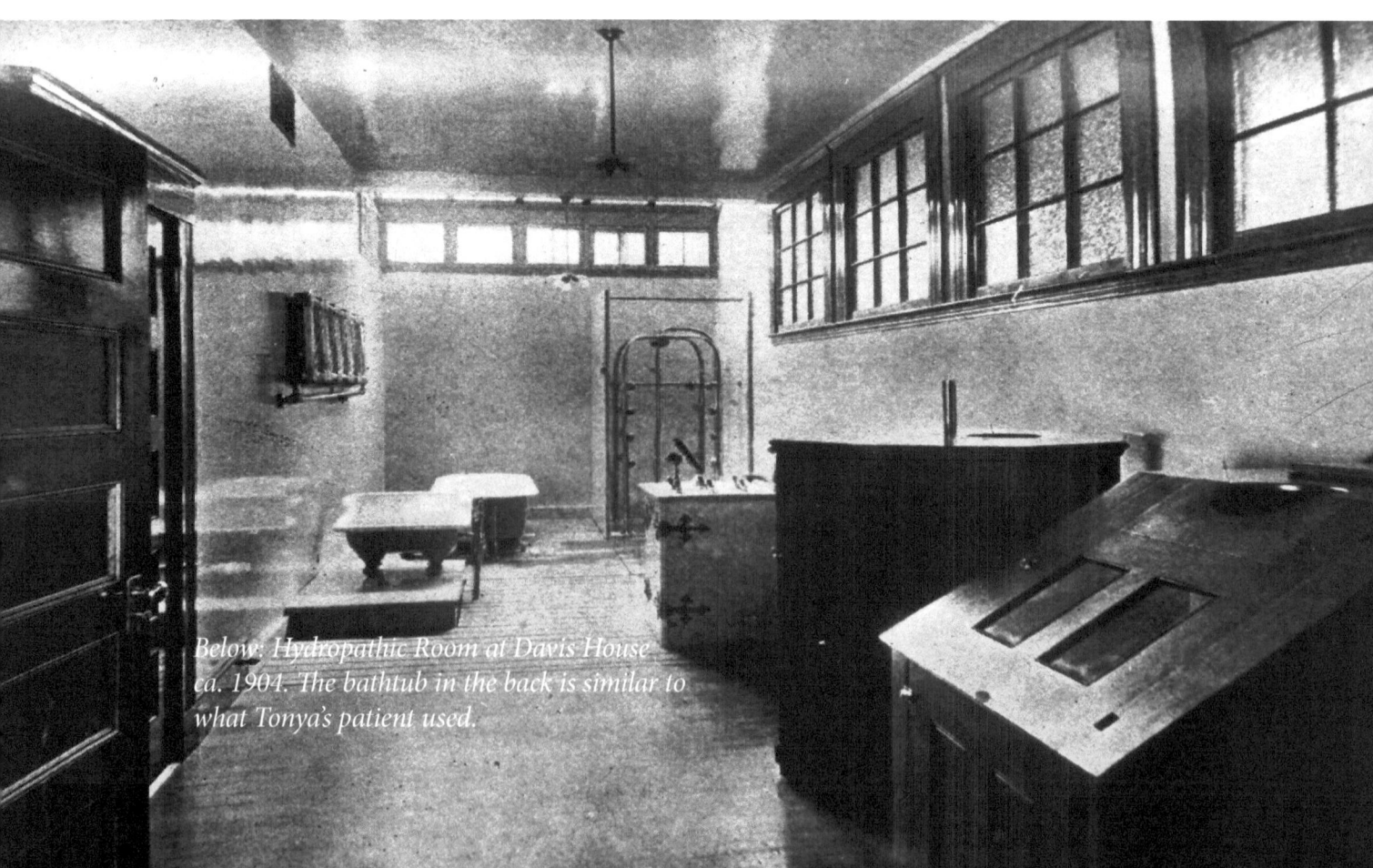

Below: Hydropathic Room at Davis House ca. 1904. The bathtub in the back is similar to what Tonya's patient used.

of those. But they [doctors] kept them so medicated, they [patients] were so mellow. "

Finally, Tonya had enough. "I never felt any violence from them towards me. but it was such a depressing place. My God, if you were depressed when you came in here, you're always going to be depressed. Depression hung like a cloud." Tonya believed the stairwells held negative energy, possibly because of the people that congregated in them. "Just heavy stuff there. And you see people lying on the steps. One person had no clothes on, lying on the cold hard steps. I couldn't take it. I had to leave. I was there maybe four or five months. The depression started affecting me."

From Central State Hospital, Tonya went to nursing home settings, where she felt she could help her patients. "I didn't feel like I could help someone or put myself into a situation where I could help in a state hospital." She believed this was mostly because of the locked area she worked in. "I couldn't reach the people, not even on a one on one basis. Because of their illness, they didn't really talk to you…I think it would have driven me crazy living there and not getting out. There were bars on the windows and you know that they [the patients] missed being out there. Up there, I felt that it was just hopeless and people gave up on them. And that made me sad."

Even her mother-in-law, left after about three years. Tonya said she believed there would have been no abuses on the wards her mother-in-law worked, "They were children to her and she was there to care for them."

WHAT KIND OF SHADY PLACE WAS I IN?

Carlos Estevez* spent six months at Central State as a musical therapy intern. Immediately he was put into "orientation", but it was for Certified Nursing Assistants (CNAs) and nurses. He worked mainly with the patient population who were going to individual and group therapies and activities.

When Carlos applied for the internship, he had no idea that Central State Hospital was on the verge of being shut down. "[After arriving] I found out a patient died of hypothermia because the restrictions were too lax on repairing a window. I was wondering what kind of shady place was I in?"

Additionally, he heard about another mishap leading to the cover up of another death. "There were some [member of the] midnight staff doing 15 minute checks. A pregnant nurse that was drowsy came back from break and missed her 15 minute checks. When the [pregnant] nurse came back, the next person who did the 15 minute checks found her [the dead patient]. They tried to revive her, [but her] lungs were filled with water. This nurse had them [the CNAs] put the patient in her bedclothes and put them (sic) to bed. They [the hospital] fired everyone who was working that shift because they [the staff] had done this cover up. I thought, 'oh my god, what is the deal with place that they [the staff covering up the death] would even think about getting away with that'?"

But for Carlos, disregard for patient's wellbeing seemed almost routine after a while, especially when it came to the social side of life at Central State Hospital. "Of course, it surprised me that residents were having sex in stairwells. It had been going on for years. I was freaked out by the whole thing."

Lax floor staff was not the only issue. Carlos heard rumors that the medical director was "shady". Internal and external accusations stated that the hospital couldn't keep track of staff. Carlos witnessed the final deterioration of the hospital firsthand. "It was frightening because the nursing stations on these wards had chicken wire to protect the nurses, who threw things at them [the patients]." He came from another organization in a similar setting and they didn't have chicken wire at the nurse stations. Sarcastically he added, "I am sure made the residents feel really, really normal- like they were in some sort of prison "

Carlos explained how patients were able to go outside or to a part time job, after certain restrictions were met. Patients had to attend a certain number of activities and achieve a certain number of points for the activities to get privileges. "If someone wasn't taking meds or achieving points, they would be in the locked day room with the chicken wire nursing station."

Security personnel at Central State Hospital had to be trained how to do take downs as "the first line of defense." A take down is getting someone on floor, applying leather restraints, get them restrained in a bed and "hope the sedatives work."

When asked if security did the best they could under the circumstances, Carlos laughed and hesitatingly said "Yes. They didn't have to intervene because of over medicating."

Additionally, Carlos' accommodations at the hospital were not up to any kind of health standard. "I had a room in the Administration building. A couple of months into living there, the Fire Marshall shut the building down saying it was uninhabitable. You had security on the first floor, some offices, and a meeting room on the third floor where I had my room. There were tiny rooms for interns and a main showering, bathing, [and] toilet area. The whole area was infested with cockroaches, had very little water pressure, and had no working shower. I did tub showers where I had the rubber hose with a shower head connected to the main faucet. The department head was shocked I would live in the Administration Building (the former Employee's Building). They'd [the hospital] only had girls before and they would stay with her [the department head] in Carmel. I had just done five years at college, and had no problem staying in the Administration Building, but it was filthy. I got to know the security guards really well."

A funny story involved the use of meeting space in the building. Once, a group of meeting participants was shocked to see Carlos come out of the bathroom in a bathrobe. "Someone lives here?" They asked.

During the day, Carlos worked with patients in groups and he felt he was adding to their quality of life. He also attended psychotherapy groups with psychologists, who were " just talking with them [the patients] about the hospital." Much of the talk about the hospital was what they wanted to see changed. And many times, the psychologist would throw it back on the patients and ask, "what do you want to see happen?"

Carlos did appreciate that the hospital had group music and occupational therapy with morning and afternoon programs. He felt it gave the patients "something to look forward to" when otherwise Carlos felt it was "just like a prison" and the patients "had nothing to look forward to. They had no one to talk to."

Meals were another matter. Carlos only went to the wards at mealtime. There, he saw people "do the Thorazine shuffle", a slow gait people do when they are heavily medicated. He also saw patients " who just liked to lay (sic) on furniture." He said the furniture was "nasty" and that it was "made so it could be cleaned." For Carlos, the wards always smelled "heavily of bleach" to the point it hurt the nose. "They didn't have to bleach as much as they did. It was inconsiderate for the people who lived there."

Carlos was to receive two meals a day, eating what the patients were served. He said he'd wait in line for a lot of "Tomatoes, succotash, mystery meat, blueberry or peach cobbler. It was really simple food. Greens, too." The water quality was an issue as well. Carlos remembered the ice tea was made with unfiltered water and that the coffee was "strong but nasty."

However, not everything seemed bad, according to Carlos. When talks of closing the hospital occurred, Carlos remembered seeing the governor at the hospital. "[Governor] Evan Bayh came to meet with the residents. I saw him

Below: view from the upper floor of the building Carlos lived in

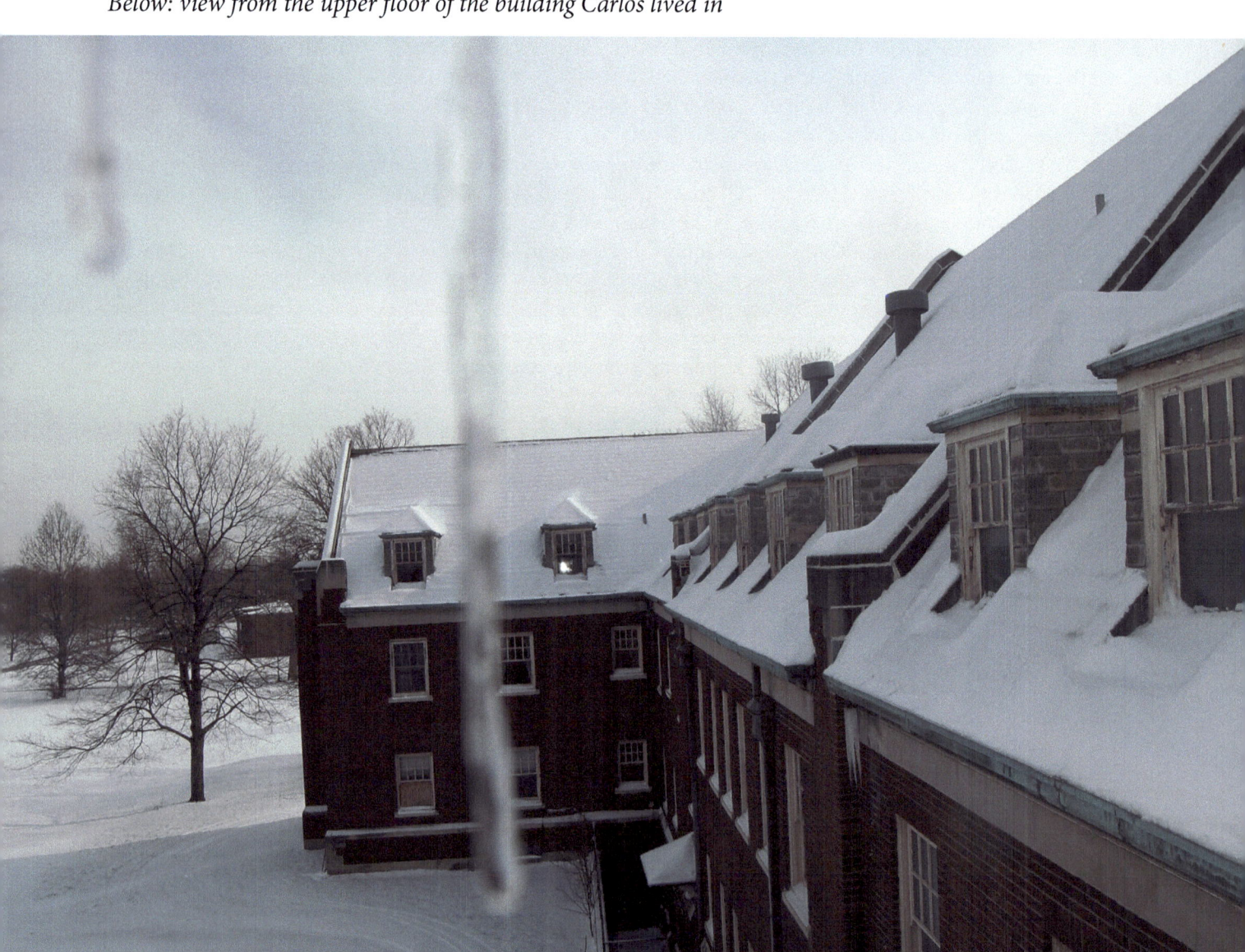

sit down and interview some teenage boys…chronically mentally ill prisoners with criminal records. He asked a kid, 'Do you like living here?' The kid said , 'It's ok.' Bayh said, "I am thinking about shutting the place down." The kid said, "Well, if I can go someplace better than here, that's great.' It was sad to see that. I was very impressed to see the governor personally talk to residents and not just the people taking him around on a tour. Very cool, very cool."

During his brief time at the hospital, Carlos saw patients transferred to the Midtown Community Health Clinic and a partial hospital setting. The chronically ill went to Logansport or Muscatatuck if they had a criminal sexual history.

"I see why it went down [the closure]. It [the hospital] was shady. And it was from another era, especially the chicken wire around nursing stations. It always surprised me, they had these big glass windows. I thought 'why are you worried about staff being in a chicken wire cage when they could easily throw a chair through the window?'"

Carlos summed up his time at Central State Hospital. "There were people who lived there most of their lives. It broke your heart. Why did they have to be here?" He thought the closing would be great for the people who were on their medications, had case manager, got housing, and would be followed and monitored. However, one patient to whom Carlos gives guitar lessons to once told him, "I like being crazy. They give me too much [medication], I am sleepy and can't get an erection. I like the feeling and energy. I like to not be on my meds. I like feeling how I am." Carlos said this was an education for him. He thought mentally ill people would be happy to be on their medications and feel better, no matter the side effects, such as the weight gain Lithium (for bi-polar disorder) causes.

Carlos still conducts music therapy with the aged population. Recently, while working in a community based program, Carlos saw one patient that murdered someone. He notified the staff and it was found that when he was registered, his first and middle name were reversed. The patient was shipped out to an appropriate facility within two hours.

The price of freedom is steep for some. Some people see patients as weak and steal their things and money or make patients victims of sexual attacks or beat them up. However, Carlos believes that their lives are overall better. "Central State Hospital's idea of shipping them off, was one way of dealing with it. I like what they are doing now [with] caseworkers checking up on people, intensive mobile team. I think Indianapolis got it right when they were doing partial hospitalization at Wishard and they'd be expected to come in and attend the different group activities and education about medication and diagnosis and of course substance abuse, I don't know how people have money for marijuana, cigarettes or alcohol, but they get it and they get educated about it the outpatient clinics."

Originally, Carlos believed the closing was just trading the larger institutional problems for smaller setting system problems. But he doesn't feel that way today. "I can tell you from the residents' perspectives, they want to have a normal life like all of us. They want money to shop and eat. They've been dealt bad cards with mental health and medications. Where Indianapolis got it wrong was the housing. They are given x amount of money and there are crooked slum lords and bad roommates. Some places will handle your rent and utilities so you know how much extra money you have. Others (the patients) will get robbed and preyed on. Midtown doesn't have the money and the city hasn't looked into making apartments for the chronic mentally ill."

As a side note, Carlos warns people who want to see the hospital to be prepared for ghosts. Carlos doesn't know if security was just "messing with" him or if it was paranormal. His hallway in the Administration Building contained several doors. Carlos heard the doors opening and closing after hours and footsteps. He finally told security, "Every time you come up, I expect you're going to knock and freak me out." Security personnel stated that no one was making rounds on his floor. "Why would we do rounds to check on one person that we know is sleeping or watching TV?"

*Note: Name changed,

Childhood and Adult Memories

Julie Rutherford spent time in the Army before she worked at Central State Hospital in the 1970s. She worked day shift as security and then as a Supervisor in the Communications Office for seven years, but her history goes back much further. "I used to tell people I grew up at Central State Hospital and they'd eye me like 'oooooh.'"

Julie's mother worked at the hospital as a recreational therapist. Julie spent a lot of time there as a kid. Many times Julie would go with her mom to help her. When the patients attended the circus, the carnival in front of the Department for Women's building, the symphony, parade and other events, Julie helped her mother "make counts" of the patients, so no one got left behind.

Julie was also able to take her pet turtle, Georgia, to the hospital and talk about her with patients. "When I think of the hospital, positive things pop up. I really like that." She described how pretty the grounds were and how the state tree and a wide variety of other trees were planted there. "If you needed a leaf collection, [you could] go get it." Julie also remembered a "beautiful walk-through garden" created by one of the staff and patients during occupational therapy. Julie thought it was ""really, really cool."

One of her biggest pleasures as a child was going to the Kitchen Building. "There was a nice library in the basement of the dining facility. I can remember thinking it was so cool that I could go over and eat with my mom and the patients. I recall the food being pretty good. I didn't think it was bad."

When Julie got out of the Army, she was looking for a job. The hospital had gotten a Federal grant to set up a security department. Working security, "was a great thing," partially because of the patients. One memorable patient was Gertrude, who would speak to Julie every day. "She'd been a fairly prominent woman. She would knock on my window every day and ask what the newspaper headlines were" July also remembered a man "who would play the piano like it was so grand." Working security during a camping adventure with patients was also a pleasant experience for Julie.

But the patients also brought some memories of sadness. "There were so many talented patients…and very, very smart. It was sad their mind had gone and they were now not functional, so they put them in a hospital."
Sad memories also surfaced of patients who would walk away from the hospital. "I remember having to go down to the Circle with another officer to get this poor little man. He'd gone to the bank to get the large sum of money he thought he had."

Patients also found themselves in unwelcome situations. Patients were allowed to walk the ground and would sometime get into trouble by getting into dumpsters. Once, Julie received a call about a patient who was masturbating by the fence line in view of houses and the road. Sometimes the troubles were more severe such as when a patient killed another patient. "As a child I felt very, very safe [at the hospital]. My mother explained a lot of things to me at a fairly young age. Some of the things they [the patients] were dealing with- [the after effect of] sexual predators and all. As a security guard I found they [the patients] had a super strength. I saw a little old lady that took five or six state troopers down. A patient reached in the window and tried to pull me out of the car by my neck."

While doing some college work, Julie used to bring teenagers out to volunteer at the hospital. Later, she received feedback from one of the teens. The teen wrote, "I remember you taking us over to volunteer and how I remember this as a good thing."

Of the hospital in general, Julie stated, "A job's a job, you gotta pay your bills, but I seen [sic] some very caring people who gave a crap about their job and what they were trying to do…I didn't see abuse in all those years. I seen [sic] a lot of people trying to do the best they could in what the State offered them." Like many others, Julie left for a "heck of a better job with insurance."

Years later, Central State Hospital was still a part of Julie. She took her great grandchildren to the hospital after it closed. "I tried to share some history with them. The kids loved the police department horses."

Julie Rutherford isn't afraid to speak her mind. "There is a thin line between sanity and insanity. We walk it every day. There is a lot of stress out there today. Jobs expect more out of you. You do the job of three people."

Julie wishes the mental health profession would have known more about mental illness earlier. Overall, she hopes the closure was a good thing. "I was sad at first when they said they were going to close it down, [but then I thought] yeah, this is a good thing. People need an environment like a home or a structured life. Working at a woman's correctional facility for seven years, it made me think it was like the hospital. The controls, the locked doors, counting patients, that's what the Department of Corrections is all about. "

"I hope the people in the group homes work. I sometime think that the hospital, reformatories and jails pick up the people who aren't in the group homes and that is a sorry thing."

BOMPA

The little girl listened in the night. What was that? Was someone coming into the house? A bird tweeted outside in the darkness. Why hadn't they taken her with her mother? And what was wrong with her daddy? He never acted so awfully towards her.

She listened again but heard nothing. Sleep came, but not for a very long time….

So it went for September Fox' mother,(1) who lived with her mentally ill father- until the night that he shot at her and September's grandmother. That night, her mother was taken away and hidden, her father arrested and sent to Norman Beatty Hospital, now a state prison and later to Woodmere (also known as Evansville State Hospital) been diagnosed as criminally insane. September's eight year old mother was left alone all night. The next day, the girl went to school and broke down, being sent home to a relative to care for her.

These events helped shape September's life. At 19 years of age, she secured a job at the Evansville State Hospital and later Central State Hospital, in part to see what her grandfather's experience was like. By this time, her grandfather, who she called "Bompa" was a "harmless old man." In the 1978 due to budget cuts, he'd been let go, without warning or communication. Bompa called the family from a pay phone. As an old man, he couldn't remember any of the events leading to his placement in the hospital.

September started at Evansville State Hospital in February 1989. During her time at the hospital, September felt a connection and it felt right for her to be at the hospital. She was paid $5 per hour as a Psychiatric Attendant V (PA-V), which was the lowest attendant category. September was happy though, because she was paid higher than minimum wage. While a PA-V, September was a primary caregiver to patients. She changed linens and diapers, gave patients baths, and handed out snacks. She also would sometimes "smoke the patients", which meant September would distribute cigarettes at specific times of the day.

Excelling at her work, September took the offer made to employees and the hospital paid for her to go to QMA classes, which allowed her to become a Psychiatric Attendant IV (PA-IV) and earn more pay.

September was assigned the Hospital ward as her home unit but she subbed all over the hospital. Normally, each unit had two people working. Generally, about ten patients were on each unit, but sometimes much less or many more would be on a unit. If patients needed help, September would do what she could to help them. For examples, one of her patients had a tracheotomy and smoked cigarettes. She and other staff members would have to clean out his tracheotomy opening. Some patients would go through a cycle where they would stop urinating for a week and the patients would have to be catheterized.

The feel at Evansville State Hospital was different than September's experiences at Central State Hospital. Many patients and staff had been at the hospital for a long time. Because of this, a rapport was established between the patients and staff. For example, one patient, "Earl" was bought a 50 year cake to commemorate the number of years he'd been in the hospital. He would say "Let's go over to Evansville in my automobile," because he didn't realize that Evansville had grown up around the hospital.

Evansville State Hospital also had mentally disabled people who had been institutionalized. Frank B. had been taught to hit himself and so he'd hit his chest. It really showed the thinking of the time he'd been institutionalized because someone had told him that hitting himself was better than hitting others. Many times he'd become upset, especially when he couldn't get a cigarette, hit his chest and say "fuck you." (2)

Another patient, Charlotte, had killed her husband. The legend stated that she'd been advised to "play crazy" instead of going to jail. Charlotte did but everyone believed Charlotte was sane when she came in but the electro convulsive therapy (ECT; also known as electroshock therapy) made her mentally ill after a while. She was a bit of an enigma as she was very wealthy, unlike most patients and her bill was always current (3).

Another difference was that September believed Evansville staff cared about patients more than the staff at Central State. For birthdays, patients received gifts and their favorite foods. Sometimes staff would sign patients out and take them different places, such as dinner or to a park. Once, September took to dinner an old German man, who was very "sweet faced". Her mother went with September. The patient had ice tea and an open faced sandwich. He ate the ice first, drank the tea then ate the sugar out of his hand. When he ate the sandwich, the man ate one side, then the other. September's mom said September should help him. September said she wanted to let him enjoy it whatever way he wanted to because it was one time that he didn't have to adhere to hospital rules. At Central State Hospital no one in her area took patients out or tried to make their day brighter or more comfortable.

The differences didn't end there. When September transitioned to Central State Hospital, she was 22 years old. She wanted to be closer to her friends and besides, she'd heard a rumor that patients had died at the hospital and that the entire second shift had been fired. September saw an opportunity for a new job and took it.

Some of the things September learned very quickly at her new job are that her coworkers were nothing like Evansville. She used to be able to count on coworkers. At Central State Hospital in the Bahr Building where she worked, she could not. September was the only Caucasian person working in the building and she was younger than most of the people. Additionally, she had been working less time in the psychiatric field than her new coworkers.

September had initiative whereas what she observed was a lot of loafing. Card playing was a common pastime when staff could have been interacting more with the patients, cleaning or making working and living conditions better. Because September didn't play by the old staff rules, she was targeted. Once she was made to work one-on-one with a violent patient when men, who were hired for the job, played cards in the women's area of the building.

Distrust for September also stemmed from her record keeping. Every month, a chart of how the patients were doing was required. Although it was impossible to keep it up every day during the month, September started working on hers half way through the month. The other staff she worked with "winged it" and worked on the chart a few days before it was due.

September was also targeted to the point of almost losing her job. Once, when she was attending a patient, a nurse, who disliked her, told her to get the other patients downstairs to the cafeteria. September left her patient and did as she was told. She stayed with the patients for dinner and upon her return, September was asked by the nurse to sign her patient's clipboard. Once she signed, the nurse told September she was writing her up for leaving her patient. When sent to the Director's office, September told him of what happened and although she was written up, she kept her job (4).

The patients were different, too. At Evansville State Hospital, patients may have hurt you, but they were sorry later. At Central State Hospital, this wasn't the case. September believes this was due to a different patient base and the attitude of the staff, which always seemed dark, unforgiving and angry.

The care of patients was different. The only time she'd ever witnessed any abuse at Evansville was when Frank B was beat by an attendant for a reason unknown to September. She took the information to another employee higher up than her, but nothing ever came of it (5). At Central State Hospital, every day was an abusive environment. Staff would curse at patients and tell them to "shut up" almost always. September remembered, "There was no kindness about the place or wholesomeness."

Cover-ups were common. In addition to the incidents that occurred before September came to the hospital, the same nurse that disliked September so much got herself in trouble. A doctor had come in and prescribed medication for two patients with very similar names. On the orders, he mixed up the medications resulting in the wrong medication being prescribed for each patient. The nurse didn't catch it and gave one patient a psychotropic drug injection in his buttocks. Instead of admitting she did it and saying she was doing what the doctor told her to do, the nurse tried to cover it up. The doctor seemed to see no repercussions.

Shortly after this incident, September moved to the Pharmacy Unit (6). At the time, a computer system had been purchased but no one had used it. As a result, all orders were hand written and mistakes were frequently made. September began staying late to enter the information necessary to begin printing the prescriptions (7).

When Central State Hospital closed in 1994, September was one of the last employees on campus. She stayed until all the patients were gone. September cleaned everything in her area and took the medications to the Drug Enforcement Administration.

Overall, September believed that the difference between the Evansville and Central State Hospitals was night and day. While Evansville State Hospital had always been open, bright, clean, and cheery, Central State was nothing but a dark, filthy, and ominous "pit." September said, "If someone pees the bed, you shouldn't have to tell someone to go change it." A feeling of "dread" hung over the entire campus. At the Evansville hospital, September had fun times and serious times. There was very little happiness at Central State Hospital.

Summing her experience up, September stated, "I am a better person for having taken care of the patients. It was evil and physically sickening to go there until I went to the pharmacy. I think the universe pushes you to do things. If that nurse hadn't done what she did, I wouldn't have gotten into computers. I can't be ungrateful."

"He was like a Zombie"

Deborah Rosenbloom worked as a social worker for two years at Central State Hospital in the 1980s. When Deborah went in for her interview, she remembered driving up to the hospital thinking, "This is a really, really strange place". When she finished her interview, she came out and an unattended patient was "messing with" one of her windshield wipers. According to Deborah, "He was like a zombie." During her time at the hospital, she saw many issues.

Deborah came to realize that Central State Hospital was "a total community onto itself." Patients, who wouldn't be leaving the hospital, seemed sequestered and didn't need to leave the hospital for any reason.

As part of her job, Deborah prepared social histories, developed treatment plans, and gave referrals for follow-up care in the community. However, because Deborah held a Master's degree in a position that required a Bachelor's degree, she felt she was not getting paid what she was worth.

Nevertheless, Deborah did her best. Deborah's supervisor was upset by how quickly Deborah made recommendations on releasing patients from the hospital. Her supervisor would say, "I think you're overdoing it." or "You're doing too much." Her supervisor was not used to such a highly productive worker.

Deborah worked on an inpatient unit where most patients were very ill. Some were schizophrenic and were not safe on the streets. Deborah's job was to monitor their progress and determine when they could transition back into the community. To do this, the patients went into a group home.

A typical day for Deborah was a round of treatment plan meetings with all disciplines present- psychologists, social workers, etc.- to go over patients' needs. The group determined if patients were meeting their goals. During the meeting participants would talk about plans for the patient, make notes and schedule group activities and therapy.

Once, Deborah was attacked by a patient while she was on a locked unit in the Evans Building. She went into a caged section where she knew she could find a psychiatrists office to finish some of her paperwork. Deborah closed the door. When D.B., the patient, entered, Deborah realized she was cornered in the room.

D.B. asked to talk and Deborah said she didn't have time. He put his right arm around the desk as he had her near the door. She screamed and Dorian told her to stop. He loosened his grip on her and moved

Below: Attendent's station in the Evans Building.

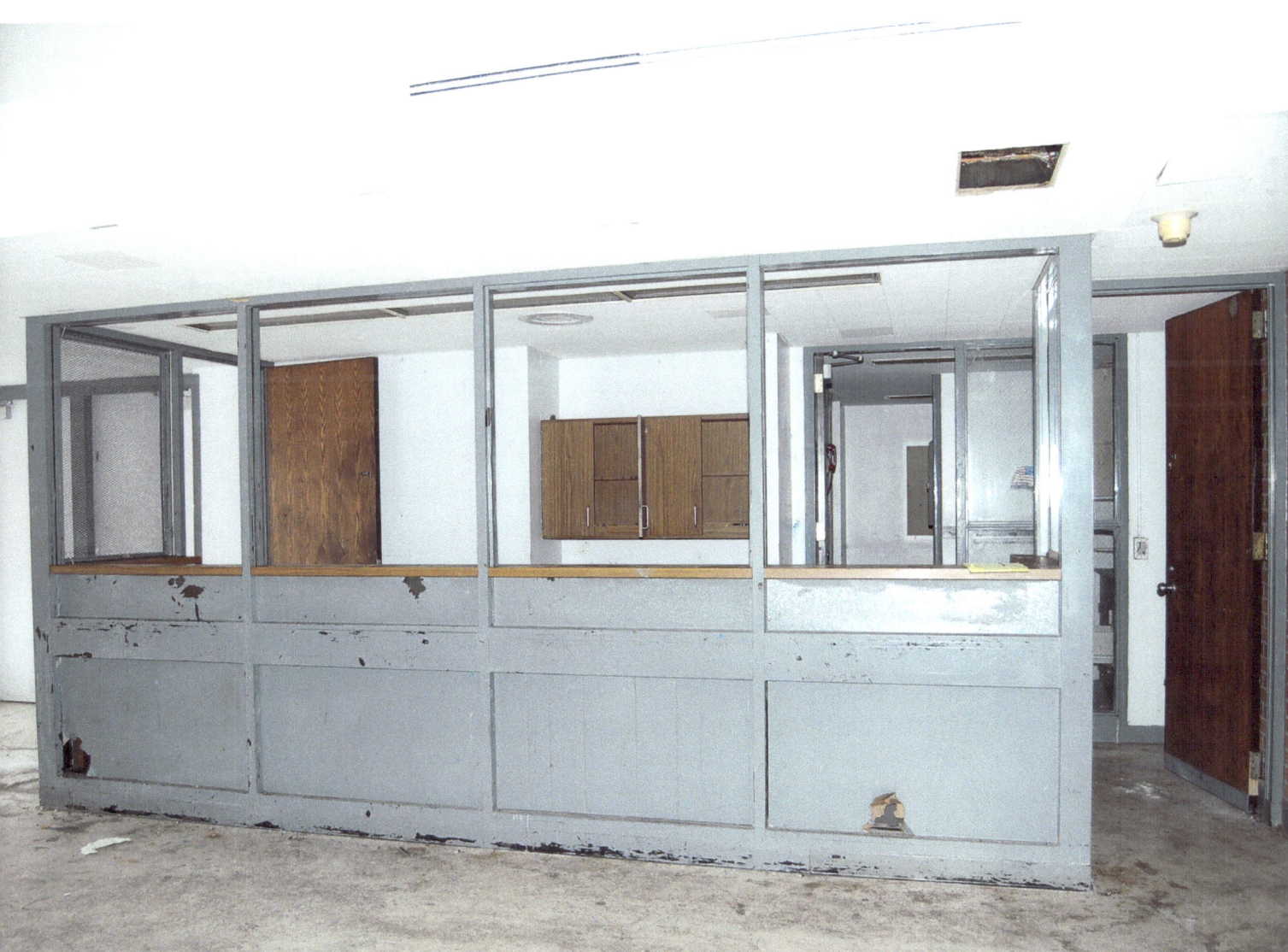

into the room, blocking her way. To Deborah, the time was a blur. She didn't realize it at the time, but he had his hand around her neck. All the sudden they were outside the room, with no one in sight to help. After what seemed like forever, an attendant showed up. D.B. growled, "You come any closer and I'll kill the bitch." D.B. took Deborah into a day room as a hostage. He told the staff he wanted off the unit with her. The staff opened the doors beside the staff cage. With his right arm on Deborah's neck, and his left on her arm against his pants, D.B. dragged her through Wards 32 and 34.

What D.B. didn't realize was that security personnel were on its way. The patient dragged Deborah through the people in the area. Before she knew it, Deborah found herself under a pile of people as she and Dorian were charged by security. A security guard, Roberta Deckard told him to let her go and run. Bill Smith, a rehab assistant grabbed D.B., who was taken to Ward 12 in the Bahr Treatment Center.

Deborah was in shock. She said all she could think of was that she had to make a chart note about the incident "like there was no problem at all." Once the patient was taken away, she did just that. Dr. B. came in and asked her what she was doing. Deborah said she needed her glasses to make the note. The doctor kept asking if she was ok. Deborah wrote the note, went to her office, and burst into tears. She was told to go home.

Instead, Deborah left the hospital and went to the doctor. She had bruises around her neck. After taking a day off, she went back. The team lead of the unit wrote up "something" and tried to get her a raise, saying what she did was commendable "because I only took a day off."

The recommendation letter from her supervisor was to Thomas Beasley, State Personnel and signed by Superintendent Ruth Stanley. Her supervisor recommended a 4% increase due to her excellent work in "preparation of admissions social service database". She had prepared more databases than any other person in her position- 31 versus numbers such as 14 or 20. It mentioned after surviving a "life threatening" situation that she didn't take a lot of time off work which "typifies devotion to work."

Deborah said Superintendent Stanley said that ward staff acted poorly. Deborah also stated there was a complete lack of "adequately trained male staff" which created a "bad situation." D.B. had a history of assaults and harassment. The day before Deborah's attack, he kicked another patient in the mouth and threatened to kill Dr. Ramus. At the time, D.B. reminded him of the policy which stated if he didn't act out in seven days, he would back to Ward 34.

Deborah said D.B. should have been in Bahr forever or in Logansport for security. The hospital wanted her to file charges. She said Brown was not psychotic, that he knew what he was doing by his words and actions. She called for additional safety measures for the Evans Building.

The event had lasting consequences for Deborah. "It made me really paranoid. I would go to a mall, see a man walking toward us, and I was convinced he was coming after me." Deborah's next job consisted of working with outpatients in a community support center- therapy activities,etc. As she helped prepare meals in a basement, all she could remember thinking was "I'm in a basement. Anyone could attack me. I am putting myself at risk." Deborah said the experience taught her not to be "naïve" because something can happen. "I could have been killed."

"Do you know what's going on at Central State?"

Many years ago, a concerned father walked into Skip Hess' office and asked him if he was aware of what was going on at Central State Hospital. That inquiry, led to an award-winning investigative reporting series from 1968-1973 about the abuses, neglect, infestation, and filth at the hospital.

Although the inquiry was luck of the draw in who it was assigned to, Skip Hess' career was no accident. When Skip graduated high school, he was drafted into the Army. During his time in the military, he was a journalist, working for the Fort Hood Sentinel, "where I learned to write." When he left the Army in 1964 the ambitious man started working as a sports writer and later sports editor. Skip worked for a morning paper in Kokomo and an evening paper in Wabash to get the experience of both types of paper. When he started at The Indianapolis News, there was no sports opening. He worked in news, hoping to eventually move into sports, but Skip found he enjoyed news more and stayed there.

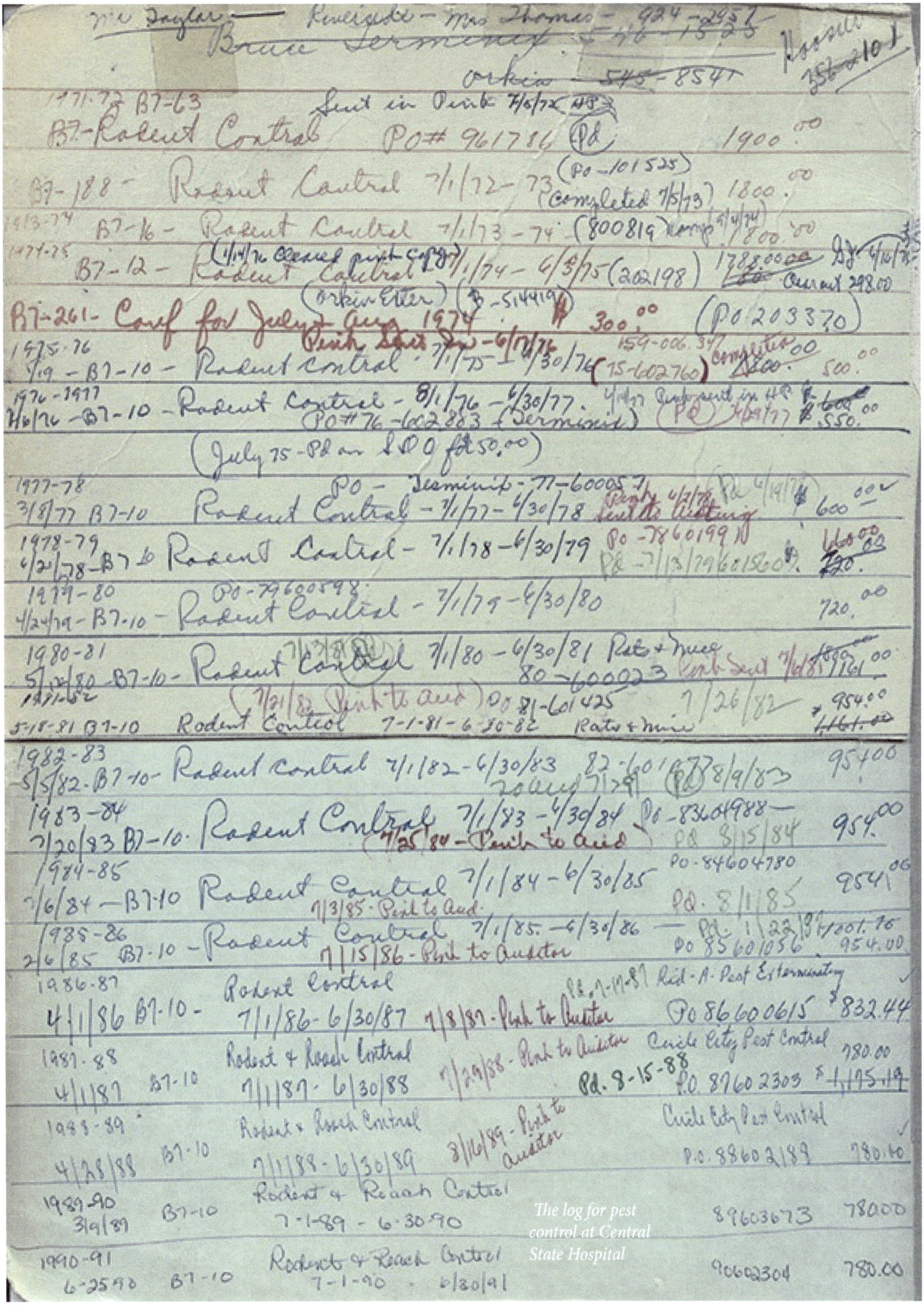

Handwritten ledger — pest control records, Central State Hospital. Partial transcription follows:

- Mr. Taylor — Riverside — Mrs. Thomas — 924-2957
- Bruce Terminix — 546-1525
- Orkin — 545-8547

Year	Acct	Description	Dates	PO#	Amount
1971-72	B7-63	Rodent Control — Sent in Quick 7/6/72		PO# 961784 (Pd)	1900.00
	B7-188	Rodent Control	7/1/72-73	(PO-101525) Completed 7/5/73	1800.00
1973-74	B7-16	Rodent Control	7/1/73-74	(800819) comp 9/4/74	800.00
1974-75	B7-12	Rodent Control	7/1/74-6/5/75	(202198)	1788.00 / Orkin 298.00
	B7-261	Conf for July+Aug 1974 (Orkin Exter)		$-514419	300.00 (PO 203370)
1975-76	B7-10	Rodent Control	7/1/75-6/30/76	(75-602760) completed	1800.00 / 500.00
1976-1977 7/6/76	B7-10	Rodent Control	8/1/76-6/30/77	PO# 76-602883 (Terminix) Pd 4/9/77	600.00 / 550.00
		(July 75-82 on S&O for 50.00)			
1977-78 3/8/77	B7-10	Rodent Control	7/1/77-6/30/78	PO Terminix 77-600057 Pd 6/19/77	600.00
1978-79 6/21/78	B7-10	Rodent Control	7/1/78-6/30/79	PO-7860199 Pd 7/13/79 601860	660.00 / 720.00
1979-80 4/24/79	B7-10	Rodent Control	7/1/79-6/30/80	PO-79600598	720.00
1980-81 5/1/80	B7-10	Rodent Control	7/1/80-6/30/81 Rats + Mice	80-600023 Sent 7/8/81	761.00
1981-82 5-18-81	B7-10	Rodent Control	7-1-81-6-30-82 Rats + mice (7/21/82 Pmt to Aud)	PO 81-601425 7/26/82	954.00 / 461.00
1982-83 5/5/82	B7-10	Rodent Control	7/1/82-6/30/83	82-601078 Pd 8/9/83	954.00
1983-84 7/20/83	B7-10	Rodent Control	7/1/83-6/30/84 (7/25/84 Pmt to Aud)	PO-83604988 Pd 8/15/84	954.00
1984-85 7/6/84	B7-10	Rodent Control	7/1/84-6/30/85 (7/3/85 Pmt to Aud)	PO-84604780 Pd 8/1/85	954.00
1985-86 2/6/85	B7-10	Rodent Control	7/1/85-6/30/86 7/15/86-Pmt to Auditor	PO 85601036 Pd 1/22/87	1001.70 / 954.00
1986-87 4/1/86	B7-10	Rodent Control	7/1/86-6/30/87 7/8/87 Pmt to Auditor — 12-1-1987 Rid-A-Pest Exterminating	PO 86600615	$832.44
1987-88 4/1/87	B7-10	Rodent & Roach Control	7/1/87-6/30/88 7/29/88-Pmt to Auditor — Circle City Pest Control Pd 8-15-88	PO 87602303	780.00 / 1,195.19
1988-89 4/28/88	B7-10	Rodent & Roach Control	7/1/88-6/30/89 8/16/89-Pmt to Auditor — Circle City Pest Control	PO 88602189	780.00
1989-90 3/9/89	B7-10	Rodent & Roach Control	7-1-89-6-30-90	89603673	780.00
1990-91 6-25-90	B7-10	Rodents & Roach Control	7-1-90-6/30/91	90602304	780.00

The log for pest control at Central State Hospital

When he was sent to the newspaper building's lobby to talk to a man about Central State Hospital, Skip believed he was just answering another inquiry. The man had a learning disabled daughter and couldn't afford a private hospital. When the man looked at Central State Hospital "he couldn't believe what he was seeing." Originally, the man went to Central State Hospital because it was something he could afford and it was closer to his home. After what the man saw, he did not put his daughter in the hospital.

Skip remembered, "I thought this guy was making up stuff, I really did. So I said,' why don't I go out there with you sometime.' He said, 'Sure.' They[The hospital] had no security, they [The hospital] didn't know who I was, they [The hospital] didn't care who I was. He [the man with the daughter] was an exterminator. That's how he was at Central State Hospital. He was hired by the state on a contract to exterminate rats. The man thought this is where I was thinking of putting my daughter. It is so hard to explain what it was like walking into that, because I could absolutely not believe what I was seeing."

Skip likened what he saw to the 1948 movie, "Snakepit."

Although Skip is very modest about his award, he admits he reported during a "terrible, horrendous" time in Central State Hospital's history. He remembered patients just wandering around and many of them would yell at him and others. "Lord only knows what I didn't uncover."

Investigative reporting was a very new concept in newspapers during the time Skip reported. He had never done investigative reporting before and described it as "incredible." Skip hoped he'd "be ok" to investigate for a long time. (Typically, early investigative reporting lasted a few months at best.) Even after everyone found out who he was, Skip was not to be silenced, "I'd been there way too long and found out too much."

"I never told anyone there I was an exterminator or a newspaper reporter. I just went with this man. Everything he told me was as bad, or worse, as he was seeing it." Skip remembered while writing the articles that he didn't think people would believe him, that they couldn't believe these things were "happening right under our noses".

When Skip went out to the hospital with the exterminator, he was privy to every place in the hospital. The exterminator took off the moulding and showed Skip the infestation. "Rats lined up head to tail in rats nests." Everyplace the exterminator pried the moulding off, it was the same result.

Skip relayed his experience in the tunnels. He'd been told that there were cells where patients used to be chained (1). Although he saw no evidence of the chains, cells remained from when the Department for Women was built. The exterminator told Skip at one point, 'I am going to show you something, don't be afraid.' He shone a spotlight in the tunnel exposing a sea of rats. There had to be hundreds if not thousands. The exterminator said ,"This is where they come from." Some of the patients would go into the tunnels, eat, leave food and crumbs and that is what attracted the rats."

He also spoke with staff. They told him they would beat the patients with soap wrapped in socks because it "wouldn't leave marks", which they would have to report. Skip went into rooms where he found mold and stinking food in cabinet drawers. He asked one patient if he brought food into the room. The patient "ran to cabinet, pulled out a terrible, stinking mess of food" and started eating it.

Eventually, the Marion County Mental Health Association "demanded" (2) to see what he was writing. A group of people went out there unannounced with Skip and a maintenance worker. The first place Skip took them was the water fountain. Taking off the back, six or seven rats scurried away. Skip also showed him the moulding and even the "filthy" kitchen where rats would invade the ovens and snack on food to be served to patients and staff.

The second floor of the Department of Women was also on the tour. There were no beds, only urine soaked mattresses. Skip stated if you pressed down on the mattresses, urine would come out. Eventually, someone in the group said "I've seen enough. I know now what I've been reading is true."

Even after the first stories and even after the Marion County Mental Health Association was informed, Skip was still able to go out with the exterminator without hindrance.

On one such visit, a woman approached Skip in the kitchen. She said, "You're not who you pretend to be, are you?" Skip asked her who she thought he was. The woman stated, "I've watched you. You are not who you pretend to be." Skip asked her again who she thought he was. The woman looked at him and said,

"I don't know but you aren't here to exterminate bugs and rats. Who are you?" Skip admitted that he was just looking around, but he knew the woman knew something was up.

After a short time, the woman said, Let me show you what this place has done to me," and she raised her gown, revealing she had no underclothes on. She asked Skip to look at her and told him, "This is what this place has done to me. It has taken all my dignity." She was a patient who had been a schoolteacher. Her family put her in the hospital. She identified herself as Dorothy S.

Dorothy said, "I can help you." I can tell you things, I can show you things." She must have known that she might not be taken seriously because Dorothy told Skip about who she was and why she was there. Skip finally told her that he was a reporter.

Dorothy's answer surprised Skip. "You're the answer to my prayers. I've tried to tell my family. You're the answer to every prayer I had and the answer to the prayers of the people in here… I know you're going to stop this, what's happening here."

Skip tried to take stock of the situation. At first he thought he couldn't use the information from her. He didn't know if it was accurate. Still, he asked her to tell him what she knew. Dorothy told Skip if he went to the top floor of the Department for Women, he would find violent patients locked in cells. She told him that the staff would slide trays of food to the patients in the cells. These people, said Dorothy, had not seen a doctor or psychiatrist in many years. She went on to disclose that there were doctors on the payroll who didn't even work at the hospital- they were in Florida. Skip followed up on these points and found Dorothy was right.

Dorothy also told Skip to go into the women's restroom and see what was going on. In the restroom Skip found the glass window broken, exposing the bars on the windows. The toilets were abysmal. They had no lids or seats. None of the toilets had toilet paper. And men and women used the facilities together at the same time. When Skip asked what the patients were doing in the restrooms, Dorothy cryptically answered, "You'll have to find out. That's how we live here. We just wipe on our socks or whatever cloth we have."

Again, Skip agreed with her, "I knew she was telling me the truth. I went to the upper floor. It was like animals, the sounds they were making. They were growling. It was really, really frightening. There was one nurse who was assigned to one unit and it was a huge unit. This nurse would go to another unit and work too."

Dorothy had an even darker, sadder secret to tell. "Did you know they pick up patients and use them as prostitutes? You stand out here along the benches on Washington Street. You'll see women at night. Cars come and pick them up. They are prostituted- they get no money- then they bring them back."

Skip found that indeed, the very staff who was to care for the patients would find the people to pick the women up and the workers got a procurement percentage of the money. Workers would target "promiscuous patients" and take them out there.

Several evenings, Skip witnessed the activity. "Again there is no security. I sit on the grounds and watch the cars come and get them [patients] and bring them back. I talked to one of the women and asked 'where do you go when the cars pick you up?' She replied, 'we have sex." Skip asked who authorized it and was told it was a medical professional for the Department of Women who lived on the grounds. The medial official was lesbian and would also take female patients back to her housing and have sex with them.

With the poor condition of the building, Skip went to the Fire Marshall to see if the building had been reported with issues. The Fire Marshall had condemned it.

Skip spent several days looking over the hospital. "Sometimes I'd go by myself and walk the grounds and see what was going on and talk to people who worked there. They had no idea who I was."

Once when Skip went to the kitchen, he noticed a huge board attached to the wall. It was about four feet wide, eight feet tall and about two inches thick. It had quite a few cut marks around the edges but not in the middle. Pointing to the board, Skip asked the butcher, "What's this?"

The butcher answered, laughing. "This is where we put patients when they don't do their work. I make them stand there and I throw a meat cleaver close to them." Skip later found out through his investigation that the butcher had a grocery store and he'd take patients to work for free at his store and then bring them back to the hospital.

The hospital wasn't the only property to be poorly run and which had abuses. The farm colony also had its share of problems. Unfortunately, by the time the abuses came to Skip's attention, he was unable to really investigate it because everyone knew who he was by then.

"I can't verify but I would see patients who were completely unaccounted for." Skip said he could find when patients were admitted but not when they were released. He was told by someone who worked there that "they [patients] were killed and buried on the grounds." He passed this information to investigators.

The investigators from the State Police asked Skip if knew anything about the deaths and he told them there was nothing he could prove. The investigators said they heard about the deaths "constantly."

During the height of his reporting about Central State Hospital, Skip asked Superintendent John Keating about the abuses, and the Florida doctors. Keating told him, "Get out of my office, you son of a bitch." Skip sat in his chair, and Keating said, rounding the desk, "I said to get out, you son of a bitch." By the time Skip got back to the office, Keating had called Skip and was apologetic. "You can't believe the pressure that's on me. Can we start the interview again?"

At one point in Keating's career, he had to release 600 people because of overcrowding. After the patients were released, Skip found many of them living in cardboard boxes on College Avenue.

Keating stated that he had complained, asked for money, nurses, and doctors but Skip believed "he [Keating] had kind of thrown up his hands and quit."

On the other hand Dr. Murray was the head of the Marion County Mental Health Association and was open with Skip. Dr. Murray stated, "Everything you're writing about is true." Skip asked, "Why would you allow this?" Murray responded, citing political influences, "You'll have to ask the governor."
Skip eventually did want to talk with Indiana Governor Roger D. Branigin by phone. After Skip stated his purpose, the governor informed skip that he was "very busy" and Skip had "one minute". When Skip started in on the highlights of the abuse and neglect, Governor Branigin said, "Your one minute is up, Mr. Hess," and hung up the phone.

In contrast, when Governor Bowen came into office, he called Skip on his first day in office and said, "I want to talk to you about Central State Hospital. We're going to investigate everything you print and more." Bowen did send investigators to the Farm Colony and initiated an investigation, but they didn't find bodies or anything buried. *

Later, Skip went to the Logansport, Evansville and Madison State Hospitals. Although he did not investigate them as closely as Central State Hospital, he was taken around to where ever he wanted to go in the hospitals. He talked to employees and patients. According to Skip, The difference between these hospitals and Central State was "night and day."

All things must come to an end. Investigative reporting was so new and the fact that Skip was allowed five years to investigate a topic was unheard of. Skip was pleased the newspaper let him run with the story.

"I felt good because I think Dorothy S. made an incredible impression on me because then I understood what she was going through, what she saw. I understood there were a lot of people in there, the people on the third and fourth floors, [living] like animals. I saw what they [the hospital] turned these people into. These doctors, psychiatrists hadn't seen anybody for years. We went on so long with the newspaper. I felt really good about what the newspaper had done. You go through life and you look back and think about what you've done good. That is one. I feel proud and I will always feel proud. I knew the terrible things going on with people. For the most part, the things stopped."

The area to which Skip was referring is where the golf course is next to the Indianapolis Motor Speedway.

Thirteen

TODAY

Over the years, the facility became a grim reminder of the recent past and less about the people who tried to help the mentally ill. The city and developers are trying hard to change that.

The buildings became useful to SWAT teams, the police, an Olympic-hopeful diving team and others after the hospital closed.

Christel House Academy, a K-12 school, has a new facility for people who have dropped out and want to obtain their GED. It opened in August of 2014 with a kindergarten to second grade reach. It plans to grow one grade each year. It is a tuition free charter school. The Administration building has been renovated and is to be used for student housing.

Apartments and mixed use commercial and entertainment venues are also slated for installation.

Additionally, Seven Steeples Farm produces fresh vegetables and chicken eggs.

And what of patients and their needs? In addition to the community mental health network, Methodist Hospital campus of the IU School of Medicine in Indianapolis contains a world class center for psychiatric and neurological disorders. Additionally a $45 million neuroscience research building was completed in 2014 to provide an "exceptional national model for the treatment of the mentally ill through modern science."

It will study and treat disorders such as schizophrenia, bipolar disorder, panic disorder, Alzheimer's dementia, alcohol and drug addiction and autism spectrum disorder using the latest technology for the human genome. Researchers hope to use MRIs and other non-invasive ways to study brain activity on live patients. Behavior observation of human volunteers and lab animals will occur.

The total cost was estimated at $53 million dollars. The State of Indiana contributed $43 million through bonds. Indiana University and the Indiana University School of Medicine contributed $5 million each.

Hopefully with these new options on the horizon patient care will improve. Time will tell.

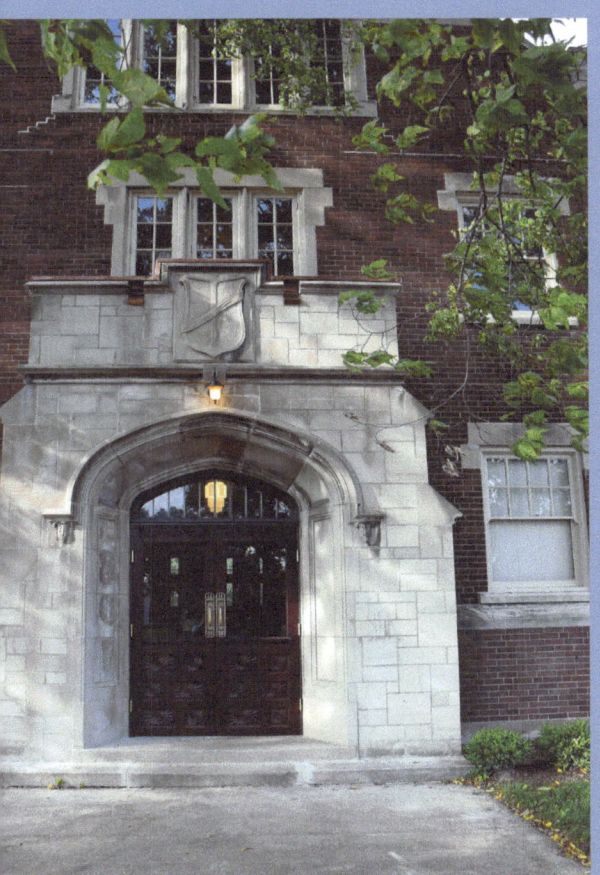

Left: The Employee Building/Administration Building, now called the Central State Mansion. You can still see the burn marks above the bottom window on the right.

Right: Sign pointing to Central State Mansion.

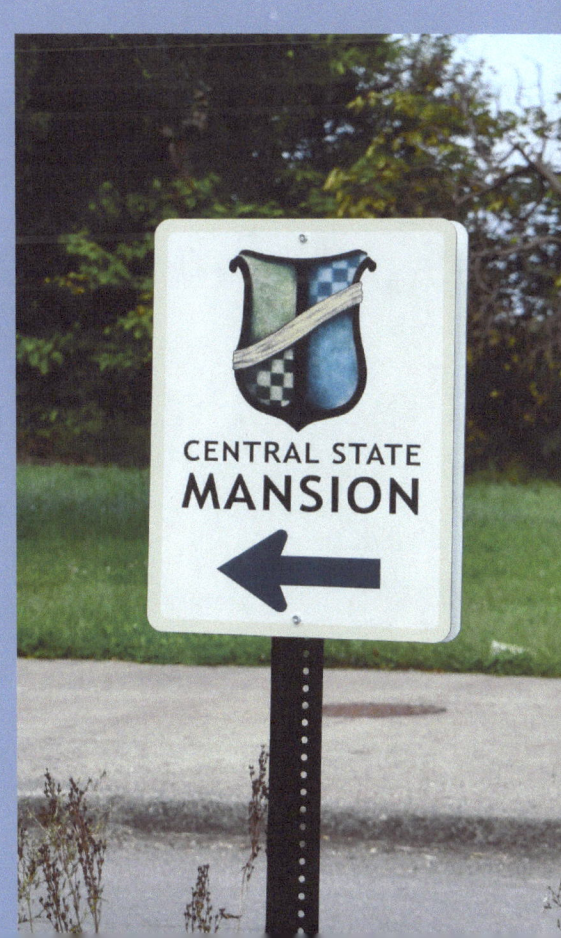

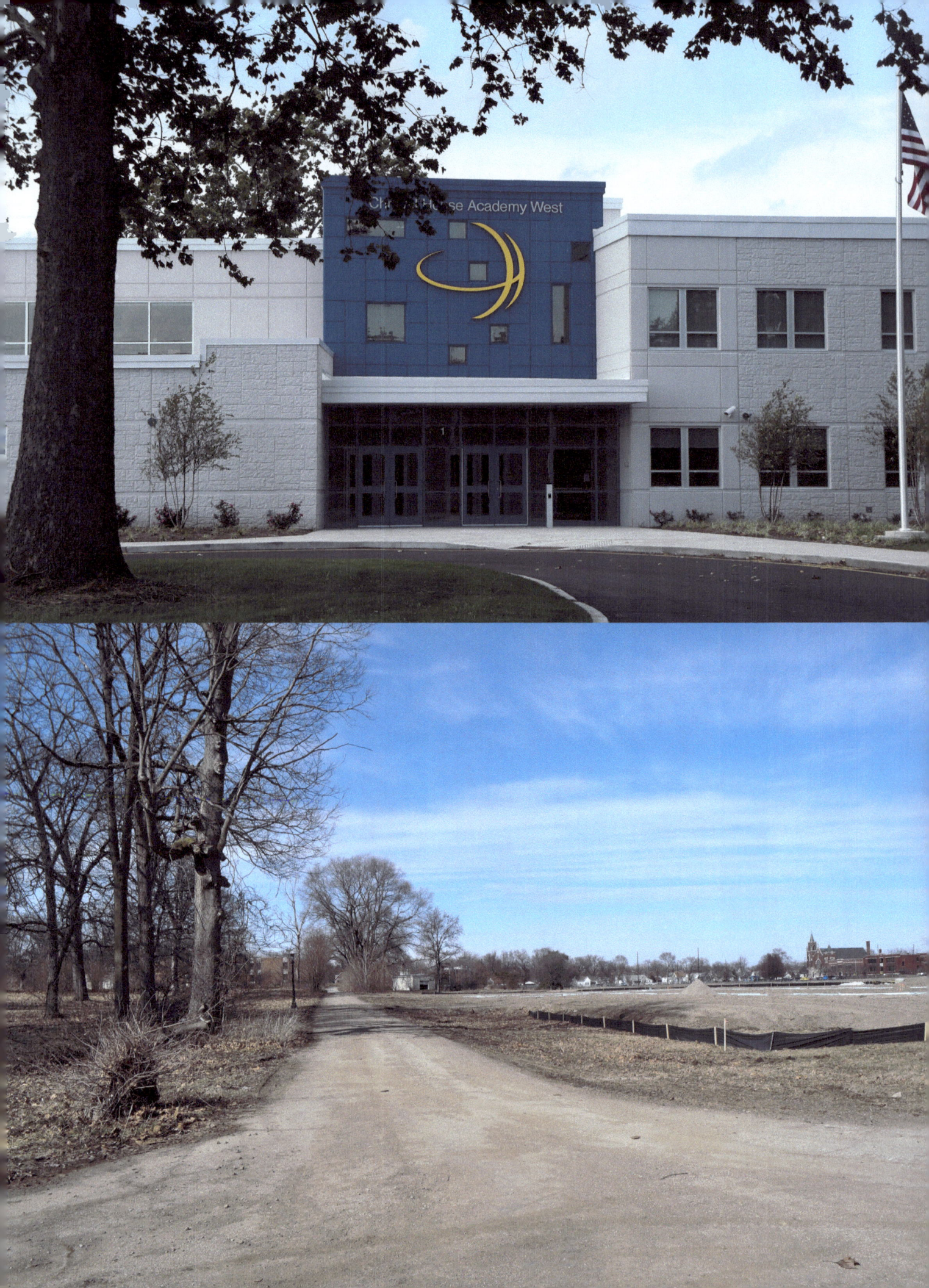

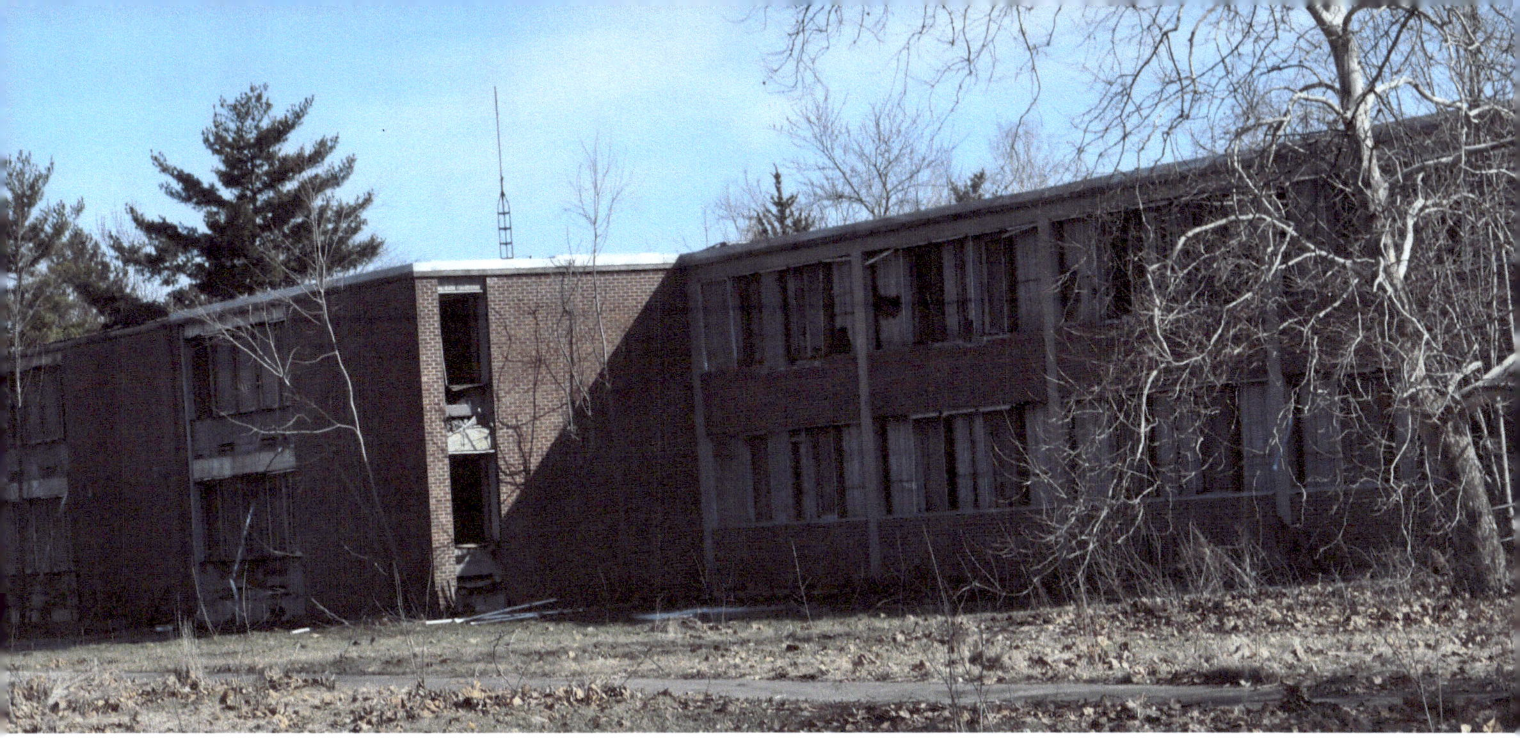

Opposite top: The new Christel House Academy West on the south west side of the hospital campus. Opposite bottom: June 2014. Road to the former Bolton and Evans buildings. This was also the road to Seven Steeples and the original Bolton Farm. Top: The Bahr Building gutted and awaiting the wrecking ball. Below: The former hospital farm site, also the Bolton Building site. Now it is under renovation with new construction.

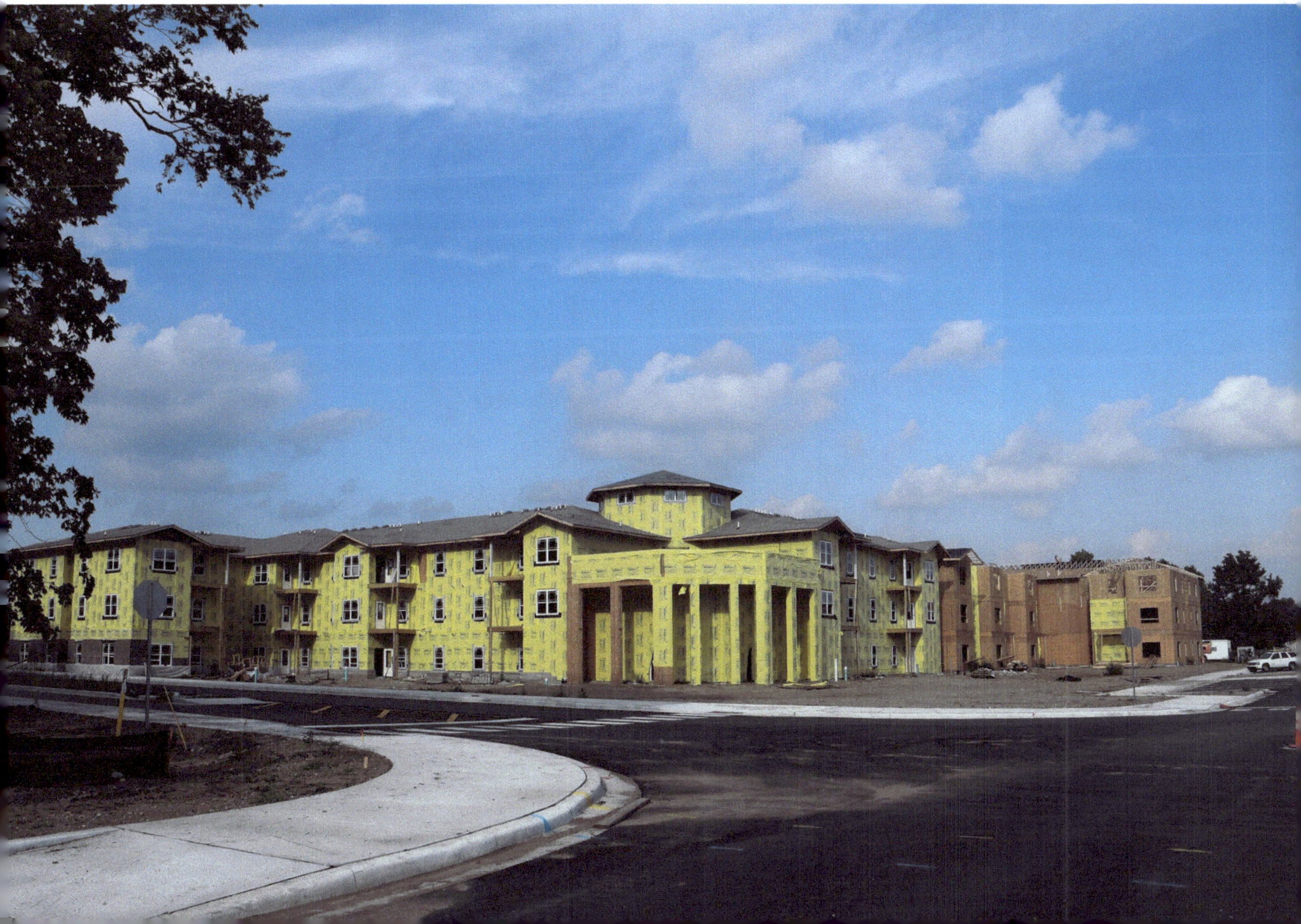

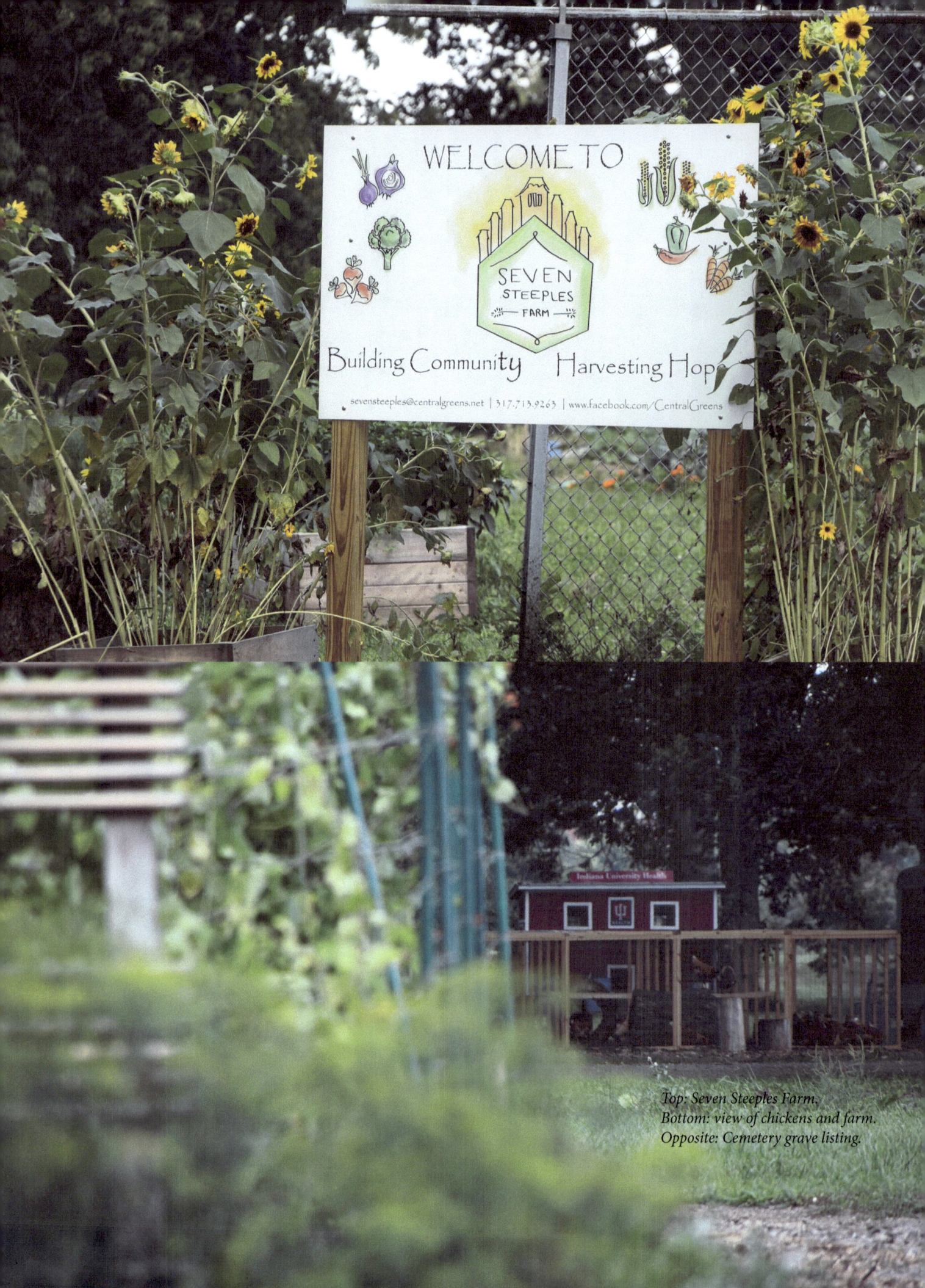

Top: Seven Steeples Farm.
Bottom: view of chickens and farm.
Opposite: Cemetery grave listing.

Fourteen

Central State Hospital Cemetery

Deaths in the yearly reports and paying for undertaker services, which was a nearly yearly expense, the final resting place of patients was not really a topic of great conversation. As a result, the cemetery, its location and purpose has always been a source of confusion and fascination.

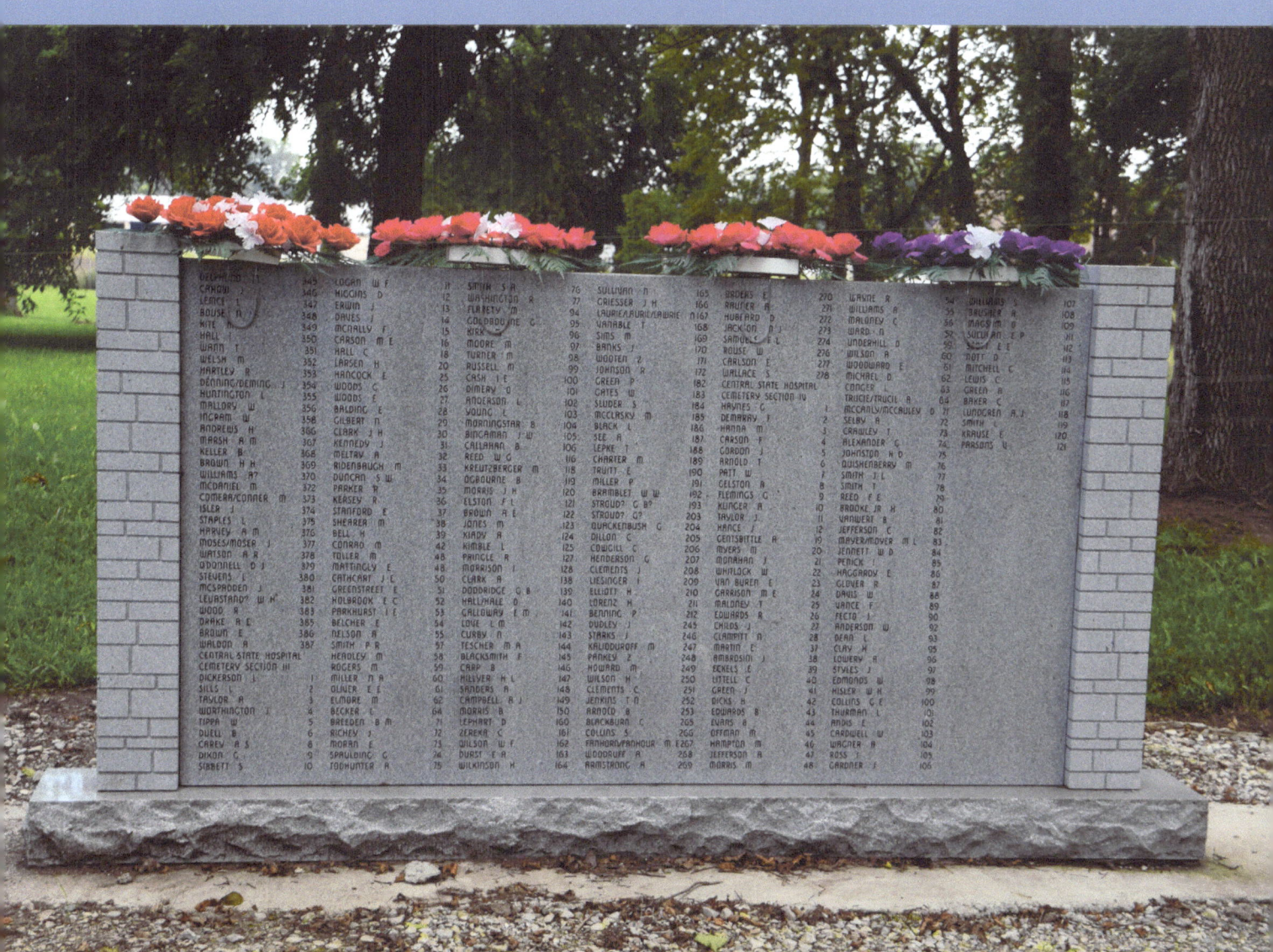

Part of the confusion stems from the 1871 yearly report, which stated Engineer Thomas Hoagland died and his remains were in "the old church yard adjoining the Hospital." Some people believed this was a church on the grounds of the hospital or the existing St. Anthony at the corner of Warman Avenue and Vermont Street. But this isn't true. Thomas Hoagland is buried in Mount Jackson Cemetery, which is on Cossell Rd. and North Tibbs Avenue.

Some of the early patient records do not indicate whether they were buried on site. A few patients were buried in unknown locations on the grounds before a cemetery was established. The 1848 annual report mentioned a cemetery was established "surrounded by a board fence." It is unknown where this section is, but many believe this is Section 1, which is on the northwest grounds of the hospital. There are no known listings for these people and no evidence of a board fence or markers having been placed on these graves.

The 1890 yearly report state that an iron post and a steel ribbon fence was placed around the cemetery. Trees and shrubbery were also purchased and were scheduled to be planted so "that proper respect may be shown to the memories of the dead." The yearly report also stated, "In case of fire, if the records should be burned, there would be no means of determining the burial place for those interred in the Hospital cemetery. That this neglect may be remedied, an iron post will be placed at the head of each occupied grave, and to these indestructible posts head boards will be affixed to indicate the name of each occupant." The report went on to talk about the aged population and the need for more burial space. "In the transfers which have been made to us from the Northern Hospital and from the jails and poor houses of the Central district, we have received a number of aged and very infirm paupers. When these patients die, they will have to be buried here. Not only will our death rate be very greatly increased within the next year or two but the space for burial purposes must, of necessity be enlarged."

We know that with the exception of very few early patients in 1848, pre-1905 burials are on Section 1, which is the northwest corner of the property at Vermont Street and Tibbs Avenue. Burials after 1905 are in the Central State Cemetery which is on the west side of Tibbs Avenue, which adjoins the south side of Mount Jackson Cemetery. Many people believe that these burials are part of Mount Jackson Cemetery, but this is not the case. Burials from 1905-1927 are in Section 2, 1928-1937 section 3 and 1938-1947 in section 4 of the Central State Cemetery.

The 1905 annual report mentions an "iron and wire fence" built on the "south side of the cemetery". Since the second section of the cemetery was opened in 1905 we are unsure which cemetery this refers to and today, there is no remnant of an iron fence.

Not all patients were buried in either cemetery or on the grounds. Some patients were claimed by family and friends and buried in other cemeteries.

The newspaper reported in 995 the graves of close to 585 patients including five Civil War veterans were relabeled. The cemetery was also cleaned up and a fence was put around it. Although some markers existed, they were moved to make way for the fence. Their whereabouts is not known.

Instead, each grave had a small concrete marker with a plastic label that included a patient number. A brick

NOTICE TO UNDERTAKERS.

The Board of Trustees of the Central Indiana Hospital for Insane will receive proposals until 2 p. m. April 25, 1901, for the burial of hospital patients from May 1, 1901, to May 1, 1902. Specifications on file at steward's office on and after April 15, 1901. The Board of Trustees reserves the right to reject any and all proposals.

By Order of Board of Trustees.

April 17, 1901 a notice from the hospital stating that it was accepting bids for undertakers to bury the hospital dead was posted in the Indianapolis Journal. April 27, 1901 the bids were awarded to Messrs. Tutewiler & Son of Indianapolis.

directory was established with the names of each person buried there put on plastic inserts. The grave markers and listing have been dismantled because the plastic, on the concrete grave markers and the listing, was brittle and easily broke during Indiana weather

Additionally, The Indiana State Department of Transportation workers used backhoes to "fill in" the southern section of the cemetery (Section 4).

New interment documentation was also found. The 1995 cleanup only guessed at where the graves were and did not follow the original documentation. Efforts are underway to correct this.

A cemetery list exists at the Indiana Medical History Museum. Additionally, autopsy records from 1899-1930 are at the museum, but are not generally available to the public. An updated listing based on the newly found records is being compiled by volunteers.

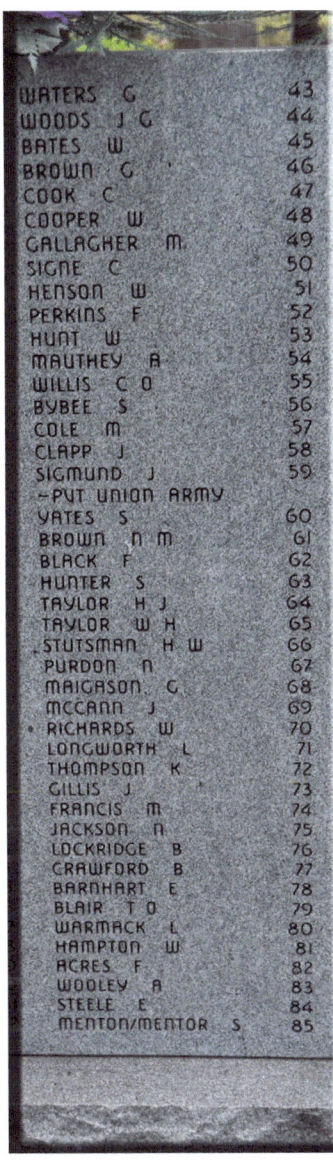

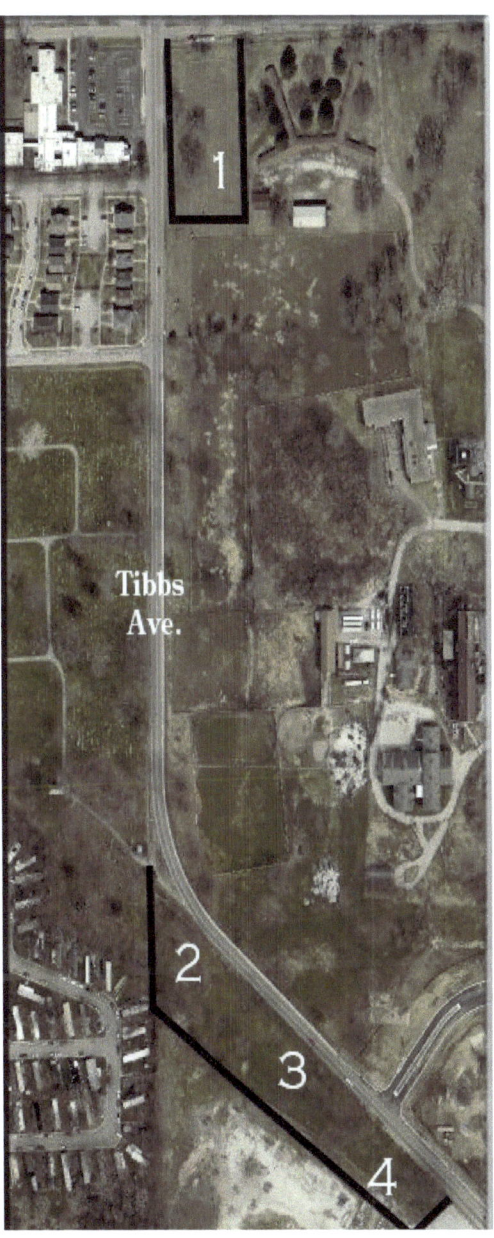

Left: The new listing where J Sigmond's name is spelled differently on the new monument. He has a different number.

Right: 2014 GIS map showing the approximate sections of the Central State Hospital Cemetery. The cemetery above Section 2 is Mount Jackson.

Below: A name plate from the old listing that was replaced by the granite monument on the previous page. His first name is John.

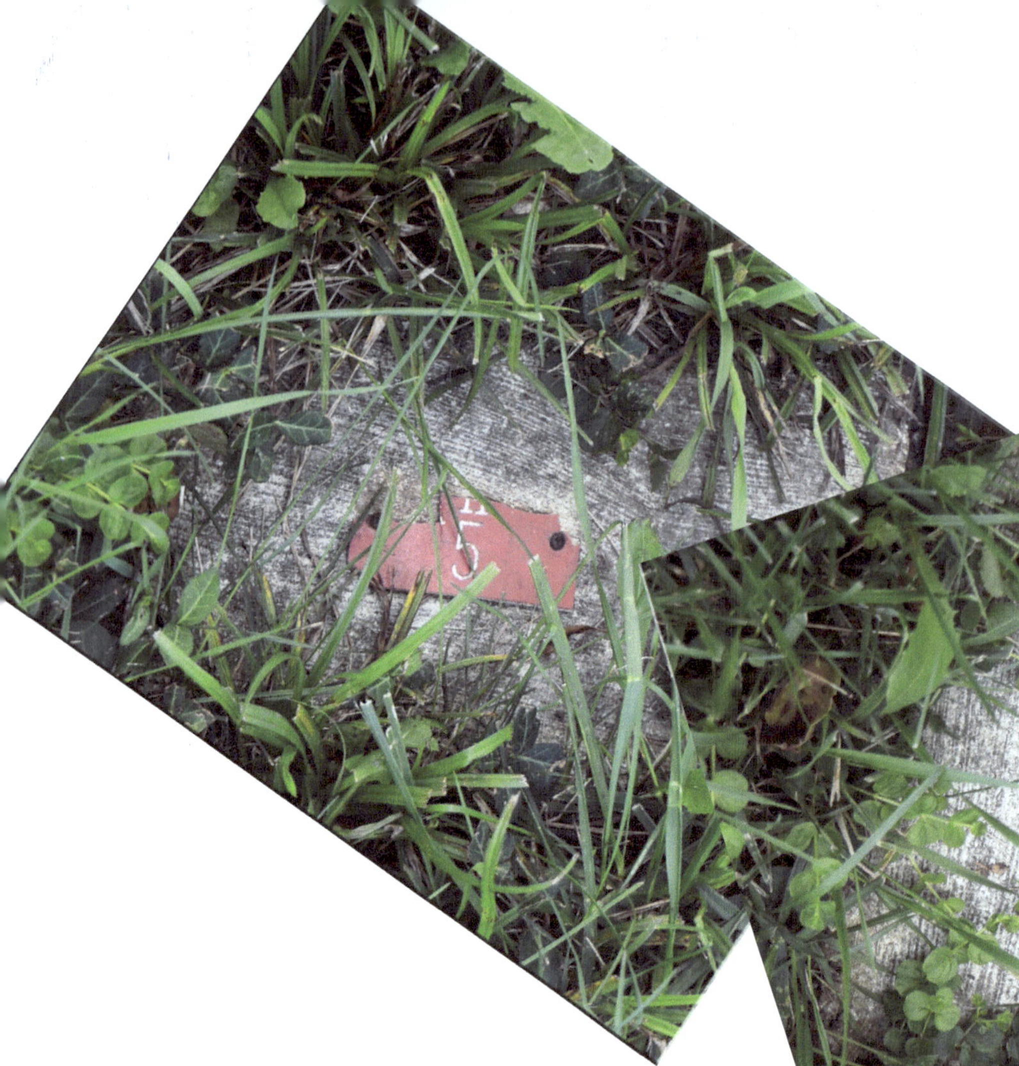

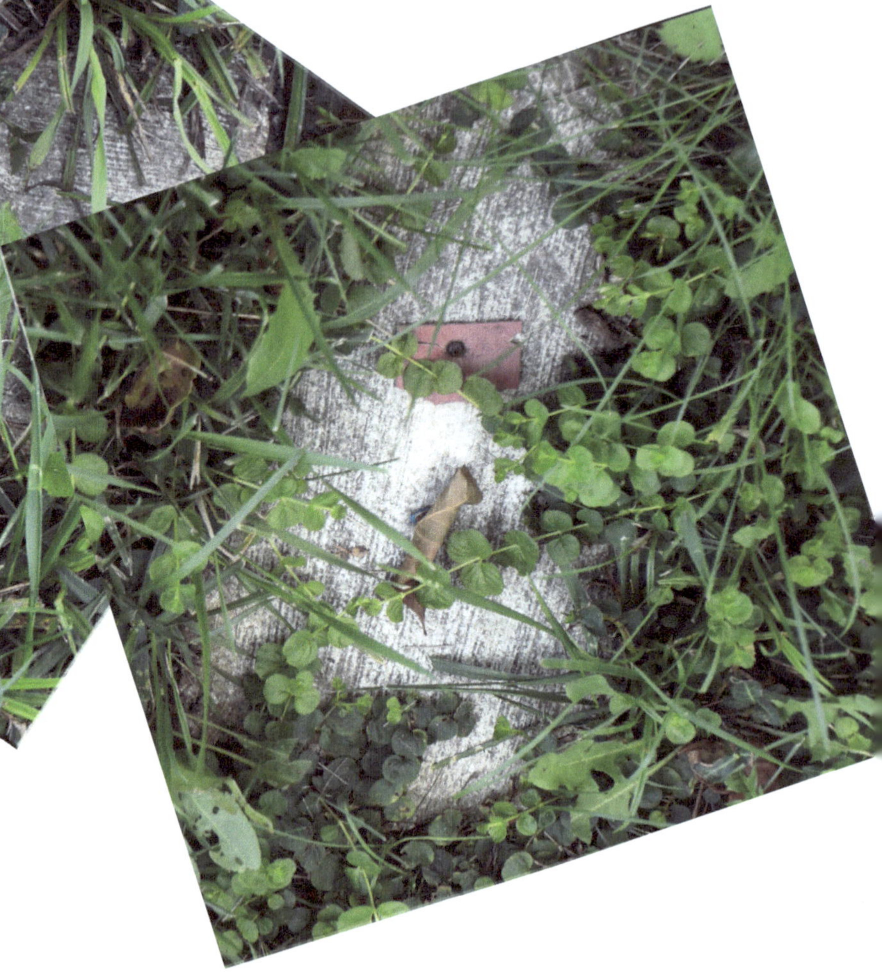

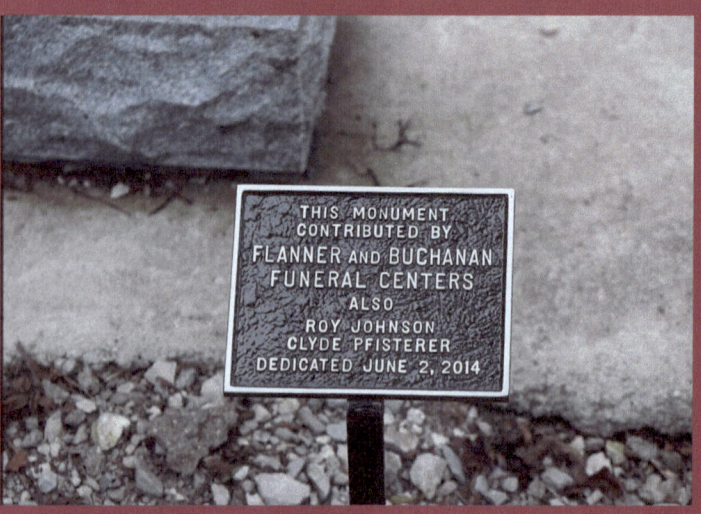

Above: Examples of grave markers in Sections 2, 3, and 4. In one you can see the remnants of "II 5", meaning section 2, number 5. The other is illegible.

Flanner and Buchanan Funeral Home donated most of the cost of the $10,000 monument. Some of the decendents of patients are putting real cemetery markers on their family memebers' graves as a remembrance of them.

One of these decendants, Roy Johnson, had a grandfather who was put into the hospital because he was too sick to be cared for at home.

Fifteen

CENTRAL STATE HOSPITAL LEADERSHIP

This list was compiled from annual reports from 1848-1948. This list is incomplete because not all the reports were available. Only the years with changes in staff are reported.

By the 1940s the key hospital staff was expanding in the post-war hospital. Some reports after 1948 are missing or do not list all staff as the hospital was very large by that time. Post-1948 staff are listed at the end of the chapter.

Note: This information appears exactly as it does in the annual reports. Some spellings in other sources or in modern English may differ.

Superintendents
1847-1847 John Evans
1848-1852 Richard J Patterson
1853-1861 James S Athon
1861-1864 James H Woodburn
1865-1868 Wilson Lockhart
1869-1878 Orpheus Everts
1879-1882 Joseph G Rogers
1883-1886 William B Fletcher
1887-1888 Thomas S Galbraith
1889-1892 Charles E Wright
1893-1923 George F Edenharter
1923-1952 Max A Bahr
1952-1966 Clifford L Williams
January 1-31, 1967 Paul D. Williams
February 1- March 31, 1968 J.V. Pace
April 1, 1968-1974 John U Keating
1974-1976 George A Teabolt
1976-1982 Eric Helmer
1982-1992 Ruth Stanley
1992 Timothy Campbell*
1992-1993 Leo Dillon
1993-1994 Diana Haugh

*Resigned after 3 weeks

Assistant Physicians *(to 1948)*
This is a list of the assistant physicians at the hospital who reported to the Superintendent. All of these doctors were formally educated medical doctors. (Sr.) and (Jr.) refer to senior assistant physicians and junior assistant physicians.

Physicians (Men and Women)
J. Nutt 1848
Thomas B. Elliot 1850-1858
Thomas P. McCullough 1853
 (Jr.) George A. Torebet 1855
(Sr.) Henry F. Barnes 1858
(Jr.) John M. Dunlap 1858
 (Jr.) J.F. Cravens 1862
(Jr.) Robert Charlton 1864
W.W. Hester 1865-1870
W.J. Elstun 1869
Charles L Armington, 3rd Assistant Physician 1871-1872

Physicians (Men)
A.J .Thomas 1879-1886
W.H. Hubbard 1879-1883
J.R. Brown 1881-1886
T. Davenport 1883
W.E. Brandt 1883
W.J. Browning, 1886
E.C. Reyer 1886-1888
J.E. Curtis 2nd assistant physician 1889
P.J. Watters 1890
F.M. Wiles 1896
J.A. MacDonald 1905
Paul M. StClair 1908
Ord Evermann 1911
Dr. Wiles 1913
John Harper 1914
P.J. Watters 1915
E. Murray Aer 1916
John M. Ladd 1916
H.J. Lemmon 1917
H.W. Trigger 1917
E.L. Ray 1917
H.J. Lemmon 1918
M.J. Silver 1918
H.H. Gordon 1918
F.J. Cayley 1919
Joseph Slattery 1919
Earl Moorman 1919
O.B. Christie 1920
Robert F. Buehl 1921
J.D. Syebert 1922
M.C. Pitkin 1922
E.O. Alvis 1922
HL Norris 1922
W.D. Wheless 1925
HH Atkinson 1927
Francis Prenatt 1928
A.M. DeArmond 1929
R.G. Thayer 1931
W.L. Sharp 1932
W.L. Sharp 1934
P.T. Lamey 1934
W.J. Dieter 1936
J.S. Skobba 1936
G.L. Sandy 1938 (killed in auto accident 12/18/1941
John R. Miller 1942
Merton A. Farlow 1943

Physicians (Women)
J.C. Walker 1879-1889
JN Smith 1879-1889
J.R. Brown 1886
Sarah Stockton 1886, returned in 1900 (female)
C.H. Wiles 1886
F.M. Howard 1887
P.J. Watters 1889
A.M. Adams 1889-1890 (female)
W.J. Browning 1889 F.M. Wiles 1890

J.D. Simpson 1890
Harvey Rainey 1896
Mary Smith 1896
Franklin E. Ray 1896
Edmund Ludlow 1897
Fred L. Pettijohn 1898
Max A. Bahr 1903
R.N. Todd 1903
A.R. Lemke 1904-1906
J.J. Hoffman 1906
Chas T. King 1908-1909
C. Stanley Aitken 1909
Edward J. Kempf 1911-1912
P.H. Weeks 1913
James S. Rushton 1913
W.S. Wentzel 1916
George E. Iterman 1916
Earl Moorman 1917
O.L. Stevens 1919
K.M. Ferguson 1920
N.W. Kaiser 1921
O.L. Stevens 1923
Elizabeth Enz Gross 1924
W.D. Wheless 1924
L.H. Gilman 1924
Clela Hull (Interne) 1924
Fross Hall 1925
Elizabeth Carroll 1925
Joseph E. Kilman 1927
Rosalie McAdams 1927
Francis Prenatt 1930
JT Tidwell 1930
R.G. Thayer 1934
M.M. Rubin 1934
F.W. Oliphant 1936
W.A. Sandy 1937
J.S. Skobba 1938
Frederic Spencer 1939
G.S. Rader 1940
John T. Slama 1940
Frank Cayley 1942
Merton A. Farlow 1942

OTHER POSITIONS *(to 1948)*

Other noted positions are below. As the years changed the institution so did the positions. In the beginning, the people holding these positions were expected to live on site at the hospital. Later, some of the positions became "non-resident" positions, meaning that the people would commute to their jobs every day.

Stewards and Matrons cared for patients and ensured supplies were ordered and used properly. They also ensured patient care met hospital standards.

These records are incomplete because the yearly records are incomplete. Additionally, not all positions were listed consistently in the yearly reports.

Note: This information appears exactly as it does in the annual reports. Some spellings in other sources or in modern English may differ.

STEWARDS
J.M.L Bradshaw 1851
Mr. Moyer (died) 1852
Isaac H. Shimer 1852
Moses Huntere 1856
W.M. French 1862
Charles Test 1869-70
George Patterson 1871
Mrs. A.J. Thomas 1881
Simon P. Neidigh 1885-1931
Mr. Stacey (assistant steward) 1887

After 1931 there was no longer a mention of stewards.

MATRONS
Mrs. Laura Ann Elliot 1848
Mrs. Mary Wright 1853
Mrs. Jane G. Shimer 1855
Miss Eleanor Lea (resigned) 1856
Mrs. Sarah G. Hall 1858
Mrs. Ester McLaughlin 1859
Mrs. Sarah J. Poage 1860
Mrs. Ellen Bigger 1862
Mrs. Mary Everts 1869-
Mrs. Margaret W Rogers 1881
Agnes O'B. Fletcher 1886
Elizabeth Galbraith 1887
Anna H. Wright 1889-1890
Mr. Kogler 1891 (worked on Men's Ward)
Marion E. Edenharter 1897-1908?

After 1908 there was no longer a mention of matrons

STOREKEEPER
Samuel McMillan 1871
M.L. Stansbury 1879-1889
R.N. Smith 1889-1895
James E. Sproule 1885
Mr. Hyde 1889
Wilbur G. Austin 1906
Peter Brown 1911
Charles M Neely 1934

Assistant Storekeeper
James M. Myers (assistant bookkeeper and storekeeper) 1879-1881; (assistant bookkeeper (1882)
B.V. Hubbard 1881-1882
L.C. Bell (assistant bookkeeper and storekeeper) 1883
J.S. Hall (assistant bookkeeper and storekeeper) 1886
W.H. Wilhelm (assistant storekeeper) 1886
H.L. Hyde (second assistant storekeeper) 1887

No assistants after 1889

BOOKKEEPER
JS Hall 1887
W.H. Wilhelm 1889
Edmund B. Noel 1900
William E. Cochran 1908
O.R. Sumner 1929
Lindsey Elder 1931
Fred Brown 1934
M.H. Alexander 1937

SECOND BOOKKEEPER
William E. Cochran 1907
Pharmacist/ Druggist
James S. Athon, Jr 1875
James C. Jameson 1886
J.M. Taylore (assistant) 1888
James C. Jamison 1895
1924 (no druggist)
Frank M Luttlitz 1931
H.R. Grant 1934

SUPERINTENDENT'S SECRETARY
Mr. John Newcomb 1881
Private Secretary
D.V. Kyte 1887
Greg C Heeb 1888
F.C. Heeb 1890

SECRETARY
Cornealius Mayer 1895-1915
E.O. Thompson 1930
John R Beasley 1936

ASSISTANT SECRETARY
Erie O. Thompson 1911
D.O. Gibson 1927
COOK
Mr. Shimmel prior to 1887

TEACHERS
Mrs. Bertha Moor (men) 1886
Miss Susie R. Wilson (men) 1886
Mrs. Sarah J. Lewis (women) 1886 (appears to be head of department)
Mrs. Marie S. Palmer (women) 1886

TIMEKEEPER (PAYROLL)
D.V. Kyte 1886

RECORD CLERK
Eva (Evangeline) M. Smith 1888-
Juliette Portteus 1911
Frank H. Ellison 1920
Nora Love Humphrey 1938

RECORD LIBRARIAN
(replaced Record Clerk)
Nadion Brandenburg 1941
Chief Engineer
Mr. Stacey (mechanical engineer) 1887
Edward Cain 1888
Edward E. Frost 1900 (died 11/20/1914)
A.L. Morgan 1916
Love Morgan 1922
Joseph Ricketts 1927
Albert Boyd 1932-?
Joe Ricketts ?-1942)
Riley Heishman 1942
George Weare 1943

CHIEF CARPENTER
T.F. Cobb 1888
William Cobb 1900
Walter D. Johnston 1913 -1941?
Chief Electrician
B.A. Hull 1934
E.V. Humphrey 1938
Pathologist

F.A. Morrison 1890
Robert Hessler 1897
Daniel Healy 1899
Charles F. Neu 1904
Frederick C. Potter 1913
Walter Bruetsch 1924

ASSISTANT PATHOLOGIST
Ernest D. Martin 1906
Clinical Psychiater
Max A. Bahr 1915

INTERNE
Edmund B. Noel 1897
Max A. Bahr 1898
M.A. MacDonald 1904
Ord Evermann 1910

EMBALMER
Dr. J. W. Hamilton 1901

SUPERVISORS
(These names came from documents used in this book.)
A.F. Schuler ?-?, 1902

ATTENDANTS (WOMEN)
(These names came from documents used in this book.)
Miss B
Miss Christie
Miss Cain
Miss Gilmour
Miss Frank
Miss DeGulyer
Miss Robbins
Miss Morsey
Miss Raeburn 1909-??*
*At some point, she became a nightwatchman.

ATTENDANTS (MEN)
(These names came from documents used in this book.)
William H. Jacobs
Columbus Talbott
Holton E. Givan
Samuel Stork
Leo E Hudson
John M Bates
Albert Bridenstine

NIGHT WATCHMAN/NIGHT USHER
Miss Raeaburn ??-1921*
Joseph Brummett

*She was an attendant who turned night watchman; year unknown

DENTIST
R.C. Akers 1925
W.E. Cochran (res) 1929 ;
R.C. Akers (non-res) 1929
O. Kemp Johnston (non-res) 1934
Charles R Gregg (res) 1941
1944 position vacant

OCCUPATIONAL THERAPIST
Bess E. Sutton 1927
Nettie Kilpatrick 1929
Clara Crooker 1934
Louise Lynch 1935

CHIEF CLERK
John R Beasley 1934
Earl Kuhn (SP Neidigh died February 21, 1942)

DIETITIAN
William Richter 1934
Charlotte Brown 1939
1943-44 vacant

PSYCHIATRIC SOCIAL WORKER FOR WOMEN, DEPT. OF PUBLIC WELFARE
Joan Wolayer 1939

PSYCHIATRIC SOCIAL WORKER, DEPT. OF WELFARE *(no men/women designation)*
Charles F Mitchell 1941
1943-44 vacant

SUPERVISOR OF FARM COLONY
Walter Lewis 1939

CHIEF LABORATORY TECHNICIAN
T.C. Brown 1939

LABORATORY AND RESEARCH ASSISTANT
T.C. Brown 1941

Laboratory Technician
Carrie McDonald 1947

X-ray Technician
E.E. Ferguson 1939
E.E. Ferguson (and supervisor) 1941

Nursing Supervisors for Women
Elizabeth Mahoney 1939 (died 8/1/1940)
Dora Taylor 1939-1942
Lulu Kennedy 1939
Margaret Peters, RN 1941
Josephine Tyrrell, RN 1941-1943
Bertha Highfill 1943
Rusie Sigler 1944
Elizabeth Schmith 1947

Nursing Supervisors for Men
George McPheters 1939
Cledith Stephens 1939-1942
William Merryman 1943

Chaplain
Rev. Almon J Coble, AB-BS Th. 1947

1949-1966 Positions

The positions listed here most closely align together during this time. During the 1960s a broader categorization was used and these are listed under separate headings: Medical Staff, Consult Staff, Hospital Service, Administrative Service and Chiefs of Service. These are listed at the end of the section.

Assistant Superintendent
Jess V. Cohn 1951

Assistant Superintendent (Medical)
Paul D. Williams 1962-1969
Donald W. Reed 1972-1975
Donald M. Jolly 1976-1983

Assistant Superintendent (Administration)
Sidney Smock 1962-1966
Irving Rosenthal 1964-1966
E. Keith Miller 1969-1987
John Newsom 1989

Psychiatric Clinical Director
Walter L Bruetsch 1951
Hans W. Freymuth 1956 *(Clinical Director)*
Paul D. Williams 1958

Pathologist
Walter L Bruetsch 1953
John S. Woodard 1956
Paul V. Evans 1961-1966

Pathologist & Director of Laboratories
Walter L. Bruetsch 1956, 1961-1966

Chief Clerk
Sidney Smock 1951

Business Administrator
Sidney Smock 1954, 1964-1966 (deceased)
Ernest R. Dunbar 1969-1975

Acting Clinical Director
Hans W. Freymuth 1954

Resident physicians
Psychiatrists (Women)
Merton A Farlow 1951
Frank Cayley 1951
Clela Harkenss 1952
June Leedy 1952

Psychiatrists (Men)
Robert D McKay 1951
Ryland Roesch *(Psychiatrist-in-Training)* 1951
Frank Cayley 1952
Margaret Hatfield 1952
Dennis E. Singleton 1952

Resident Psychiatrists
Merton A Farlow 1953
Frank Cayley 1953
Clela Harkenss 1953
June Leedy 1953
Eric Otten 1954
Herbert Fleischel 1954

Non-Resident Physician, Ft. Harrison Colony
Charles T. Knowles 1951

Chief Psychologist
Morton Wiener 1954

Resident Dentist
Charles R. Gregg 1951

Dentist (Non-Resident)
O. Kemp Johnston 1952

Dentist
Wallace E. DeWitt 1956-1964
Wallace C. Sechrest 1961-1966
Stuart R. Loft 1966

Pharmacist
Homer Roy Grant 1951

Head Nurse
Eunice Wood, RN 1951
Vacant 1952

Chief Psychologist
Winifred S. Graves 1951

Psychologist
Wynne Arnholter 1951

Supervisor, Psychiatric Social Services
Ellafrank Sikes 1951
Edith J. Beatty 1954

Psyciatric Social Workers
C.L. Wallin
Hazel Funk *(resigned March 10, 1951)*

Chaplain
Rev. Albert Ashley 1951-1956
Rev. William L Peterson 1956
Rev. Robert C. Alexander 1958-1966
Rev. David Richards 1970s)
Rev. Earl Hoppert 1975
Rev. Benjamin Friend 1975
A rabbi was on call in the 1970s

Director of Occupational Therapy
Clara Crooker 1951

Director of Music Therapy
Carl S. King, Jr. 1953

Director of Recreational Therapy
Evelyn Calhoun 1954

Director of Dietetic Department
Phyllis McKay 1951

Dietitian
Wilma J. Palmer 1952

Steward of Dietetic Department
J.A. Douglas 1951

Chief Laboratory Technician
T.C. Brown 1951

Laboratory Technician
Carrie McDonald

XRay Technician
Vacant 1951

Medical Records Librarian
Edna Fager 1951

Administrator of Ft. Harrison Colony
Fay W. Hall 1951

Supervisor of Farm Colony
Walter Lewis 1951

Director of Nursing
Martha Rogers 1953

Instructor of Nurses
Opal H. Bradley 1953
Alice M. Nixon 1954

Supervisor of Nursing
Wilbert E. Yates 1953

Nursing Supervisors (Women)
Lulu Kennedy 1951

Attendant Supervisors (Women)
Elsie King 1952
Lulu Kennedy 1952

Nursing Supervisors (Men)
E.E. Ferguson 1951
Wiilliam Merryman 1951
Joseph J. Leonard 1951

Attendant Supervisors (Men)
E.E. Ferguson 1952
Wiilliam Merryman 1952
Edward Harlow 1952
Joseph J. Leonard 1952

Nursing Supervisor, Farm Colony
Fred LaHue 1951

Nursing Supervisor, Ft. Harrison Colony
Charles McCafferty 1951

Plant Maintenance Engineer
E.V. Humphrey 1951
John Ricketts 1953

Chief Engineer
George Weare 1951

Manager of Laundry
Lawrence Saudners

Superintendent Secretaries
Nora Love Humphrey 1951
Elise R. Smock 1951

Assistant to the Chief Clerk
Sylvia Landers 1951

Chief Clerk Secretary
Isabelle Mink 1951

Director Volunteer Services
A.H. Rittenhouse 1953

Beauty Operator
Ruth R. Young 1953

Farm & Garden Supervisor
Walter Lewis 1953

Sewing Room Supervisor
Gladys Kellams 1953

Mattress & Upholstery Shop Supervisor
Oliver J. Sprinkle 1953

Consultant, Eye Clinic
G.S. Rubin 1954

The names listed in the following sections can be confusing because some are listed in the previous section as well. Use the index to see all the pages on which the names appear.

MEDICAL STAFF

Clela Harkness 1956-1966
June Leedy 1956
Herbert Fleischl 1956-1966
Ernest A. Kellen 1956
Erich Otten 1956
Everett L. Hays 1956-1962 (resigned)
John D. Ralston 1956-1966 (resigned)
Edwin L. Libbert 1956
John A. Standard 1956
William DeMyer 1956
H. Dean Hartvigsen 1958
Dale S. King 1958
Otto W. Wickstrom, 1961-1963
John W. Lowe 1961-1962 (resigned)
John R. Crise 1961
John W. Reuter (part time) 1961-1962 (resigned)
Karl R. Sturckow 1961
Thomas P. Rogers 1961-1962 (resigned)
Harold N. Jones 1961
Edward J. Armbruster 1961
Charles R. Bonsett, Neurology & Electroencephalography 1961-1966
Claude M. Lowe 1962 (resigned)
Joseph M. Parker 1962-1963
Phillip Holmes 1962-1964
Dorothy C. Heinz 1962-1964 (resigned)
Gabra Gachaw 1962 (deceased)
Frank Fischer 1962
Jerome V. Pace 1963-1966
Phillp Hennessee 1964-1976
Lowel C. Becker 1964
Julia Thom 1964-1966 (resigned)
Ralph W. Taraba 1964 (resigned)
Nicholas Pappas 1966
Thorndike C. Toops 1966
Aida Alar 1975
Roshdi Azzam 1975
E.V. Ganaden 1975
Susan Ganaden 1975
Charles Hazelrigg 1975
Narendra Markand 1975
Virginia Ramos 1975-1987
Kenneta J. Shaffer 1975-1989
Harold Stoner 1975-1987
Rosendo Tansinsin 1975-1989
Dolloros Adeva 1976-1983
Lynn Anderson 1976
William Binkley 1976
Charles Bonsett 1976-1987
Suzanne Combs 1976
Rhonda Fogle 1976
Leslie Friedman 1976
Pamels Godley 1976
Derinda Radjeski 1976
Cecil Rhoads 1976-1987
Jack Ross 1976
Rouhana Rouhana 1976
Patrick Tidman 1976-1983
James Wright 1976-1983
Natwerlal Jani 1976-1988
Dale Giolas 1978
Rosita Cua 1983-1989
William Darroca 1983-1989
Orlando Gustilo 1983
Linda Burrows 1987
Pamela Drapeau 1987
Irvin Epstein 1987
Donald Jolly 1987-1989
Robert McDaniel 1987
Jashbhai Patel 1987
Israel Rosales 1987-1989
Andrew Wachtel 1987
Purushothama Iyenger 1987
Steven Brant 1987
Teresita Ramilo-Briones 1987-1989
Douglas Mullinix 1987-1989
Carlo Ronzoni 1989

CONSULT STAFF

John R. Melin, Gynecology 1956-1966
Charles A. Fisch, Internal Medicine 1956-1966
Gerald S. Rubin, Ophthalmology 1956-1961
Robert J.W. Kinzel, Orthopedics 1956-1964
John A. Campbell, Radiology 1956-1966
Harold S. Aron, Podiatry 1956-1966
James H. Stygall, Chest Diseases, 1958
Charles R. Bonsett, Electroencephalography 1958
Paul F. Benedict, General Surgery 1958-1963
Edward L. Dreyer, Laboratory Technology 1958-1966
Fred H. Priebe, Chest Diseases 1961-1966
Benedict Abreu, Psychopharmacology 1961
Theodor H. Barrett, Psychology 1961-1966
Lawrence H. Baker, Psychology 961-1966
Dwight W. Schuster, Psychiatry 961-1966
Jack I. Taube, Opthalmology 1962-1966
Austin L. Gardner, General Surgery 1964-1966
James H. Gosman, Dermetology 1964
Donald C. McCallum, Urology 1964-1966
Schlaegel Optical Service, Optical 1966

Clinton S. Wainscott, Orthopedics 1966
Robert A. Toal, Psychology 1966

Hospital Service
Jean Hiliard, Librarian 1956-1966
Homer Roy Grant, Pharmascist 1956-1962 (resigned)
James Poston, Director Industrial Therapy 1956-1966
Herbert Guy, Director Nursing Services 1956-1966
Martha E. Rogers, Director Nursing Services 1956-1966
Sophia R. Lindahl, Director Occupational Therapy 1956-1958
Morton Wiener, Director Recreational Therapy 1956
Don A. Miller, Director Recreational Therapy 1958-1966
Pauline A. Scholfield, Director Social Services 1956-1966
Glenna Bolstad, Director Volunteer Services 1956-1958
Director of Psychology *(vacant)* 1958
Werner F. Kuhn, Director of Psychology 1961-1966
Rachel T. Bash, Director Volunteer Services 1962-1966
Elmer A. Crews, Pharmacist 1962-1966
Charles C. Carter, Dietitian 1962-1966
Catherine Yoder, Director Occupational Therapy 1963-1966
Charles Sides, Pharmacist 1963-1964
Janatha Ashton, Medical Records Librarian 1966
Paul Neely, School Administrator 1966

Administrative Services
Chester C. Fields, Personnel Officer 1956
Ernest R. Dunbar, Personnel Officer 1958-1966
Wilma Jean Bloom, Dietitian 1956
John Ricketts, Plant Maintenance Engineer 1956-1964
Walter Lewis, Farm & Garden Supervisor 1956
James Dunlevy, Farm & Garden Supervisor 1958-1966
Raymond Fleck, Storekeeper 1956
Flora Benefiel, Housekeeper 1956-1962 (resigned)
Lawrence L. Sanders, Laundry Manager 1956
Ross Wickliff, Laundry Manager 1958-1966
Gladys Kellems, Sewing Room Supervisor 1956-1962
Mabel Kellems, Sewing Room Supervisor 1958-1966
Gladys Allen, Canteen Manager 1958-1964
Raymond E. Short, Supervisor Storeroom 1961-1966
Effie Thomas, Acting Housekeeper 1962-1963
Imo Gene Cunningham, Housekeeper 1964-1966
Eloise Bays, Canteen Manager 1966
William Holgate, Engineering Supervisor 1966
Dalen V. Shank, Personnel Director 1969-1983
Ernest Dunbar, Business Officer 1983
R. Robert Kenner, Medical Director 1983-1986
Kenner R. Robertson. Medical Director 1986
James Donahue, Medical director 1987-1989

Chiefs of Service
Bolton
Werner Kuhn 1976-1983
Evans
Blas Davila 1976-1983
Bahr
Charles Hazelrigg 1976-1983
Exit Unit
Rosa Harding 1976-1982

Epilogue

Funny farm, nut house, loony bin ,crazy house. Crazy, psycho, nuts, cuckoo, mental, weird, strange, bonkers, certifiable, cray, cra cra, freaky-deaky, have a screw lose, one brick shy of a full load, the barn lights on/door's open but no one's there, kooky, mad, off one's rocker, out of your mind, out to lunch, screwy, wacked out, batty, bats in the belfry, berserk, lunatic, maniacal, nutty as a fruitcake, out of one's tree, touched (in the head), unbalanced, unglued, unhinged, cockeyed, eccentric, idiotic, peculiar, dotty, demented, go postal.

Sixty one thousand, eight hundred and fifty nine (61,859) patents were admitted to Central State Hospital and not one of them was any more <insert derogatory word of choice here> than the rest of us. Don't believe it? Think about it. Do you have a fear, phobia, intense dislike, get stressed out, or have PMS? Then you are mentally ill. What makes you, different from them?

The overarching word I have for mental health issues is hope. My hope is that research to find and treat mental disorders includes non-drug treatments, or if drugs are found to be the key, that researchers create drugs with fewer side effects. In my life, I know many people who would at one time been put into Central State. Today, they live their lives to varying degrees of success by a cocktail of psychotropic drugs, therapy and sometimes sheer will.

While I don't believe that what is available today is the right answer, I don't claim to have all the answers. People who are far more skilled and knowledgeable than I am have the ability to research and find the answers. Since 1956 the IU School of Medicine Department of Psychiatry's Institute for Psychiatric Research has had a mission to "understand the neurobiological origins and treatment of psychiatric disorders and to communicate this understanding to all interested persons."

Despite organizations such as this, the fact is that fewer doctors are going into psychiatry. Currently there are about 50,000 in the United States, which is too few to serve the mentally ill. Half of those doctors are over 55 and will soon retire. The American Psychiatric Association states that medical schools need to show potential doctors that psychiatry can be a "rewarding and profitable career." However, according to information compiled by Medscape, psychiatrists rank in the bottom third for doctor salaries, with an average of $186,000 per year. Nineteen percent earn over $300,000 per year and 13% earn less than $100,000 per year. Women psychiatrists earn 20% less per year than their male counterparts.

In 2014 only 1,300 residencies opened for students who wanted to be psychiatrists. According to the Association of American Medical Colleges, with the current number of psychiatrists, there is a 3,900 doctor shortage just by Federal government standards.

In my experiences, it seems that people are almost in the same situation as the patients who were moved out of Central State. The mental health system has some good professionals in it- doctors, nurses, therapists, social workers and others - but it also contains burnt out, underpaid, undereducated, and sometimes uncaring and greedy individuals who prey on the patients. For all the requirements that professionals in the field obtain continuing education credits (CEUs), many of these workers feel they "know what they know" and don't want to take the initiative to learn more. Undoubtedly, this occurs in all professions. Sure, there are channels to lodge complaints. But how many years does it take to resolve them and how many years will it take for someone to look at the issues seriously? To me, this screams of the unhealthy cycle of Central State Hospital.

I have to live with the direction science is going. Mental health will progress, it will just take time with bumps along the way. What we all need to do during this journey is show compassion, give assistance when we can, find better systems for helping mentally ill people, and work with researchers to help find better ways to manage these conditions.

I hope for the best.

Chapter Notes

Chapter 2: Hospital Life
1. Medical condition where the foreskin becomes trapped behind the glans penis, and cannot be reduced (pulled back to its normal flaccid position covering the glans penis
2. Prior to working at the hospital, the attendant had been a farmer.
3. It was not clear the exact cause, but it may have been stress on family members left behind to handle day to day life and finances
4. If anyone knows where this is, let the author know!
5. She died there in 1936. Her son had been in and out of various Indiana and Ohio hospitals for a better part of his life. Frederick Macomber, Jr. died in Richmond State Hospital in 1944

Chapter 3: Patient Life
1. A quilt
2. These were made from old clothing that was no longer suitable for wear. Patients would cut or tear the longest piece to make strips. These were rolled into balls and later made into braided and woven "rag rugs".
3. This is wool from Cheviot sheep.
4. Paraldehyde has been used in treatment for alcoholics, nervous, and mental conditions. It has a calming effect on patients. Although still used somewhat today, better medications exist for the treatment of these conditions.
5. Beef essence was and still is used for patients who are ill and need a lot of nutrients in a small, powerful meal. It consists of pure juices from beef. The meat should be very lean with as much fat removed as possible. Broiling the meat is preferable until it begins to give juices. The meat is then cut into small pieces and the juices squeezed from the meat into a bowl. It was served alone or sometimes over a piece of dry hot toast.
6. He was learning German (Deutsch), but in earlier times, "Dutch" was used to refer to the Dutch (Netherlands) and German (High and Low) languages.
7. It is unclear whether he killed himself or died through some other means such as alcoholism due to depression.

Chapter 5: Staffing
1. This was during a time in which the building was recommended as demolished per the hospital and the Fire Marshall.
2. Many people don't realize that Thomas Kirkbride's methodology was much more popular in the early 1850s than in the 1880s when most people associate with him the beautiful Victorian architecture to him.
3. One exception to this is Dr. Clifford Williams who was reported to have slept on the grounds of the hospital in a small cottage.
4. He retired in 1923 and three weeks later, he died.
5. Janitorial and laundry staff
6. The Psychiatric I and II designations are higher than attendants are assigned and have more responsibility and were usually assigned and sometimes were supervisors. Later the III and IV were for supervisors.
7. Although not mentioned in every report Australia Armour won the CSH Psychiatric Aide of the Year award and was honored with the runners up at Claypool Hotel on 4/10/62.
8. She died in from a heart attack in 1924.
9. Seven Steeples
10. Although by this time it was illegal to use patients as labor even as part of therapy without pay, it seemed

it was in full force at the hospital.
11. By the 1970s the hospital received many more visitors than in the early days. Much credit can be given to community education and advances in therapies.
12. Formerly the Chaplain Department

CHAPTER 6: TREATMENTS AND RESEARCH
1. Note: A Utica crib created in the 1840s named after the Utica State hospital in New York state. The facility, which was also known as the NY State lunatic Asylum at Utica and the Utica Psychiatric Center, was the first of New York's state mental health facilities. The crib was an approximately 2 feet tall by 2.5 feet by 5 or six foot cage with a hinged lid that patients would live in.
2. Although other hospitals would put them in comas for up to 50 hours!

CHAPTER 8: INVESTIGATIONS
1. Rothman, D.J, (2002). Conscience and Convenience: The Asylum and Its Alternatives in Progressive America (2nd Edition). Hawthorne, NY: Aldine Transaction.
2. Ibid
3. However, in 1885 a newspaper investigation stated that everything was "in order" in the Department for Men.
4. Central State Hospital had gotten rid of all except mitts made of bed ticking by 1887.
5. In fact, although Dr. Harrison was later acquitted, he was accused of being an "abortionist for hire." He boasted of having sex with many "respectable" women in Lebanon, a small town north west of Indianapolis in Boone County, where he made his home. He also spoke not unsurprisingly bad to his patients. His acquittal was the result of many political friends coming to his rescue and testifying as to his moral character. Shortly before the investigation into the hospital in 1887, Dr. Harrison was seen intoxicated on the streets of Lebanon.
6. Replacing the Board of Trustees took two years.
7. This is a report that was written by a group (mostly the hospital administration and the Board of Trustees, who disagreed with the investigative findings.
8. It is unknown if these were announced visits.
9. Notice that Gapen had not been fired after the 1887 debacle
10. This is believed to be a typographical error. The doctor was Dr. PJ Watters.
11. Interestingly, this was dictated and the testimony was signed by Charles Young with an X because he could not write.
12. Kempf went on to a distinguished career and died in 1971.
13. The Board asked Mr. Rawley if he thought his wife was feeble minded when he married her. He said she wasn't.

CHAPTER 9: PATHOLOGY DEPARTMENT
1. Andrew Carnegie donated the money for the New York laboratory. In addition to the burgeoning laboratory sciences, psychotherapy was rising, which meant long term treatment. In its infancy, psychotherapy was all but dismissed as ineffectual. However, this type of treatment continued and by the mid-1900s, it was beginning to gain widespread popularity and its effectiveness was beginning to be seen by the medical community. During the 1890s, most doctors believed treatment should consist of biological assessment or psychotherapy, and the two disciplines didn't interact much together.
2. Since 1937 the malarial study was done with the United State Public Health Service, to which Bruetsch was a consultant, and with the Cooperative Clinical Group. It is unclear where this group was located or what its affiliations were.
3. Many of the reasons people were admitted to CSH were later to be found symptoms of syphilis.
4. This is ironic as he was highly influenced by Hitler's teachings and supported the Nazi invasion of Austria

in 1938, even though his application to the Nazi party had been denied because his first wife was Jewish. He was also an advocate of eugenics, especially in regard to Jews and mental illness. He was also the President of the Austrian League for Racial Regeneration and Heredity, which advocated sterilization for inferiors.
5. This was an in-depth study of medical education in the United States published in 1910 by its author, Abraham Flexner, and underwritten by the Carnegie Foundation
6. After the war, this program was discontinued.
7. Stockton left for a while due to health issues and also exploring different work. However, she came back and worked until her death in 1923.
8. Students were required to take a semester of courses focused on mental illness for many years.
9. Legend has long stated that this building was built without permission and the money used to build it was taken from hospital funds. As of this time, no proof has been found to the contrary.
10. A block of ice was put in the cistern behind the wall. As the block melted, it provided drinking water.

Chapter 11: Final Decline and Closure
1. Central State participated in using drugs as part of patient therapy and in clinical studies with Eli Lilly. The staff continued to participate in studies for inoculation and other items.
2. Assumed because it would be within 3 days.
3. Steve Leonard, maintenance chief was fired June 1992.
4. Not including 9 other state hospitals- 3 for developmentally disabled, 6 for developmentally disabled, mentally ill patients.
5. The state paid $60,000 of the research bill plus $2.3M in grant money.
6. Knapp, M., Beecham, J., Anderson, J., Dayson, D., Leff, J., Margolius, O., O'Driscoll, C., & Willis, W. (1990). The TAPS Project 3: Predicting the community of costs of closing psychiatric hospitals. The British Journal of Psychiatry, volume 57.

Chapter 12: Interviews
Skip Hess:
1. Chained people-someone from mental health association gave background. Said that was in the history. SH said there were some cells in the men's and women's. Didn't see chains.
2. Bill Hudnut was a president of the association before he was governor.
3. Perhaps the governor was too busy running as a stand in for Lyndon B Jonson in the 1968 Indiana Democratic primary and later running against Robert Kennedy.

September Fox
1. September said her mother heard the bullet go past and felt like her body was lead. September's mother also said that her dad was a crack shot, and could have killed them if he wanted.
2. Today he probably would have been considered autistic, but back then, he was called "retarded."
3. Many patients would be upset when they got the bills. It all seemed a bit cruel to September. Reminding patients of bills was one of the least pleasant tasks of September's job. Every month she had to give the patients their bills. Some bills were $100,000. When September received a bill for her grandfather, the hospital threatened to take away their family's land. They went to court and asked for it to be itemized. They couldn't.
4. Whereas at Evansville she'd been commended for saving patient lives! Whereas at Evansville she'd been commended for saving patient lives!
5. The worst thing she witnessed during an emergency was a "Paging Dr. Jack Armstrong", which meant all hands on deck to help a patient. One patient that couldn't stop drinking water drank herself to death. When September went to the call, the staff was pumping her and water came out like she drowned.

6. In the middle of Bahr.
7. As a result, working in the system afforded her an opportunity to become a trainer for the software company, which helped launch September in the direction of her current role as a corporate software trainer.

Photo Credits

Images in this book are property of Unseenpress.com with the following exceptions:

p1 Dr. Pinel in the courtyard of the Salpêriere] Gravure by Goupil after painting by Robert-Fleury. Retrieved April 1, 2014 from http://ihm.nlm.nih.gov

p3 Dr. Phillippe Pinel/Dr. Pinel in the courtyard of the Salpêriere. Retrieved April 1, 2014 from http://ihm.nlm.nih.gov

p4 Dr. Benjamin Rush. Retrieved April 1, 2014 from http://ihm.nlm.nih.gov/; "The Tranquilizer. Retrieved April 1, 2014 from http://ihm.nlm.nih.gov/

p5 Bolton homestead. Undated photo from Indiana State Library

p6 Dr. John Evans Retrieved April 1, 2014 from http://commons.wikimedia.org/wiki/File:John_Evans.gif; Dorothea Dix Retrieved April 1, 2014 from http://www.loc.gov/pictures/item/2004671913/

Pp 8 Sarah T. Bolton, from "The Life and Poems of Sarah T. Bolton" Retrieved April 1, 2014 https://archive.org/stream/lifepoemsofsarah00boltrich#page/n7/mode/2up

p16 East Haven 1930, From "Indiana". State Board of Printing.

pp18,25, 28-31, 36-37 Indiana State Archives, Commission on Public Records

p39 1937 Overhead view of Central State. Marion County GIS. Retrieved April 1, 2014 from http://maps.indy.gov/MapIndy/

p40 1972 Overhead view of Central State Farm Colony. Marion County GIS. Retrieved April 1, 2014 from http://maps.indy.gov/MapIndy/

p43 From "On the Construction, Organization and General Arrangements of Hospitals for the Insane with Some Remarks on Insanity and Its Treatment"

p44 WB Fletcher . 1907. Indiana Medical Journal Vol XXVI No 3

pp 50-51 Depaw University Nurses, Indiana State Library

pp 56-57 Application rules Indiana State Archives, Commission on Public Records

pp 59-60 Picture plates from "On the Construction, Organization and General Arrangements of Hospitals for the Insane with Some Remarks on Insanity and Its Treatment"

p61 Photo from Traité. Retrieved April 1, 2014 from http://ihm.nlm.nih.gov/

p64 Edinburgh, Constable, 1893; Secondary Syphilis (man), and Secondary Syphilis (woman) From Bramwell, Byrom "Atlas of Clinical Medicine" v. II, pl. XLII, P. 69 Edinburgh, Constable, 1893.

p64 Ecthyma Syphilitica Secondary Syphilis From "Bramwell, Byrom Atlas of Clinical Medicine" v. II, pl. XLV,

P69 Dr. Egas Moniz; Dr. Pedro Almeid Lima; Dr. James W. Watts Dr. Walter Freeman. Retrieved April 1, 2014 from http://ihm.nlm.nih.gov/

p70: Surgical Catalogue from Wm. Hatteroth's Surgical House (2nd Edition)

p83 Letter from Dr. WB Fletcher's Sanitorium Indiana State Archives, Commission on Public Records

pp84, 92 Indiana State Archives, Commission on Public Records

p96 Adolph Scherrer 1899. "Men of Progress. Indiana. McGraph, HJ and Stoddard, W.

p97 George Edenharter. 1893. Pictorial and biographical memoirs of Indianapolis and Marion County. Chicago: Goodspeed Brothers

p98 Floor plans of Central State Hospital Pathology Department Retrieved April 1, 2014 from http://www.loc.gov/pictures/item/in0058.photos.065147p/

p104 Max Bahr. (1930), Indiana. State Board of Printing.

p106 Indiana University School of Medicine . Walter Bruetsch. (1955). Bloomington, IN: Indiana University School of Medicine

pp 109,111 Indiana State Archives, Commission on Public Records

pp112-113 Sanborn Map 1915 Personal Collection

pp 116, 117, 118(B), 123, 125, 129 (b) Indiana State Archives, Commission on Public Records p162 Hydropathy room. Retrieved April 1, 2014 from http://ihm.nlm.nih.gov/

p180 Notice to Undertakers. April 17, 1901. Indianapolis Journal p.6

p181 2014 GIS map. Marion County GIS. Retrieved April 1, 2014 from http://maps.indy.gov/MapIndy/

BIBLIOGRAPHY

This section contains the items used to write this book. They contain books, documents, interviews and newspaper articles.

Agnew, A. 1887. From Under the Cloud. Cincinnati: Robert Clarke & Co.

Bahr, M.A. 1927. Letter and documentation to John Brown about the malarial treatment.

Board of State Charities. Legal document concerning the discharge and abuse of ME Miller.

Board of State Charities. 1901. Insanity trust report t Governor of Indiana. Indianapolis: State of Indiana.

Bodenhammer, D.J & Barrows, R.G. 1994. The Encyclopedia of Indianapolis. Bloomington, IN: Indiana University Press.

Browning, OE Letter to Governor Warren T McCray Bedford, IN 1921

Carroll County. 1872. Transcript to f proceedings William Harter.

Central Greens LLC. Central State Development Land Use Plan.

Central State Hospital. (1847-1859, 1861-1867, 1869-1871, 1873-1876, 1878-1881, 1883-1887, 1889-1890, 1895-1896, 1898-1899, 1902-1903, 1905-1906, 1908-1909, 1911-1915, 1920-1922,1924-26. 1930-44. 1947, 1949, 1951-55, 1958, 1961-64, 1966, 1969, 1971-72, 1975-1976, 1978.1983, 1986-90). Annual Report to the State of Indiana. Central State Hospital. Indianapolis, IN: State Contracted Printer

Central State Hospital. (n.d.) Inquiry concerning death of Clinton Martz Cooperider.

Central State Hospital County Book 1848-1883 Indianapolis: State of Indiana.

Central State Hospital. 1861 Bylaws. Indianapolis: Indianapolis Journal Company.

Central State Records, Department for Men, Pre-1900. pp 67, 78, 79, 213, 281 89, 185, 105, 79, 69, 22, 103, 139, 104, 141, 62, 207.

Central State Records, Department for Women. Pre-1900. pp 1, 7, 19, 23, 143, 162, 188, 198.

Central State Records by County, Pre-1900. pp 66, 90-92, 121, 131, 157, 266, 296.

Central State Hospital. (1904 May 17). Statement of Mr. JP Morphew .

Central State Hospital. 1917-1918. Annual report from the Department of Pathology. Indianapolis: State Printing Contractor.

Central State Hospital. (1918 January 16). Visit of JA Brown Supervisor of field work.

Central State Hospital. 1948. Pamphlet Centennial Anniversary of Central State hospital Indianapolis Indiana Indianapolis: State of Indiana.

Central State Hospital. 1985. We Care for People. Indianapolis: Central State Hospital. City of Indianapolis and Ball State University, College of Architecture and Planning, Indianapolis Center. Central State Workshop & Reuse Study. City of Indianapolis

Central State Hospital for Insane Statement of Miss Nora Raeburn regarding her discharge from the service.1921

Central State Hospital. 1879. Report of the Provisional Board of Commissioners for the Indiana Hospital for the Insane (Department for Women): March 20 1875, to October 31, 1878 to the Governor. Indianapolis: State of Indiana

Central State Hospital. 1890. Report of Officer of the Day: WO Weekly.

Central State Hospital. (1908, 1917, 1918, 1919) Report from the Pathological Department, Central State Hospital. 1992. Central State Hospital Exit Unit: community re-integration services.

Indianapolis: State of Indiana.

Central State Hospital. 1992. Quality improvement task force report on the treatment planning process at Central State Hospital. Indianapolis: State of Indiana.

City of Indianapolis & Ball State University , College of Architecture and Planning, Indianapolis Center. 2004. A Framework Discussion for the Future. Indianapolis: City of Indianapolis.

City of Indianapolis. (2004 Summer). Summary of Findings & Conceptual Recommendations. City of Indianapolis.

City of Indianapolis. 2004. Central State Reuse Study Appendix B: Public Workshop Information & Images. City of Indianapolis.

City of Indianapolis. 2004. Central State Reuse Study Appendix A: Project Demographic and Site Information. City of Indianapolis.

Conrad, P. & Scheider, J.W. 2010. Deviance and Medicalization: From Badness to Sickness. Philadelphia: Temple University Press.

Coons, P.M, & Bowman, E.S. 2010. Psychiatry in Indiana: The First 175 Years. Bloomington, IN: iUniverse.

Curtis, JE. 1891. Letter to Charles E Wright, MD regarding WO Weakly.

Curwen, J, Nichols, C.H., & Callender, J.H. 1885. Memoir of Thomas S. Kirkbride, M.D., LL. D. Warren, PA: E. Cowan & Co. Printers.

Davies R. 2001 Doubles: The enigma of the second self. London: Robert Hale

Day, TC 1912. Letter and documentation to Amos Butler, Sec BOSC regarding Mrs. Jacob Schmidt and Mrs. AE Cory.

Dean, E.T. 1997. Shook Over Hell: Post-traumatic Stress, Vietnam and the Civil War. Cambridge, MA: Harvard University Press.

Division of Mental Health. (1993 December) Closing Central State Hospital: Why the Decision was made.

Dunn, JP. 1919. Indiana & Indians. Chicago: American Historical Society.

Drenovsky, R.L. (n.d.) Humanities Bonfire: William B. Fletcher, M.D.

Ellison, TE. 1901. Insanity Trust letter and documentation to the Board of State Charities.

Estevez*, C. 2014. Personal Interview. Westfield, Indiana: Unseenpress.com, Inc.

Family and Social Services Administration. 1993. Central State Closure plan; Commitment to Community Based Care. Indianapolis: State of Indiana.

Family and Social Services Administration. 1994. Central State Hospital Report Indianapolis: State of Flexner, A. 1910. Medical Education in the United States and Canada Bulletin Number Four (The Flexner Report). The Carnegie Foundation for the Advancement of Teaching.

Fox, S. 2014 Personal Interview. Westfield, Indiana: Unseenpress.com, Inc.

Grob, G.N. 1973. Mental institutions in America. Piscataway, N.J: Transaction Publishers.

Hess, S. 2014. Personal Interview

Hurd, H. M. 1916. The Institutional Care of the Insane in the United States and Canada. Baltimore: Johns Hopkins Press.

Indiana Historical Society. 1976. Indiana Medical History Quarterly. Indianapolis: Indiana Historical Society. 2(3) pp 48-49.

Indiana Historical Society. (1983 March). Indiana Medical History Quarterly. Indianapolis: Indiana Historical Society. 9(1).

Indianapolis Journal. 1880. Sarah T. Bolton, Poetess. Indianapolis: Fred L Horton & Co.

Indiana State Board of Charities. (1897, 1917, 1918, 1903, 1920) Annual Report of the Board of State Charities. Indianapolis: Indiana State Board of Charities.

Indiana Board of State Charities. 1899. Proceedings of the Annual State Conference of Charities and Correction, Indianapolis: State of Indiana.

Indiana State Board of Charities. 1916. Mental Defectives Indiana. Indianapolis: Indiana State Board of Charities.

Johnson, A. 1923. Adventures in Social Welfare. Fort Wayne, IN: Ft. Wayne Printing Company.

King, L.J. (2001 Spring). The Seven Steeples. Indianapolis: Traces.

King, L.J. 2013. Under the Cloud at Seven Steeples: The Peculiarly Saddened Life of Anna Agnew at the Indiana Hospital for the Insane Carmel, IN: Hawthorne Publishing.

King, L. J. & Schmetzer, A.D. 2012. Dr. Edenharter's Dream: How Science Improved the Humane Care of the Mentally Ill in Indiana 1896-2012.

Kirkbride, T.S. 1880. On the Construction, Organization, and General Arrangements of Hospitals for the Insane: With Some Remarks on Insanity and Its Treatment. Philadelphia: J.B. Lippincott.

Knapp, M., Beecham, J., Anderson, J., Dayson, D., Leff, J., Margolius, O., O'Driscoll, C., & Willis, W. 1990. The TAPS Project 3: Predicting the community of costs of closing psychiatric hospitals. The British Journal of Psychiatry, volume 57.

Knight, P.S. 1827. Observations on the causes, symptoms and treatment of derangement of the mind. London: Longman, Reese, Orme, Brown and Green

Lawson, A. H, Wright, E.R., Jaeger, S., McGrew, J., Pescosoido, B. (2005 March). The Central State Hospital Discharge Study Tracking Report. Indiana Consortium for Mental Health Services Research, Institute for Social Research, Indiana University.

Mahtesian, C. (1993 March 1). The Last Days of the Asylum. Governing.

McGrew, J.H., Wright, E.R., & Pescosolido, B.A., (1999 Aug) Closing of a State Hospital: An overview and framework for a case study. The Journal of Behavioral Health Services & Research. 26(3). pp. 236-245.

McGrew, J.H., Wright, E.R., Pescosolido, B.A., & McDonel, E.C. 1999. The Closing of Central State Hospital: Long-term outcomes for persons with severe mental illness. The Journal of Behavioral Health Services & Research. 26(3). pp. 246-261.

McMechen, E.C. 1924. Lie of Governor Evans. Denver, CO: The Walgreen Publishing Co.

Mesch, D.J., McGrew, J.H., Pescosolido, B.A., & Haugh, D.F. E. 1999. The Effects of Hospital Closure on Mental Health Workers: An overview of employment, mental and physical health, and attitudinal outcomes. The Journal of Behavioral Health Services & Research. 26(3). pp. 305-317.

Niccum, T. 2014. Personal Interview. Westfield, IN: Unseenpress.com, Inc.

Pescosolido, B.A., Wright, E.R., Kikuzawa, S. E. 1999. "Stakeholder" Attitudes over Time toward the Closing of a State Hospital. The Journal of Behavioral Health Services & Research. 26(3). pp. 318-328.

Pescosolido, B.A., Wright, E.R., Lutfey, K. 1999. "Stakeholder" Attitudes over Time toward the Closing of a State Hospital. The Journal of Behavioral Health Services & Research. 26(3). pp. 276-288.

Purchasing Files. 1920. The Hospital Purchasing File.

Rice, T.D. "Founding of Central State Hospital for the Insane. Monthly bulletin of Indiana

Rosenbloom, D. 2011. Personal Interview. Westfield, IN: Unseenpress.com, Inc.

Rothebard, A.B., Kuno, E., Schinnar, A.P., Hadley, T.R., Turk, R. 1999. Service Utilization and Cost of Community Care for Discharged State Hospital Patients: A 3-Year Follow-Up Study. American Journal of Psychiatry 156:920-927.

Rothman, D.J. 1990. The Discovery of the Asylum (2nd Ed). Hawethorne, NY: Aldine De Gruyter.

Rothman, D.J. 2002. Conscience and Convenience: The Asylum and Its Alternatives in Progressive America (2nd Edition). Hawthorne, NY: Aldine Transaction

Rutherford, J. 2014. Personal Interview. Westfield, IN: Unseenpress.com, Inc.

Sanborn Map Company. 1898. Map. Sanborn Map Company

Sanborn Map Company. 1914. Map. Sanborn Map Company

Sanborn Map Company. 1915. Map. Sanborn Map Company

Sanborn Map Company. 1956. Map. Sanborn Map Company

Scull, A. 1981. Madhouses, Mad-Doctors and Madmen. Philadelphia: University of Pennsylvania Press.

Smith, SE Letter to Board of State Charities from Dr. WB Fletcher's Sanatorium regarding Miss Catherine Taylor. 1893

State of Indiana. 1887. Journal of the Indiana State House of Representatives. Indianapolis: State of Indiana.

State of Indiana. 1887. Report of Committee of the House of Representatives on the Management and Affairs of the Indiana Hospital for the Insane Indianapolis: State Printing Contractor

State of Indiana. 1890. The Indiana Yearly Bulletin of Charities and Correction. Indianapolis: Wm. B. Buford.

State of Indiana. 1918. Yearbook of the State of Indiana. Indianapolis: Wm. B. Buford.

State of Indiana. 1926. Record of inquest for Mary Cox, Boone Co. Indianapolis, IN: State of Indiana.

Thayer, A. 1886. The Rough Diamond Indianapolis: Albert Thayer.

Williams, C.L. (n.d.) A History of Mental Hospitals in Indiana.

Wright, E.R. 1999. Fiscal Outcomes of the Closing of Central State Hospital: An Analysis of the Costs to State Government. The Journal of Behavioral Health Services & Research. 26(3). pp. 262-275.

Wright, E.R., Avirappattu, G.A., & Lafuze, J.E. 1999. The Family Experience of Deinstitutionalization: Insights from the closing of Central State Hospital. The Journal of Behavioral Health Services & Research. 26(3). pp. 289-304.

Wright, E.R, Gronfein, W.P, & Owen, T.J. (2000 March). Journal of Health and Social Behavior. 41(1) pp. 68-90.

Wright, E.R., Jaeger, S., Lawson, A. H, Kooreman, H., McGrew, J., Pescosoido, B. (2005 January). The Central State Hospital Discharge Study Reports to the Indiana Division of Mental Health and Addiction 2004-2005. Indiana Consortium for Mental Health Services Research, Institute for Social Research, Indiana University.

Wright, C.E. 1891. Letter to W.W. Weakley regarding WO Weakly. 1891

Wright, C.E. 1891. Letter to Alexander Johnson Sec BOSC Indianapolis regarding W.O. Weekly.

United States Public Health Service. 1921. Letter to Amos Butler

United States Bureau of the Census. 1914. Summary of state laws relating to the dependent classes, 1913 Washington, DC. United States Government.

United States Bureau of the Census. 1923. Patients in hospitals for mental disease. Washington, DC. United States Government.

The newspaper articles were so numerous they have been put into a table sorted by newspaper. The newspapers on the following pages represent many years of media coverage for the hospital. The author hopes they are useful to future research.

Paper	Date	Title	Byline	Page
Indianapolis News	3/23/1965	Gladys Roberts Likes Work In Gloomy Mental Infirmary	Evie Birge	19
Indianapolis News	5/12/1949	State Hospital Tour Sickens Legislators	James Newland	1
Indianapolis News	5/12/1970	Central State Asks Better Fire Security	Skip Hess	39
Indianapolis News	1/13/1982	Even Psychiatrist Can't Tell Players Without A Program	David McCarty	18
Indianapolis News	5/17/1982	Outpatient Program For Alcoholics Closing	Jane Stegemiller	19
Indianapolis News	5/24/1973	Patient Abuse Probe		1
Indianapolis News	6/14/1971	Work To Start July Or August	Skip Hess	1
Indianapolis News	8/13/1927	New Figures Confirm Malaria Germs As Brain Diseases Cure		
Indianapolis News	12/19/1959	Patient' Is Freed After Two Years		
Indianapolis News	10/7/1972	Keating Improves Central State	Skip Hess	19
Indianapolis News	8/21/1973	Sanitation Force Inspects Hospital	Skip Hess	1
Indianapolis News	1/12/1972	State Hospital Programs Reorient Patients Sooner	Bob Jareczek	7
Indianapolis News	6/1/1973	Bowen Deplores Facilities In Visit To Central State	Skip Hess & Reginald Bishop	1
Indianapolis News	9/7/1971	Patient Unit Under Way At Central State		21
Indianapolis News	5/22/1973	Abuse At Central State		2
Indianapolis News	7/17/1973	Bowen To Probe		2
Indianapolis News	9/4/1973	Central To Move Patients	Skip Hess	1
Indianapolis News	5/25/1943	Central Hospital Additions Urged		
Indianapolis News	8/8/1973	County Grand Jury To Assist In Probe of Central State		1
Indianapolis News	8/10/1961	Seven Steeples' Make Impression	William C. Kassebaum	54

Paper	Date	Title	Byline	Page
Herald Bulletin	2/24/1995	Forgotten Cemetery upgraded		C4
Indianapolis Journal	Nov-Dec 1885	The Home of the Insane	NA	NA
Indianapolis News	3/16/1978	Herman Hoglebogle Column		56
Indianapolis News	6/12/1953	Conditions at '7 Steeples' Anger Craig	Edward Ziegner	21
Indianapolis News	4/3/1968	Fire Peril At Central Cited	Skip Hess	57
Indianapolis News	7/10/1973	Central State Blame Accepted	Skip Hess	1
Indianapolis News	8/18/1990	Agency to develop guidelines for mental hospitals	Linda Gillis	A1
Indianapolis News	10/11/1968	Education Head Removes 'Bars' Of Bahr Center	Skip Hess	37
Indianapolis News	4/10/1968	$4 Million Ready To Begin Work	Skip Hess	1
Indianapolis News	8/3/1960	Mental Hospital Lab Is Milestone	Hortense Myers	
Indianapolis News	6/16/1973	Conditions 'Filthy' At Central State, Probers Tell Bowen	Skip Hess	1
Indianapolis News	7/24/1973	Supervision Lack Alleged In Central State Deaths	Skip Hess	p1c1
Indianapolis News	2/16/1972	Chaplain Trains Seminary Students In Patient Concern	Bob Jareczek	p33c1_7
Indianapolis News	9/15/1959	McCarty - Fellow Taxpayers	Mickey McCarty	
Indianapolis News	5/7/1971	Oldest State Medical 'School' Is Revived	United Press International	34
Indianapolis News	9/19/1968	Men's Security Ward To Lose Locked Doors, Bars	Skip Hess	p35
Indianapolis News	2/7/1969	State Hospital Plans $10 Million Project	Skip Hess	1
Indianapolis News	10/13/1970	Central State Program Better Prepares Patient	Robert Jareczek	23
Indianapolis News	7/12/1973	Patient Beating Report At Central State Probed	Skip Hess	1
Indianapolis News	1/12/1982	Central State Has Changed	David McCarty	2

Paper	Date	Title	Byline	Page
Indianapolis News	1/16/1982	Chaplains Aid The Mentally Ill	Diane Fredrick	6
Indianapolis News	4/16/1948	Psycho Colony to break "bottleneck"		Part 2 p1
Indianapolis News	9/9/1983	Central State Criminial Charges 'Unwarranted'	Art Harris	17
Indianapolis News	9/27/1973	Central State Employees Indicited In Hospital Thefts	Skip Hess	1
Indianapolis News	6/11/1968	Patients, Ordered	Skip Hess	1
Indianapolis News	9/8/1973	Central State Patients To Move	Skip Hess	1
Indianapolis News	7/27/1966	Red Tape Ties Up Plan At Hospital	Fremont Power	4
Indianapolis News	8/4/1960	Needle, Thesis Aid Muscle Research	Hortense Myers	
Indianapolis News	6/10/1966	Gun-Shy Officials Bog Aid To Kids	Fremont Power	33
Indianapolis News	7/9/1973	Treatment Quality At Central State Blamed On 'Politics'	Skip Hess	1
Indianapolis News	2/15/1968	990 Rats Killed At Hospital In 3.5 Mos	Skip Hess	1
Indianapolis News	8/17/1939	Hospital Employes' Home Nears Completion		
Indianapolis News	2/1/1961	Musician Aids Mental Patients	Charles Staff	16
Indianapolis News	7/17/1973	Bowen To Probe Story Of Central State Fatal Beating	Skip Hess	1
Indianapolis News	1/11/1982	Ann Heard Voices And Couldn't Sleep	David McCarty	11
Indianapolis News	2/20/1968	State At Fault At Hospital, Branigin Says	Skip Hess	1
Indianapolis News	5/22/1973	Central State Patient Abuse Revealed	Skip Hess & Reginald Bishop	1
Indianapolis News	11/2/1955	Feminine Fourth Estaters Lend Their Talents To Worthy Cause	Myrtie Barker	10
Indianapolis News	7/11/1990	Central State Hospital wants to demolish historic building	Paul Bird	Section E p2
Indianapolis News	2/17/1968	Recommendations Made To Remedy Hospital Plight	Skip Hess	3

Paper	Date	Title	Byline	Page
Indianapolis News	1/16/1982	Chaplains Aid The Mentally Ill	Diane Fredrick	6
Indianapolis News	4/16/1948	Psycho Colony to break "bottleneck"		Part 2 p1
Indianapolis News	9/9/1983	Central State Criminial Charges 'Unwarranted'	Art Harris	17
Indianapolis News	9/27/1973	Central State Employees Indicited In Hospital Thefts	Skip Hess	1
Indianapolis News	6/11/1968	Patients, Ordered	Skip Hess	1
Indianapolis News	9/8/1973	Central State Patients To Move	Skip Hess	1
Indianapolis News	7/27/1966	Red Tape Ties Up Plan At Hospital	Fremont Power	4
Indianapolis News	8/4/1960	Needle, Thesis Aid Muscle Research	Hortense Myers	
Indianapolis News	6/10/1966	Gun-Shy Officials Bog Aid To Kids	Fremont Power	33
Indianapolis News	7/9/1973	Treatment Quality At Central State Blamed On 'Politics'	Skip Hess	1
Indianapolis News	2/15/1968	990 Rats Killed At Hospital In 3.5 Mos	Skip Hess	1
Indianapolis News	8/17/1939	Hospital Employes' Home Nears Completion		
Indianapolis News	2/1/1961	Musician Aids Mental Patients	Charles Staff	16
Indianapolis News	7/17/1973	Bowen To Probe Story Of Central State Fatal Beating	Skip Hess	1
Indianapolis News	1/11/1982	Ann Heard Voices And Couldn't Sleep	David McCarty	11
Indianapolis News	2/20/1968	State At Fault At Hospital, Branigin Says	Skip Hess	1
Indianapolis News	5/22/1973	Central State Patient Abuse Revealed	Skip Hess & Reginald Bishop	1
Indianapolis News	11/2/1955	Feminine Fourth Estaters Lend Their Talents To Worthy Cause	Myrtie Barker	10
Indianapolis News	7/11/1990	Central State Hospital wants to demolish historic building	Paul Bird	Section E p2
Indianapolis News	2/17/1968	Recommendations Made To Remedy Hospital Plight	Skip Hess	3

Paper	Date	Title	Byline	Page
Indianapolis News	5/21/1955	New Home Plan for Mental Patients	Jackie Freers	5
Indianapolis News	9/2/1971	Hospital Building Begins Tuesdaya		1
Indianapolis News	8/19/1967	Camp For Disturbed Children Moves Ahead	John Flora	3
Indianapolis News	1/4/1952	Mental Hospital Handcuffs Laid to Lack of Help		9
Indianapolis News	12/23/1958	Mental Patients Get Annual Bahr Gifts	Hortense Myers	
Indianapolis News	3/12/1968	Hospital Lacks 303 Employes	Skip Hess	23
Indianapolis News	5/23/1973	State Mental Health Group Asks Patient Abuse Probe	Skip Hess & Reginald Bishop	1
Indianapolis News	1/7/1953	Mental Hospital Hopes You Get Mad	Bruce Hilton	9
Indianapolis News	9/22/1966	Hospital In Dire Need Of 'Crutch'	Fremont Power	39
Indianapolis News	1/12/1940	State Hospital Staff Reorganized on Q. T.	Bill Wildhack	15
Indianapolis News	4/4/1893	Catherine Taylor's Disappearance		
Indianapolis News	4/5/1893	Catherine Taylor Returned		
Indianapolis Star	10/19/1958	Ceramics Interest Aids Mental Patients	Genell Jackson	
Indianapolis Star	2/23/1995	Mending a Grave Injustice	R. Joseph Gelarden	A1
Indianapolis Star	8/8/1938	General Central State column	With pictures	
Indianapolis Star	5/19/1940	First Building Used as State Hospital for Insane Soon to Be Razed; Once Center of Modern Psychiatry		
Indianapolis Star	5/13/1976	NY Psychologist Will Head Central State	William M Shaw	67
Indianapolis Star	9/27/1990	Central State's head nurse quites over conditions	George Stuteville	A1
Indianapolis Star	11/14/1948	Public Invited To Open House Next Sunday		Secion 2 p2
Indianapolis Star	11/26/1972	Patients Relearning Skills In Central State Hospital Program	Donna Knight	Section 1 p1
Indianapolis Star	7/5/1944	The Day In Indiana	Maurice Early	
Indianapolis Star	8/16/1953	State Hospital Gets Screens		Section 2 p1

Paper	Date	Title	Byline	Page
Indianapolis Star	10/10/1971	He Finds Someone Cares	Myrta Pulliam	1
Indianapolis Star	9/13/1959	Central State Hospital Wins International Kitchen Best In Nation	Advertisment	Section 1 p20
Indianapolis Star	6/18/1961	Piano Teachers Volunteer Hospital Services	Donna Snodgrass	Section 5 p6
Indianapolis Star	7/23/1989	Troubled woman's time capsule	Kathy Whyde Jesse	Section H p1
Indianapolis Star	9/20/1981	Suicides at Central State Hospital riase alarm	Mark Nichols	Section 2 p12
Indianapolis Star	10/14/1990	Tragic	?	Section A p1
Indianapolis Star	9/9/1983	No basis found for charges in 22 deaths at Central State	Eric C Rodenberg	p1c1_3
Indianapolis Star	6/9/1983	Goldsmith vows review of deaths at Central State	Richard D. Walton	1
Indianapolis Star	2/18/1968	Dr. Sheeley And Staff Defended By Leader For Mental Health	Michael P. Tarpey	Section 2 p4
Indianapolis Star	8/28/1975	Fourth Escape Was Final One	Thomas R. Keating	69
Indianapolis Star	8/7/1978	Central State Uneasy	Thomas R. Keating	19
Indianapolis Star	12/20/1974	Old Main Doomed		6
Indianapolis Star	2/19/1976	Central State Hospital Head Resigns Under Pressure	William M Shaw	39
Indianapolis Star	9/11/1959	Central Hospital Kitchen Gets International Honor		
Indianapolis Star	9/10/1957	Central Hospital To Get New Treatment Facility		1
Indianapolis Star	10/14/1990	Family decries patient's tragic chain of events	Richard D. Walton	Section A p1
Indianapolis Star	11/7/1971	2 New Buildings to Aid Care At Central State		Section C p14
Indianapolis Star	5/29/1938	Central State Hospital Mattress Maker Enjoys Work After 63 Years' Service		
Indianapolis Star	10/29/1972	Mentally Ill Patients Find A Special Kind Of Love	Isabel Boyer	9
Indianapolis Star	9/11/1973	Five-Step Mental Health Plan, Firm Warning On Poor Management Issued By Governor		16
Indianapolis Star	10/29/1974	Demoltion Of Old Central State Administration Building Planned		22
Indianapolis Star	5/20/1990	Investigation of prcedures at mental hospital stalls	Richard D. Walton	Section B p1

Paper	Date	Title	Byline	Page
Indianapolis Star	1/26/1958	Central State Hospital Drama Group Rehearses mondays	Dotty Steinmeyer	Section 6 p2
Indianapolis Star	6/8/1983	Error' cited in 15-18 Central State deaths	Richard D. Walton & Eric C. Rodenberg	1
Indianapolis Star	9/9/1973	Central State Hospital To Open New Buildings	Isabel Boyer	Section 2 p1
Indianapolis Star	5/16/1973	Sexual Deviant On Hospital Leave Charged In Beating Of Housewife	Star State Report	6
Indianapolis Star	1/29/1952	Help Poses Problem For Beatty Hospital	Charles G. Griffo	1
Indianapolis Star	8/18/1990	Mental patients at risk at Central State, panel reports	George Stuteville	Section A p 1
Indianapolis Star	8/12/1980	Modern Michelangelo		11
Indianapolis Star	7/21/1988	Inside Looking Out	Kathy Whyde Jesse	Section A p12
Indianapolis Star	3/6/1983	Central State patients suffer from lack of staff	Eunice McLayea	Section 1 p1
Indianapolis Star	9/21/1973	Serious Questions about Murray	Staff	Section 2 p6
Indianapolis Star	11/6/1943	Reroofing Job Will Erase Historic Seven Gables at Central Hospital		
Indianapolis Star	11/30/1965	Disturbed Children's Center Being Set Up		21
Indianapolis Star	7/25/1971	State Hospital's Historic Edifice To Be Restored	Leila Holmes	20
Indianapolis Star	11/21/1938	91st Year of Caring for Mentally Ill Is Started by Central State Hospital		
Indianapolis Star	6/19/1983	Ex-Central State chief saw problems coming		
Indianapolis Star	6/9/1994	Central State settles wrongful death suit for $210,000	Linda Graham Caleca	A1
Indianapolis Star	6/24/1992	Central State ordered to close in '94	Linda Graham Caleca	A1
Indianapolis Star	7/1/1993	Central State throws last bash	Rececca Buckman	B1
Indianapolis Star	9/6/1992	Facing closing, Central State proceeds with improvements	Jeff Swiatek	A1
Indianapolis Star	12/24/1995	Program provides ex-mental patients a working solution	Joe Fahy	7

Paper	Date	Title	Byline	Page
Indianapolis Star	1/27/1994	Releases from Central State bring violent consequences	Linda Graham Caleca	A1
Indianapolis Star	9/1/1993	Central State patients go to court in bid to halt out-of-county moves	Janel E. Williams	B3
Indianapolis Star	10/8/1005	Taste of freedom has a tragic ending	Linda Graham Caleca	C1
Indianapolis Star	1/1/1994	Central State girds itself for the end of an era	Linda Graham Caleca	p1
Indianapolis Star	12/18/1994	The secret shame of Central State	R. Joseph Gelarden	A1
Indianapolis Star	5/18/1993	State, families seek to get grand jury evidence	Linda Graham Caleca and Janet E Williams	A4
Indianapolis Star				
Indianapolis Star	12/10/2013	New hospital needed for mentally ill	Opinion: Marvine Miller, MD	
Indianapolis Star	9/16/2013	Will Indy charter schools boost former Bush Stadium, Central state sites?	Scott Elliot	
Indianapolis Star	5/30/2014	Remembering forgotten patients	John Tuihy	A1
Indianapolis Star	4/15/1992	Assault allegedly left patient pregnant	Linda Graham Caleca	A1
Indianapolis Star	5/19/1993	2 officials resigning state mental health jobs	Linda Graham Caleca	A2
Indianapolis Star	1/23/1993	Central State receives high inspection marks despite bleak future	Linda Graham Caleca	C2
Indianapolis Star	2/2/1992	Health care inspectors pass Central State	Linda Graham Caleca	A2
Indianapolis Star	10/14/1993	Popular executive at Central State to be reassigned	Linda Graham Caleca	C3
Indianapolis Star	4/26/1994	Central State patients losing an oasis of artistic expression	Dan Carpenter	A1
Indianapolis Star	4/26/1994	Smooth Central State shift exceeds officials' expectations	Linda Graham Caleca	A1
Indianapolis Star	11/4/1994	City, state join forces in plan to convert Central State	Larry MacIntyre	C3
Indianapolis Star	8/11/1994	Draft plan for Central State draws criticism	Larry MacIntyre and Andrea Neal	A1

Paper	Date	Title	Byline	Page
Indianapolis Star	8/11/1992	Union has Central State plan	Barb Albert	B1
Indianapolis Star	2/4/1992	Republicans seek dialogue on closing of Central State	William J Booher	C3
Indianapolis Star	6/14/1994	Central State staffers sued over death	John R. O'Neill	C3
Indianapolis Star	5/16/1993	A brief look at Central State and two decades of problems	Linda Graham Caleca and Janet E Williams	A1
Indianapolis Star	5/16/1993	Central State indictments expected Monday	Linda Graham Caleca and Janet E Williams	A1
Indianapolis Star	3/16/1993	Sprucing up and closing down	Linda Graham Caleca	A1
Indianapolis Star	10/7/1993	Latest round of Central State layoffs bring the total so far to about 90	Nancy J Winkley	D3
Indianapolis Star	11/14/1993	Central State workers are told 75 will be laid off next month	Nancy J Winkley	B3
Indianapolis Star	6/7/1993	Report details plans to close Central State	Linda Graham Caleca	A1
Indianapolis Star	8/26/1993	Central State to lay off scores of workers	Linda Graham Caleca	B1
Indianapolis Star	5/28/1992	Inquiry covers 24 deaths at Central State	Barb Albert	A1
Indianapolis Star	5/29/1992	Bayh orders study of future of Central State	Bill Theobald	C1
Indianapolis Star	2/12/1993	Central State must stay open parents say	William J Booher	D1
Indianapolis Star	6/30/1992	Families jam meeting, urge Central State be left open	Linda Graham Caleca	A1
Indianapolis Star	4/25/1992	Questions shroud drowning at Central State, coroner says	Linda Graham Caleca	E1
Indianapolis Star	8/11/1993	Central State sending 35 patients elsewhere	Nancy J Winkley	B1
Indianapolis Star	6/25/1992	Central State decision leaves many uneasy	Linda Graham Caleca	A1
Indianapolis Star	6/25/1992	Health officials support closing hospital	William J Booher	A8
Indianapolis Star	4/7/1993	Ministers want Central State to be kept open	Robert N. Bell	C5

Paper	Date	Title	Byline	Page
Indianapolis Star	6/3/1993	Neighborhood association and activists share worries about Central State closing	Kevin Morgan	B3
Indianapolis Star	8/25/1992	Family to try to salvage Central State despite death	Linda Graham Caleca	B4
Indianapolis Star	4/1/1992	Special jury to convene on Central State	Barb Albert	B1
Indianapolis Star	1/20/1994	Central State not best site for youth groups say	Nancy J Winkley	B1
Indianapolis Star	9/3/1992	Central State layoffs may affect patients' safety, doctors charge	Linda Graham Caleca	A1
Indianapolis Star	7/17/1992	Funds allocated to transfer patients from Central State	Linda Graham Caleca	B1
Indianapolis Star	7/20/1993	Researchers log experiences of ex-Central State patients	Nancy J Winkley	B3
Indianapolis Star	2/5/1994	Office tracks those who have left Central State	Linda Graham Caleca	A1
Indianapolis Star	5/17/1994	An Uncertain Prognosis: Hospital's decay rooted in Indiana's neglect of mentally ill	Linda Graham Caleca	A1
Indianapolis Star	9/3/1993	Central State to give patients costly new drug	Janet E. Williams	C1
Indianapolis Star	4/10/1994	Dream House	Linda Graham Caleca	A1
Indianapolis Star	5/18/1993	Five Indicted in Central State Probe	Linda Graham Caleca and Janet E Williams	A1
Indianapolis Star	3/30/1992	Central State Position Tough to Fill	Linda Gillis	C1
Indianapolis Star	4/18/1992	Central State Chief Resigned, but State Says She was Fired	Linda Graham Caleca	A1
Indianapolis Star	12/2/1994	Ex-Central State Duo get Probation for Part in Death of Patient	Janet E Williams	D1
Indianapolis Star	12/14/1991	Nurse Suspended in Patient's death at Central State	S. Hanafee	A1
Indianapolis Star	3/29/1992	Central State's History Keeps on Repeating	S. Hanafee	A1
Indianapolis Star	3/25/1992	Hospital Suspends 7 after Patient Dies	S. Hanafee	A1
Indianapolis Star	3/26/1992	Hospital to Fire 7 in Wake of Patient Death	S. Hanafee	A1

Paper	Date	Title	Byline	Page
Indianapolis Star	4/3/2003	Graves may be issue in deal-possible unmarked sites could complicate Central State Plan	J. Fritze	B1
Indianapolis Times	3/6/1949	Legislators Walk Among The Living Dead At Central State	Richard Lewis	3
Indianapolis Times	8/4/1954	Ed Sovola Inside Indianapolis	Ed Sovola	21
Indianapolis Times	3/31/1947	After 40 Years, Indiana Can Help Mentally Unfit	Robert Bloem	
Indianapolis Times	7/23/1958	Bahr Honored In Rite Opening Mental Center	John V. Wilson	p17
Indianapolis Times	8/16/1959	Central State Hospital Is Age 81 This Year	Nancy Lowe	
Indianapolis Times	2/9/1955	Ed Sovola Says: Do-It-Yourself Plan Helps Mental Patients	Ed Sovola	p30
Indianapolis Times	9/11/1960	Is Escape Too Easy From Central State Hospital?	Don Baker	3
Indianapolis Times	11/20/1957	New Mental Treatment Center		p18
Indianapolis Times	1/18/1955	Burn It', Report Says of Building		1
Indianapolis Times	12/1/1957	Central State Officials Ponder Problem of 10-Year-Old Patient	John V. Wilson	12
Indianapolis Times	8/21/1947	Central State Hospital Cans Food Grown On Its 200-Acre Farm	Robert Bloem	Section 1 p19
Indianapolis Times	8/3/1961	There's No Other Place for These 38 Children	John V. Wilson	15
Indianapolis Times	12/2/1958	Budget Those Hats Under 'Therapeutic'	Hortense Myers	
Indianapolis Times	10/19/1937	Beauty Treatment Held Safer and Better Than Insulin in Mental Cases		10
Indianapolis Times	11/24/1959	Art League's Special Project Is Exhibited	Jan Colcord	7
Indianapolis Times	9/20/1956	Music Guides Mental Patients Over Barrier		30
Indianapolis Times	5/29/1953	State hospital plans Motels		1
Indianapolis Times	8/3/1952	63 years behind bars at State institution	Donna Mikels	1

Paper	Date	Title	Byline	Page
Indianapolis Times	1/31/1960	Floors Crack in New 1.5 Million Hospital	John V. Wilson	2
Indianapolis Times	8/3/1960	Muscle Lab thrives at Mental Hospital	Hortense Myers	4
Indianapolis Times	8/17/1960	Time and tender Treatment help the human "whirlwind"	James Rourke	17
Indianapolis Times	4/22/1905	Transplanting of Six Million Trees Planned		
Indianapolis Times	12/14/1951	Mental Patients' play brings out their best	Robert Newell	1 and 19
Indianapolis Times	12/21/1956	Union Gives Charter at Central State		15
Indianapolis Times	7/20/1958	Self-Government Group Is Proving Successful	Mary Black	9
Indianapolis Times	8/2/1960	Central State Aided by Deceased Patient	Hortense Myers	
Indianapolis Times	7/19/1959	What Are We Feeding Our Mentally Ill?	John V. Wilson	
Indianapolis Times	5/25/1956	Volunteer 'Gold Ladies' Help Put Patients In Touch With The World Outside Hospital chambers		8
Indianapolis Times	6/19/1953	State Hospital To Receive a Face-Lifting		5
Magazine Star	7/30/1978	Renewed Doses of Old Medicine	Fred D. Cavinder	16
Magazine Star	4/3/1977	The Apartment	Fred D. Cavinder	8
Magazine Star	11/9/1952	Worth Their Weight In Gold	Paul N. Janes	
Magazine Star	5/3/1953	Not Forgotten	Kenneth Hufford	42
Marion County Mail	8/20/1964	First Insane Asylum And Earliest Apartments In Log Cabin Complex		3
News	3/4/1970	Rumors At Central		4
Nuvo	12/12/1990	Gridlock	Diane Brandt	10
Post-Tribune	10/15/1987	Former Mental Hospital Patients Pleased with Pay Ruling	R.A. Krause	B1

Index

A

abuse 11, 47, 51, 63, 74, 83, 85, 86, 89, 142, 143, 165, 166, 168, 174, 198
Administration Building 5, 38, 45, 110, 117, 124, 125, 151, 156, 164, 165, 175, 207
African American 30, 31, 102
Agnew, Anna 78, 198, 199
alcohol 4, 44, 67, 68, 83, 94, 143, 153, 165, 175
almshouse 2
Artificial lake 111
Assistant Physician 44, 184
astral projection 77
Asylum 6, 11, 16, 62, 66, 72, 77, 88, 195, 200, 213
Attendants 10, 42, 45, 46, 47, 48, 74, 88, 145, 187
autopsies 44, 91, 96, 98, 101

B

Bahr 24, 31, 34, 38, 40, 44, 45, 49, 52, 53, 54, 66, 67, 71, 92, 98, 101, 102, 104, 105, 108, 111, 116, 119, 132, 135, 138, 142, 147, 149, 151, 157, 167, 170, 177, 184, 185, 187, 192, 197, 198, 203, 206, 212
Bahr Building 31, 38, 71, 111, 135, 147, 149, 157, 167, 177
Bahr, Max 44
Bake House 110
baker 42
Beers, Clifford 76
Bellevue Hospital 95
Bid Rigging 89
Board of Commissioners 7, 22, 42, 43, 44, 76, 96, 198
Board of Trustees 42, 43, 87, 88, 89, 108, 195
Body Shop 111, 132
Boiler House 110
Bolton 5, 8, 9, 10, 109, 111, 115, 117, 132, 135, 138, 142, 151, 177, 192, 197, 199
Bolton Building 111, 132, 135, 177
Bolton, Sarah T. 5, 8, 9, 30, 44, 45, 51, 80, 90, 93, 97, 132, 184, 185, 186, 197, 199
Browning, Otis E. 51, 92, 93, 184, 198
Bruetsch, Walter L. 98, 101, 102, 104, 105, 106, 108, 187, 188, 195, 197
building 5, 6, 7, 8, 9, 10, 13, 14, 17, 18, 21, 22, 23, 24, 26, 35, 40, 42, 44, 45, 46, 49, 58, 59, 74, 80, 81, 84, 96, 98, 101, 105, 109, 110, 111, 114, 115, 116, 117, 119, 120, 122, 124, 131, 132, 134, 136, 138, 139, 140, 143, 155, 156, 162, 163, 164, 165, 167, 168, 172, 173, 175, 194, 196, 204, 205

C

Canning plant 111
carpenter 14, 42, 66, 128, 160
Carpenter's Shop 110
carriage driver 42, 46
Car Storage 111
Car Wash 111
cemetery 31, 130, 136, 139, 179, 180, 181, 182
Central State Hospital 4, 5, 4, 5, 8, 11, 12, 14, 16, 17, 18, 20, 21, 23, 27, 32, 33, 34, 38, 39, 42, 45, 50, 51, 54, 58, 59, 63, 65, 66, 68, 70, 71, 72, 75, 77, 78, 79, 80, 81, 82, 83, 86, 94, 95, 96, 98, 101, 102, 104, 109, 124, 126, 131, 138, 139, 141, 142, 143, 144, 145, 146, 147, 149, 150, 151, 152, 153, 155, 156, 163, 165, 166, 167, 168, 170, 171, 172, 174, 179, 181, 193, 195, 197, 198, 199, 200, 201, 204, 205, 206, 207, 208, 212
Central State Hospital for the Insane 17, 66, 200
Chaplain 42, 55, 58, 188, 189, 195, 203
child 27, 93, 146, 166
children 4, 8, 9, 26, 30, 63, 71, 78, 79, 81, 86, 94, 143, 144, 145, 150, 151, 163
Christel House Academy 175, 177
Civil War 7, 8, 14, 26, 27, 75, 78, 79, 94, 180, 199
closure 13, 40, 82, 141, 143, 145, 147, 149, 150, 151, 152, 153, 154, 155, 165, 166
Closure Plan 145
Coal Room 110, 120
colored 30, 31
Columbus Hospital for the Insane 11
Consulting physicians 42
cook 42, 43
crime 2, 104, 144

D

Danvers State Hospital 11
death 9, 13, 21, 34, 55, 63, 65, 66, 74, 78, 79, 80, 84, 90, 97, 101, 144, 145, 148, 155, 163, 180, 196, 198, 208, 210, 211
Deep pump house 111
Department for Men 9, 16, 17, 18, 22, 23, 34, 41, 45, 74, 75, 85, 111, 114, 115, 116, 119, 126, 136, 137, 195, 198
Department for Women 16, 21, 30, 34, 38, 44, 84, 85, 92, 96, 108, 109, 110, 115, 116, 122, 137, 138, 165, 172, 173, 198
Dix, Dorothea Lynde 7
domestic 26, 41, 46
drugs 3, 20, 21, 35, 44, 45, 54, 63, 67, 71, 102, 122, 142, 193, 196
Dyer, Robert 144, 145, 151, 152

E

East Haven) 14
Edenharter, George F. 30, 38, 44, 45, 70, 96, 97
   Edenharter 30, 38, 44, 45, 51, 58, 68, 70, 80, 83, 90, 91, 92, 93, 96, 97, 184, 185, 197, 199
Edward J. Kempf 90, 91, 185
electro convulsive therapy 27, 65, 167
Employee Housing 111, 130
Employees Building 5, 45
engineer 42, 120, 186
Estevez, Carlos 163, 199

Ethics 71, 88, 89
Eugenics 71
Evans Building 111, 122, 130, 132, 156, 169, 170
Evans, John 6, 131, 184, 197
Evansville 14, 15, 20, 149, 154, 167, 168, 174, 196
Exit House 111, 132

F

families 12, 53, 54, 75, 79, 101, 144, 145, 149, 150, 209
farm 8, 9, 10, 16, 17, 22, 23, 24, 27, 33, 37, 38, 40, 63, 88, 94, 174, 177, 178, 193
Farm and Garden Barn 110
Farm Colony 38, 40, 72, 139, 174, 187, 190, 197
farmer 12, 42, 77, 194
Fayette Hospital 11
fire 16, 17, 18, 20, 23, 116, 117, 118, 119, 123, 126, 143, 144, 149, 180
firemen 42, 46
first patients 10
Fletcher, William B. 30, 44, 70, 79, 97, 199
forensics 98
Fort Benjamin Harrison Colony 24
Fox, September 167, 196, 199
Freeman, Walter 69, 197

G

Garbage Furnace 111
gardener 42
Gas House 111, 136
gatekeeper 42, 46

H

Hess 170, 174, 196, 199, 202, 203, 204, 205, 206
Hess, Skip 170
Hicks, Tonya Niccum 162
Highsaw, June Christy 13, 145, 148
hospital 2, 3, 4, 5, 6, 7, 9, 10, 11, 12, 13, 14, 16, 17, 18, 20, 21, 22, 23, 24, 26, 27, 28, 30, 31, 33, 34, 35, 38, 39, 40, 41, 42, 43, 44, 45, 46, 47, 48, 49, 50, 51, 52, 53, 54, 55, 58, 59, 62, 63, 64, 65, 66, 67, 68, 70, 71, 72, 73, 74, 75, 76, 77, 78, 79, 80, 81, 82, 83, 84, 85, 86, 87, 88, 89, 90, 91, 92, 93, 94, 96, 97, 98, 101, 102, 104, 105, 108, 109, 114, 116, 117, 119, 122, 123, 126, 130, 132, 138, 139, 142, 143, 144, 145, 147, 150, 151, 152, 154, 155, 162, 163, 164, 165, 166, 167, 168, 169, 170, 172, 173, 174, 175, 177, 180, 182, 183, 184, 185, 194, 195, 196, 198, 201, 207, 209, 210, 212
Hospital for the Insane 3, 4, 8, 9, 11, 12, 14, 16, 17, 23, 42, 43, 44, 45, 63, 66, 77, 79, 86, 97, 198, 199, 200
Hydrotherapy 63
hypnotics 66

I

Ice House 110
Illegal Loans 89
Indiana Hospital for the Insane 8, 9, 11, 12, 16, 17, 44, 45, 97, 198, 199, 200

Indiana Medical History Museum 105
industrial therapy 63, 124
Infirmary No 1 110, 126
insane 1, 2, 3, 4, 5, 6, 7, 9, 12, 14, 16, 22, 23, 26, 27, 34, 42, 43, 45, 46, 59, 62, 63, 68, 72, 78, 83, 86, 90, 91, 94, 104, 114, 167
Insanity 2, 3, 42, 59, 90, 93, 197, 198, 199
Insanity Trust 90
Insulin Therapy 65
investigation 84, 86, 87, 89, 92, 93, 144, 173, 174, 195
ironers 42, 46

J

jobber 42
Junk Shop 111

K

Kempf, Edward J. 90, 91, 92, 185, 195
Kentucky Lunatic Asylum 11
Kirkbride 14, 23, 38, 42, 43, 46, 47, 49, 59, 114, 115, 124, 194, 199
Kirkbride, Thomas 42, 43, 194
Kitchen 36, 110, 111, 127, 134, 166, 207

L

Laundry 110, 111, 118, 119, 131, 190, 192
leucotomy
 lobotomy 68
Lima, Pedro Almeid 68, 69, 197
Lively, Carrie 46, 80, 81
Logansport 14, 15, 18, 34, 81, 154, 165, 170, 174
Longcliff 14

M

machinist 42
malaria. 65, 101
masturbation 66
Matron 42, 44, 46
Mattress factory 110
Mayer Hall 45, 110, 124, 137, 138
meals 33, 43, 47, 48, 75, 162, 164, 170
Men's Cottage 72, 110, 127
Men's Recreation Hall 17, 110, 127
menu 33, 81
money 3, 9, 10, 11, 14, 16, 17, 18, 22, 23, 26, 35, 38, 40, 43, 45, 55, 71, 74, 75, 85, 87, 88, 89, 90, 96, 116, 124, 134, 142, 143, 145, 147, 149, 150, 151, 153, 165, 166, 173, 174, 195, 196
Moniz, Egas 68, 69, 197
moral therapy 3, 4, 26, 33, 62, 63
Morgue 110, 136
Motel 111, 130
Music therapy 67

N

Negro 31, 76, 80

neurology 96, 98, 101
New York State Lunatic Asylum at Utica, 11
night watchers 42, 48
North Dining Room 110
North Infirmary 110
nurse 21, 49, 79, 93, 143, 144, 145, 149, 151, 162, 163, 168, 173, 206

O

occupational therapy 18, 35, 45, 52, 108, 115, 164, 166
Officer's barn 111
Oil House 111
Old Main 21, 49, 52, 54, 55, 110, 115, 116, 207
Overcrowding 23, 24

P

Paint Shop 110, 111
Pathology Department 95, 96, 97, 98, 101, 102, 105, 108, 110, 134, 136, 139, 195, 197
Pavilion 111
Philadelphia 2, 30, 199, 200
Physician in Chief 42
Pinel, Philippe 3, 114
Pipe shop 110, 120
poor house 6, 62, 79
Power Plant 110, 111, 134
prison 2, 4, 16, 21, 24, 80, 86, 151, 163, 164, 167
psychiatry 2, 4, 20, 96, 98, 101, 104, 193
psychotherapy 35, 65, 66, 68, 164, 195
Pump house 111
Pump House 110, 137

R

railroad 17
Ray, Issac 3
Record Keeping 88
Recreational therapy 35, 66
Refrigeration 111, 134
Restraints 45, 70
rheumatic disease 104, 106
Richmond 14, 34, 80, 81, 83, 154, 194
Rogers, Joseph G. 12
Rosenbloom, Deborah 168, 200
Rush, Benjamin 2
Rutherford, Julie 165, 166, 200

S

Scherrer, Adolph 96, 197
school 4, 7, 8, 17, 25, 34, 35, 80, 83, 104, 105, 167, 170, 175
seamstresses 42, 46
Segregation 26
Seven Steeples 44, 81, 84, 92, 96, 110, 115, 116, 117, 156, 175, 177, 178, 194, 199, 202
Seven Steeples Farm 175, 178
Shelby, Linda 145, 146
Shock therapy 65

Sick Hospital 17, 68, 82, 110, 131, 137, 138
South Dining Room 110, 137
Sparke, Mary Jo 6
spirit rappings 67
Staff 13, 22, 41, 50, 52, 54, 86, 87, 144, 149, 168, 188, 191, 204, 205, 206, 207, 208
Steward 42, 44, 46, 87, 189
Stockton, Sarah 30, 44, 45, 51, 80, 97, 184
Storage 110, 111, 138
Store and Supply House 110, 120
suicide 13, 14, 45, 75, 78, 79
Superintendent 9, 12, 20, 22, 23, 24, 30, 34, 35, 38, 42, 44, 45, 47, 48, 49, 50, 54, 58, 66, 67, 70, 71, 77, 79, 80, 83, 85, 87, 88, 89, 91, 92, 96, 97, 114, 116, 143, 144, 145, 152, 170, 174, 184, 186, 188
supervisors 42, 48, 194
surgery 13, 18, 72, 91, 101
syphilis 35, 53, 63, 64, 65, 67, 101, 102, 104, 106, 195

T

teachers 25, 35, 42
teaching 7, 10, 11, 20, 45, 96, 98, 101, 105, 151
Thayer, Albert 74, 200
therapy 3, 4, 18, 20, 22, 26, 27, 33, 35, 38, 45, 52, 53, 58, 62, 63, 65, 66, 67, 68, 71, 72, 102, 108, 115, 124, 132, 134, 142, 143, 156, 162, 163, 164, 165, 166, 167, 169, 170, 193, 194, 196
Tin Shop 111
tours 5, 52, 63, 105
Treatments 11, 63, 195
trustees 12, 20, 33, 86, 87
Tuberculosis 17
tunnel 138, 139, 140, 172

U

Utica 11, 70, 86, 195
Utica crib 70, 86, 195

V

veterans 18, 79, 130, 180
volunteer 52, 166

W

ward 13, 16, 18, 20, 27, 44, 50, 53, 55, 59, 74, 75, 76, 77, 78, 79, 80, 81, 82, 83, 91, 92, 93, 116, 117, 122, 138, 143, 145, 156, 162, 167, 170
warehouse 11, 142
washer 43
Washhouse 111
Watch house 111
Watts, James W. 68, 69, 197
William B. Fletcher
  Fletcher 17, 22, 30, 35, 44, 45, 70, 74, 75, 79, 83, 86, 87, 88, 94, 97, 184, 185, 197, 199, 200
Woodmere 14, 167
Worcester State Hospital, 11
workhouse 2
World War I 17
World War II 18, 20

www.ingramcontent.com/pod-product-compliance
Lightning Source LLC
Chambersburg PA
CBHW060811010526
44116CB00003B/42